Patients, Power and Responsibility

The first principles of consumer-driven reform

John Spiers

Visiting Professor
School of Humanities and Social Sciences
University of Glamorgan

Foreword by
Professor Karol Sikora

In association with the
Institute of Economic Affairs

RADCLIFFE MEDICAL PRESS

Radcliffe Medical Press Ltd
18 Marcham Road
Abingdon
Oxon OX14 1AA
United Kingdom

www.radcliffe-oxford.com
The Radcliffe Medical Press electronic catalogue and online ordering facility.
Direct sales to anywhere in the world

British Library Cataloguing in Publication Data

A catalogue record for this book is available from the British Library.

ISBN 1 85775 924 9

Typeset by Advance Typesetting Ltd, Oxfordshire
Printed and bound by TJ International Ltd, Padstow, Cornwall

Openeth the window, to let in the light; that breaketh the shell, that we may eat the kernel; that putteth aside the curtain ... that removeth the cover of the well, that we may come by the water.

King James Bible

He that will not apply new remedies must expect new evils; for time is the greatest innovator.

Francis Bacon

The society which scorns excellence in plumbing because plumbing is a humble activity and tolerates shoddiness in philosophy because it is an exalted activity will have neither good plumbing nor good philosophy. Neither its pipes nor its theories will hold water.

John Gardner

There would be more loose ends. But it is out of loose ends that freedom and progress are made.

DS Lees

History will not stay written.

William Sloane

In the life of a nation, to dispose of one problem is to start another.

GM Young

Without will and freedom there can be no virtue and vice.

Gertrude Himmelfarb

Life is not a splendid romance ... [but] a true history.

Hannah More

We must be serious and decided – for, after all, the person who has contracted debts must pay them ...

Jane Austen

For Byron
(born Sydney, Australia, 22 August 2001)
and Oscar
(born Singapore, 17 March 2003)

Contents

Foreword

Professor Karol Sikora MA, PhD, FRCR, FRCP, FFPM is a leading cancer specialist. He is an adviser to a major multinational pharmaceutical company on the development of new cancer drugs, and is creating, with HCA International, an innovative centre of excellence for cancer care in London which will bridge the private–NHS divide. He is Professor of Cancer Medicine at Imperial College, Hammersmith Hospital, London.

Every healthcare system around the world is struggling with change. Unprecedented demand, empowered patients, ageing populations, novel technologies and huge shortages in care staff due to the changing role of women in society have led to an almost constant crisis in many countries. This has been fuelled by politicians seeking to use health as a political football – promising all, but delivering nothing. Rationing, distrust and quick-fix solutions abound in Britain's NHS, which hurtles from crisis to crisis incessantly. I was there when Tony Blair promised to fix the NHS by the next election. It's just not possible – even though a large amount of my tax will be wasted in the attempt. Instead, we will be drip-fed endless propaganda about casualty waiting times improving, cancer mortality falling, cancelled operations falling – all easy-to-collect but also easy-to-manipulate statistics. Healthcare's journey in Britain has come from the charitable–religious foundation of the early hospitals through the militaristic hierarchy of the post-war NHS. We are now in a Stalinist period with modernisation plans, collaboratives, networks, frameworks and commissioners. This communist vocabulary comes with an expensive and never-ending propaganda machine and the installation of a culture of fear of speaking out against the apparatchiks of Richmond House.

Against this background, how refreshing it is to read John Spiers' latest offering. Basically, its main premise is attractively simple. If you want to give patients real power, then they have to own the resources to pay for their care. This is how consumerism works in other walks of life, whether one is choosing an insurance policy, a holiday or a car. 'Money talks, preference walks', as John puts it. 'Patient fundholding' is the key theme. Achieving some sort of equity using this system then becomes the role of the politicians. There is an information asymmetry in health purchasing but, as John shows, this is neither inevitable nor beyond correction. Deciding on core services, here called 'patient guaranteed care', organising effective public health and regulating novel delivery systems will become the role of UK Health. But the politicians must be kept well away from running the day-to-day operation of healthcare delivery with its inevitable use as an arena for vote catching.

John's background is ideal for this whirlwind tour of consumerism and health. He was Chairman of the Patients' Association and of a major hospital trust board, and a founding member of Reform. He has written extensively on the problems surrounding the delivery of the medical care that we actually want. I frequently travel abroad for work and, as he points out, British Airways doesn't demand my time in planning or rationing its services. Instead, it offers me a service, and if I don't like it because of timing or cost, I can use another carrier. Heightened levels of local political activity along with consumer representation through professional patients – mainly white, vocal, female and middle-class – are no substitutes for individual patient fundholding. Market mimicry, where the appearances of a marketplace are created but the reality is little shift in the balance of power, is the current emphasis.

Existing providers, new investors and entrepreneurs need to be encouraged to offer differentiated services. Only then can consumers choose where they spend their health credit. John considers the UK optics market as an example of one system for all. It has not levered down standards to the lowest possible level. The revolution in eye care has led to no elitism in private care – everyone goes through the same door. The patient, rich or poor, is seen as an opportunity, not a nuisance. Contrast this with a busy outpatient clinic in the NHS, the waiting times for elective surgery and the inequality of being able to go down the road for private care delivered by the same doctor if you have money.

The lack of credible opposition to our current Government means that John's concepts deserve widespread dissemination and debate. If we are to get out of the current rut in healthcare delivery we need visionaries to point the way. This book is an inspirational guide to a potential way forward.

Professor Karol Sikora
January 2003

Preface and acknowledgements

This book could not have been completed without the enormous support, encouragement and creativity of my wife, Leigh, with whom I have spent many hours discussing the themes and problems. As ever, I am deeply grateful for the time, patience and thought she has brought to bear over nearly a decade together now in clarifying and sharpening my arguments, extending and deepening my thoughts – and for all indispensable and necessary help with complex machinery, from paper clips to computers. As always, she is my first and best reader. She has made many invaluable suggestions. Let me say here, in the hope that she believes me, that I do not take for granted the time she gives from her own work in art history. I have, too, had the advantage of access to the special insights and knowledge she gained in directly managing several very large specialist departments within the NHS over more than 20 years.

I am also indebted to friends and colleagues for their comments on earlier sketches and explorations of these ideas, in particular to Professor Karol Sikora, who has also kindly contributed the Preface, and to Professor Michael Connolly and Professor Jim Mansell, for giving their valuable time to close readings of my text, and for their challenges in putting awkward questions. I am also grateful to Dr William Pickering, the late Glynn Vernon, John Simmonds, Dr Robert Lefever, Stephen Pollard, Geraint Day and John Blundell and Philip Booth of the Institute of Economic Affairs. Gillian Nineham, Editorial Director of Radcliffe Medical Press, has been a very supportive publisher and I am as ever grateful to her; to my editor, Jamie Etherington; and to Gregory Moxon, who finds an audience for the work. I thank, too, Rebecca Connorton for her aid.

My warmest thanks are also due to Lord Howe of Aberavon CH, QC, and to Doug JD Perkins (Managing Director and co-founder, with his wife, of Specsavers) to whom I am indebted for discussion of the eye care market as the successful model of competition with the poor and the rich all in *one market*. My stepdaughter, Lorna Richardson, has been very informative in her capacity as a successful practising optometrist. I am most grateful for her professional advice.

Few things are entirely new under the sun. I have been fundamentally influenced in framing my approach to stasism and dynamism as alternative ways of looking at the possibilities by my reading of Virginia Postrel's superb and important book on the sources of dynamism in society, *The Future and Its Enemies*.[1] I draw in detail on Postrel's analysis, which illuminates the choices we face in England concerning healthcare. The two concepts of order – one of control and premeditated design, the other of adaptive voluntary exchange – are Mill's and Hayek's. I am indebted, too, to the work of Professor Alain C Enthoven[2] and for his comments on the first part of this book, and Dr DS Lees,[3] and to Dr David Misselbrook's remarkable book, *Thinking About Patients*.[4]

In seeking out the history of the prescriptive bureaucracy of the NHS – and how and why we got where we are now – I am also indebted to the historical and theoretical works of my former tutor and old friend, Professor Stephen Yeo. In particular for my discussion of 'needs', 'wants' and the 'Webbian' intellectual basis of the NHS itself as it replaced working-class self-organisation with bureaucratic/elitist direction and professional 'Webbian' management by a professional and managerial class, with a specific culture of control from above. In my analysis, they have – damagingly – become the fulcrum of 'health politics'.[5]

I am not trained as an economist. And so I lack what Professor Martin Ricketts has called 'the penchant of economists for setting themselves theoretical puzzles'. But I do deploy economic concepts, and necessarily make use of numbers, at least in outline. My chief concern, however, is with principles and their operation, and with vested interests and their insistence, endurance and resistance. For, as Matthew Arnold tells us, we 'must begin with an idea of the world in order not to be prevailed over by the world's multitudinous'.[6] The bulk of the figures cited can be found in the electronic publications of the Organisation for Economic Co-operation and Development (OECD). The OECD is the notary of competing notions about what works best where.[7]

We learn much from international comparisons, although Dr Heinz Redwood has warned of the difficulties posed by them. They are indeed fraught with difficulties, even considering the fact that – in the absence of a state monopoly of funding – people in many overseas countries clearly do prefer to spend more of their income on healthcare when the approach is governed by the private decisions of individual citizens. Dr Redwood's words bear repetition at this juncture, even though we must seek to make comparisons if we are to learn from others. And if we are to understand why, despite rising prosperity, we have not devoted more of our GNP to health services. This despite the new opportunities and new knowledge, and the fact that as incomes rise demand for healthcare has risen elsewhere in proportion.

Dr Redwood has written that 'International comparisons are rarely based on precisely comparable statistics. Countries vary in their definitions of "health care" and data can be changed prospectively and retrospectively if terms are re-defined or reviewed. Often, the same parameters are reported with quite different numbers in a variety of sources.' His suggestion is that the health database of the OECD is, more than most sources, the result of deliberate efforts to achieve comparability between countries.[8]

Statistics prove little about individual men and women. But the English Government's own current figures are on its website (www.doh.gov.uk). They remind us that those who insist on continued NHS monopoly have somehow to dispose of the result.

The opinions expressed here are, of course, my own and not necessarily those of my friends and colleagues, or of those organisations with which I am associated. Errors of fact or tact are mine alone. I would like to stress, too, that I am not now a member of any political party. I am an independent contributor. But I declare an interest. I seek to be loyal to ideas which I believe are relevant to achieving a guarantee of high-quality healthcare for all in a society of liberty and justice. Unanswered questions – perhaps unanswerable ones – remain. For some quandaries are a matter of permanent doubt and discussion. Michael Oakeshott 'always insisted that explanation ends in the unexplained or (more likely) the inexplicable'. This is Kant's view, too: 'It is very absurd to expect enlightenment from reason, and yet to dictate to her in advance upon which side she must necessarily determine.'[9] And so there is plenty of scope for further work, not least by economists, in confronting ideals with facts. Napoleon famously said that the test of a plan is in its execution. There is no way to skip the groundwork, to set in progress a maturing process of evolutionary change, if we are to discover that changes are practicable and how they are practicable.

Ultimately, however, in the words of the early co-operative leader, JTW Mitchell, 'Not only must we bear our own burdens, but each other's burdens'.[10] And perhaps the key messages of this book are to raise suspicions about final answers, to diminish both faith in and expectation of 'Government', to replace 'representative agencies' with personal self-reliance, and to urge every patient and professional to ask their *own* questions. Thus, we can avoid confusing a specific instrument – the NHS – with the end of better outcomes. We can, too, distinguish results from activities (or mere volume).

Much of the book concerns risk. Macneile Dixon hands us the compass:

> *It may be that I am wrong. It may be that the world is on the way to become what it has never been, a home of rest for the gentle and the timid, a sequestered garden for those who hate the turmoil of the seas. I can well understand the religious fear, the humanitarian horror of its sullen skies, its mounting waves and devouring storms, the disrelish for battle, murder and sudden death, the war in nature and the war in man. Life, as Christianity has always taught, as all clear-eyed observers have known, is a perilous adventure, and a perilous adventure for men and women it will, I fear and believe, remain.*

As he says, 'It is not the lofty sails but the unseen wind which moves the ship.'[11]

John Spiers
Twyford, Sussex
January 2003

Notes

1 Postrel V (1998) *The Future and Its Enemies: the growing conflict over creativity, enterprise and progress.* The Free Press, New York. I am grateful to Steve Buckstein, Director of The Cascade Policy Institute, Portland, Oregon, who drew my attention to this critically important book when I was an Adjunct Scholar there in 1999. On Postrel's themes see also, especially, F Hayek, *The Constitution of Liberty* (University of Chicago Press, Chicago, 1960) and DS North, *Understanding the Process of Economic Change* (Institute of Economic Affairs, London, 1999). The most articulate statist alternative is offered by J Gray, whose work Postrel critiques. See, for example, J Gray, *Beyond the New Right. Markets, Government and the common environment* (Routledge, London,

1993), as well as J Mander and E Goldsmith (eds) *The Case Against the Global Economy* (Sierra Club Books, San Francisco, CA, 1996). Postrel's website can be found at www.dynamist.com

2 Enthoven AC (2002) Introducing market forces into health care: a tale of two countries. Paper delivered to Fourth European Conference on Health Economics, Paris, 10 July 2002. I am grateful to Professor Enthoven for sending me this paper. See also his 'Consumer Choice Health Plan' (*NEJM*. **298**: 650–58, 709–20, 1978), 'History and Principles of Managed Competition' (*Health Affairs*. **12 (Supplement)**: 24–8, 1974), *Theory and Practice of Managed Competition in Health Care Finance* (Amsterdam, North Holland, 1988), AC Enthoven and SJ Singer, 'The Clinton Health Plan. A single-payer system in Jackson Hole clothing' (*Health Affairs*. **Spring issue**: 81–95, 1994), 'Why not the Clinton Health Plan?' (*Inquiry*. **32**: 129–35, 1994), 'Why managed care has failed to contain health costs' (*Health Affairs*. **12**: 27–43, 1993), *Reflections on the Management of the National Health Service: an American looks at incentives to efficiency in health service management in the UK* (Nuffield Provincial Hospitals Trust, London, 1985), *In Pursuit of an Improving National Health Service* (Nuffield Trust, London, 1999), 'In pursuit of an improving NHS' (*Health Affairs*. **19**: 102–9, 2000), 'Commentary: competition made them do it' (*BMJ*. **324**: 143, 2002), AC Enthoven, HH Schauffler and S McMenamin, 'Consumer choice and the managed care backlash' (*Am J Law Med*. **27**: 1–15, 2001), *Health Plan*, reprinted by Beard Books, Washington, DC, 2002. See also G McLachlan and A Maynard, *The Public/Private Mix for Health* (Nuffield Provincial Hospitals Trust, London, 1993), Browne A and Young M, *NHS Reform: towards a consensus* (Adam Smith Institute, London, 2002).

3 Lees DS (1961) *Health Through Choice. An economic study of the English National Health Service*. IEA, London.

4 Misselbrook D (2001) *Thinking About Patients*. Petroc Press, Newbury.

5 This is an important body of work, but with whose increasingly 'hard' Marxist analysis I fundamentally disagree. See CS Yeo, *Religion and Voluntary Organisations in Crisis* (Croom Helm, London, 1976), 'A new life: the religion of socialism in Britain, 1883–1896' (*History Workshop*, Autumn, 1977), 'Working-class association, private capital, welfare and the state in the late nineteenth and twentieth centuries' in N Parry, M Rustin and C Satyamuri, *Social Work, Welfare and the State* (Edward Arnold, London, 1979), 'Towards "making form of more moment than spirit": further thoughts on Labour, Socialism and the New Life from the late 1890s to the present' in JA Jowitt and RKS Taylor, *Bradford 1890–1914: the cradle of the Independent Labour Party* (University of Leeds Centre for Adult Education, Bradford, 1980), 'State and anti-state: reflections on social forms and struggles from 1850' in P Corrigan (ed.) *Capitalism, State Formation and Marxist Theory. Historical investigations* (Quartet Books, London, 1980), 'Socialism, the State and some oppositional Englishness' in R Colls and P Dodd (eds) *The Idea of Englishness: politics and culture, 1880–1920* (Croom Helm, London, 1986), 'Notes on three socialisms – collectivism, statism and associationism – mainly in late-nineteenth and early-twentieth-century Britain' in C Levy (ed.) *Socialism and the Intelligentsia, 1880–1914* (Routledge, London, 1987), 'Three socialisms: statism, collectivism, associationism' in W Outhwaite and M Mulkay (eds) *Social Theory and Social Criticism* (Blackwell, Oxford, 1987), two essays in S Yeo (ed.) *New Views of Co-operation* (Routledge, London, 1988), *Who Was JTW Mitchell?* (CWS Membership Services, Manchester, 1995). Also see 'Co-operative and mutual enterprise, the co-operative movement and the learning and skills agenda', Evidence

to Co-operative Commission, June 2000, Co-operative Wholesale Society, Lough-borough. But see TW Heyck, *The Transformation of Intellectual Life in Victorian England* (Croom Helm, London, 1982). A different historical account is offered by Lawlos S (2001) *Second Opinion? Moving the NHS monopoly to a mixed system* (Politiea, London).

6 Arnold M, cited in Trilling L (1936) *Matthew Arnold* (Unwin University Books edition, London (1963)) p.32.

7 Organisation for Economic Co-operation and Development (OECD) (1998) *OECD Health Data 1998: a comparative analysis of 29 countries*. OECD, Paris. Also see OECD (2001) *OECD Health Data 2001: a comparative analysis of 30 countries* (10e). OECD, Paris.

8 Redwood H (2000) *Why Ration Health Care? An international study of the United Kingdom, France, Germany and public sector health care in the USA*. Civitas, London.

9 Minogue K (1993) The history of political thought seminar. In: J Norman (ed.) *The Achievement of Michael Oakeshott*. Duckworth, London, p.91; Kant cited, Macneile Dixon, op. cit., p.119.

10 Quoted in Yeo, *Mitchell*, ibid., p.72.

11 Macneile Dixon W (1938) *The Human Situation. The Gifford Lectures delivered in the University of Glasgow, 1935–1937*. Longmans Green, New York, p.50.

About the author

Professor John Spiers is a well-known independent commentator on healthcare in the UK and abroad. He is not a member of any political party. In 2001 he was appointed to the board of the new National Commission on Care Standards, where he has continued to pursue his chief interest of urging improved quality and individual empowerment from the consumer's point of view. He has particularly urged financially empowered choice, the encouragement of co-operative and self-governing mutual-aid organisations, and the protection of individual choice and of provider competition. He is descended from a grandfather who was born in the Hoxton Workhouse (in the poorest district of the nineteenth-century East End) and from a great-great-grandmother who died there with two of her 13 children. His family were nineteenth-century stonemasons and marblemasons, and his great-grandfather was a Windsor chairmaker. He is now working on their history for a new book, *Land of Promise*.

John Spiers has consistently urged that consumers will only be empowered when economic purchasing power is returned to them. And that equity, fairness, access, social solidarity and personal responsibility can only be achieved by ensuring that everyone, including the poor, has the cash which makes the difference. For him the key issue is how to equip both the poor and everyone else to be individually empowered buyers of healthcare, just like the middle class.

His mother was disabled, and her youngest brother (now 89 years of age and still living independently) has been seriously visually impaired all his life. John once toured a Brighton hospital in a wheelchair, with a wheelchair-bound woman and her virtually blind husband, in order to dramatise with them and to management what he called 'the invisible hospital'. This is the institution which managers too often overlook, but which is the awkward and unwelcoming reality for the disempowered patient. He appointed the first ever Patient's Advocate in an NHS hospital in 1991. This became a model for the NHS. He also established the first Clinical Performance Improvement Unit in an NHS hospital in 1993. After he had left, the Chief Executive referred to him as 'just an ordinary member of the public'.

John Spiers took a First Class Honours degree in History at the University of Sussex, where he has been Chairman of the Alumni Society since 1983. In 1969, while a graduate student there, he founded the book publishing firm The Harvester Press, which he ran for nearly 20 years. The firm won the Queen's Award for Export Achievement in 1986.

Since the late 1980s, John has devoted his time to writing and lecturing in various public roles in health and education. Since 1998 he has been a Visiting Professor at the University of Glamorgan. He is a Visiting Fellow of the Centre for Health Leadership, and in 1999 he was an Adjunct Scholar at the Cascade Policy Institute, Portland, Oregon (where he was studying US healthcare). In 2001, he became a founder member of the Advisory Council of 'Reform', campaigning for new directions in public policy. He has been Chairman of Brighton Health Authority, Brighton Health Care NHS Trust, the David Salomons Management Centre, and the Patients Association, whose re-launch he led in 1995. He was also a member of the Prime Minister's Citizens' Charter Advisory Panel.

His other interests are in education, where he has held senior posts in public service. He is a Trustee of the Ruskin Foundation, John Ruskin's charity The Guild of St George, the English Schools Orchestra, the Shakespeare Authorship Trust, the Francis Bacon Society and the League of Mercy (which awarded him its Companion's Cross in 2002). For 8 years he was Vice-Chairman of the Grant-Maintained Schools Foundation. He is now organising the 2003 Centenary Conference, 'Gissing and The City', at the University of London, commemorating the nineteenth-century novelist George Gissing.

By the same author

- Spiers J and Sinkins P (1994) *'Things to Fix': an initiative using the best ideas of Brighton Health Care staff to help patients, staff and the organisation.* Brighton Health Care NHS Trust, Brighton.
- Spiers J (1995) *The Invisible Hospital and the Secret Garden. An insider's commentary on the NHS reforms.* Radcliffe Medical Press, Oxford, and Institute of Health Services Management, London.
- Spiers J (1996) *An Innocent Elopement. Patients and empowerment* (lecture). The Patients Association, London.
- Spiers J (1996) *Sense and Sensibility in Health Care.* M Marinker (ed.). BMJ Publishing, London.
- Spiers J (1997) *Who Owns Our Bodies? Making moral choices in healthcare.* Radcliffe Medical Press, Oxford, and Institute for Health Policy Studies, Southampton.
- Spiers J (1997) *User Involvement in Health Care: what next?* Association of Charitable Foundations Fourth Annual Lecture on Philanthropy, London.
- Spiers J (ed.) (1997) *Dilemmas in Modern Health Care.* Social Market Foundation/ Profile Books, London.
- Spiers J (1999) If this is a question, is this an answer? Patients and empowerment: first principles, moral problems, and patient benefit. In: T Ling (ed.) *Reforming Health Care by Consent.* Radcliffe Medical Press, Oxford.
- Spiers J (1999) *The Realities of Rationing. 'Priority setting' in the NHS.* Institute of Economic Affairs, London.
- Spiers J (2002) Safe in *whose* hands? Effective consumer power in health care. In: E Vaizey (ed.) *The Blue Book On Health.* Politicos, London.
- Spiers J (2002) *'Coming, Ready or Not!' The present, politics and future of health care. Essays on the potential of consumer power to renovate health care.* Edward Everett Root, Brighton.
- Spiers J (in preparation) *Land of Promise. Being the memoirs of A.J.Root, an Edwardian North London boy. Or, it's a long way from Shipway Terrace!*

Part 1

Patients: some introductions

Chapter 1

Must reform always be like trying to knit with water?

There are two great principles – demand –
'*A cup of tea if you please, dear,*' interrupted Tibbs.
And supply.

(Charles Dickens)

We are considering the scarcest thing in the world – the days of our lives, their quality, and the extent of our control over them. Health is one of the keys to a good life, as is self-responsibility, self-restraint and self-discipline. The fundamental concept and concern of this book is to explore how to place consumers in charge, in order to guarantee good patient care for all.

To find good answers to the perennial problems of UK healthcare, it is vital to ask the right questions. The answers that this book offers revolve around the radical notion of putting consumers in charge of their own healthcare. This model proposes that individuals should have control – voluntarily grouped in purchasing co-operatives. And that competitive forces be released to spur innovation, integrate services, improve productivity and drive change in our producer-dominated, tradition-bound healthcare system. Believable answers must carry both philosophical and emotional weight if we are to achieve democratic rationality.

The fundamental concept and concern of this book is to explore how to place consumers in charge, in order to guarantee good patient care for all on the basis of first principles of justice and equity. The word *guarantee* figures largely, and deliberately. I propose a legally-enforceable guarantee of a 'core' package of care. For this constitutes a vital re-assurance. Here, 'guarantee' is a prismatic word which makes an emotional appeal – and one of moral, philosophical, practical and political significance. It is a crucial evaluative reference for any policy change. It offers the fundamental and explicit promise to provide what people want from the health system. It is, too, the necessary re-assurance of justice and social unity at a time of change. It is, fundamentally, a demonstration that it is within our capacity to realise justice in healthcare. This means a clear guarantee of good services for all. For we must ensure that the poorer and weaker are not left behind in any financial re-structuring. This ambition is intended to appeal to the commonality – to a nobility of sentiment that takes liberty as its ideal and humanity as its spirit. And it seeks to inspire a new confidence in the availability of appropriate services, and to transmit a promise that will be believed.

So the guarantee of patient care – and of how to achieve it in reality – is at the heart of my proposals. We need to discover terms and language which will encourage the discussion. For language, style, and practice – or content together with the descriptive words and the force of their relation one with the other – are inextricably linked. Disraeli once said, 'We govern men with words.' But we do so, too, with moral concepts, reason, and common sense which that language must encapsulate. And, too, by referring actions to fixed and fundamental first principles which reflect a profound national moral sense. We should be aware, too, in addressing the necessities of good presentation of ideas and policies, of the benefits of being alert to the rhythm of sentences, to the tone of voice, to the ways in which ideas are heard (*and mis-heard*), and to the expression of will and imagination which can deliver democratic objectives. To achieve real change we should remember that one of Winston Churchill's greatest achievements was to have 'mobilised the English language and sent it into battle'.[1]

Today, the presumption in healthcare is all in favour of change. But to find good answers to the perennial problems of UK healthcare – and answers which secure emotional and political legitimacy – it is vital to ask the right questions, so as to reveal the cardinal realities beneath. The answers you get depend on the questions you ask, and how you ask them. And, too, some questions may be more easily asked than answered. But unless we realise that there are insistent questions which need answers – and unless we reconsider answers which have been marginalised for half a century – we have little chance of making progress, or of understanding the problems which prompt the questions. This requires us, also, to be conscious of the genuine concerns people have about change, and to address these concerns.

New questions are being asked, and old ones revived. For example, is it really true that public spending *is* the only way to improve services? Why not a smaller State, and competitive choice instead? Is it really essential that the State provides services, rather than provides *for* services? Why not the State acting as an enabler which makes *sure* it happens? Why not recover a system of genuine individual empowerment and self-responsibility? Why not think more radically on how to encourage both doctor-led and patient-led reform in healthcare delivery systems and a re-engineering of care processes? Why not look again at motivation, and at structures which were swept aside by a focus on long-term, inanimate personal social forces and 'the logic of history' – and which has proved elusively illogical and frustrating, notably to the poor whose gains from the NHS have been disappointing and to medical professionals, whose morale is disturbingly low.

Cultures and context exert a massive grip. Yet, vibrant leadership matters in determining the course of events – notably in refusing to elevate 'the system' above the patient. Here, too, I explore the idea that there are enduring truths and first principles which transcend race, gender, class, and temporary and unenduring events – and which can be set out clearly.

Significantly, the problems are cultural. They are about self-belief, by patients and by staff. I argue that unless patients have to take charge of their lives there will be too little self-responsibility. And that unless doctors are better motivated, better rewarded, and have higher morale there will not be better outcomes. There must be job satisfaction, with people who know they are doing a good job and are being appreciated. This is not just about pay. It is about the broad cluster of feelings summed up in the phrase 'job satisfaction'. And of how each individual can add value *by their own actions.* Staff and patients have got to believe in the possibilities of doing better, and not have their hopes and ambitions so easily squashed. It is no good constantly reforming healthcare if large numbers of staff continue to go home in a state of nervous exhaustion.

Individuals (patients and staff) owning change can only come about by a cultural transformation – one which shifts the entire axis of the system. This will turn on how things and people are managed, so that all involved are made to feel that they can do more, achieve more, work harder, and produce better results. A necessity is constant feedback and regular appraisal (including personal contracts for all), which is checked. A different ethos is possible, as continental experience shows (and as UK experience in some other areas of public services which are changing, such as the results achieved with 'average' intakes by City Technology Colleges, where levels of achievement are significantly greater). The issue is for every individual consciously and willingly to batten down for quality and outcomes. Then we can achieve the objectives which are supposed to be on the social agenda, but which are not achievable by centralisation and control from above. We can show what can be achieved by vision, clear management, and clear responsibility. But the trigger must be individual responsibility – *starting* with the patient.

The message here is a simple one, but one which is often overlooked by management. It is this: we need to catch people doing things right, as well as catch people doing things wrong. Good doctors must be properly rewarded, whereas they are poorly rewarded in the NHS. Good doctors must be enabled to do medicine, and not be social cogs in everyone else's Ferris wheel. Good doctors create something in their own right, which is good care and faith in care itself. Yet if this goes unrecognised then good people will remain poorly motivated and patients feel stranded. This does not mean there must be little or no accountability. Such an idea is absurd, and now hardly canvassed. But it must be accountability for *outcomes.*

One imperative is to stop the forces trying to stop change and drag us back – and some doctors are among them – in a deft rallentando. One example concerns the role of so-called 'public sector unions'. Historically, it was important for trade unions to help create better conditions for workers. But we cannot remain locked into problems by changes made for previous generations, and now entrenched by sea-dog opposition and special interest. No doubt change will involve some hardship and agony, but it needs to be explained in terms of first principles, and with sunshine and hope and the promise of conquest and victory – even in Churchillian terms – if the vital energy of the community is to be successfully concentrated.

The proposal to put the consumer in charge – with services for all still to be mainly funded by central taxation (which of course I recognise is coercive) – offers the potential for much better and essential partnerships between consumers and providers, for better, more responsive, better-funded care and higher morale and reward for those delivering good care. And for outcomes relevant to, and significantly defined by, individual consumers themselves. If the structure offers incentives for better services to be offered, the State should empower individuals to use them and contribute towards their cost, in whole or in part. I offer the concept of patient fundholding, with the individual owning a specific healthcare fund, empowering choice. This can have many benefits, not least in educating consumers about the cost of health services, prompting individuals to seek information about those services they consume, and – perhaps – evolve more cost-effective patterns of use. Informed purchasing decisions will not necessarily be inexpensive decisions, but the provision of cost and quality information will educate and perhaps amend some behaviours.

As Professor Regina Herzlinger of Harvard University recently said of the US system, which is in no less difficulty than our own:

> When consumers apply pressure on an industry, whether it's retailing or banking, cars or computers, it invariably produces a surge of innovation that increases productivity, reduces prices, improves quality and expands choices. The essential problem with the health care industry is that it has been shielded from consumer control – by employers, insurers and the government. As a results, costs have exploded as choices have narrowed.[2]

This book examines some very difficult problems of policy and conscience, and different theories of 'community' in the functioning of the State. These dilemmas are not easily simplified by rough-hewn labels and abstractions like 'collectivist' or 'individualist' as we seek to distinguish what we think should be 'class actions' to be taken by the State and what should be specific actions to be taken by the individual. This discussion will, however, inevitably lead us from the present State monopoly of funding, purchasing and providing, into a more subtle if more complex approach which combines the remedial action of the State, the actions of the self-responsible individual, and voluntary or 'community' effort. Reform will need the State to occupy a supervisory role rather than an incessantly directive role, and this itself will evolve in self-adjustment.

This is an approach which co-ordinates all three elements – the State, the individual, and voluntary effort. It offers great operational as well as moral value, with self-responsibility in the foreground. The individual seeking the best, including *from themselves* in self-responsibility. The mutual-aid organisation offering leadership and incentive to persuade people to do some things or stop doing others. The State as rule-maker, with the power to enforce patient guaranteed care by law but encouraging the spontaneous discipline of the individual and the family. In this description, the 'individual' never constitutes a uniform pattern, the more so in an increasingly diverse society. And so we should seek an approach which employs organisations that stand separately both from the State and the individual. This can enable time and money to be marshalled by which to investigate individually (and empower financially) the hidden and deeply personal reasons for individual action. These should be assessed by the patient and the adviser in a necessarily delicate balance of risk and opportunity, and with an approach which ensures that everyone gets their chance. The adaptive patchwork this constitutes can reflect many of the characteristics of mutual-aid: stable but adaptive, ingenious and innovative, transparent and often inexpensive.

The trend of modern healthcare is towards more complex and more highly individualised care, which improves outcomes and the quality of life as determined by the patient.

Here, choice and control are the essential elements for successful change. In the UK we have made virtually no progress towards either. This, despite Mr Alan Milburn's drive to focus the system on the individual. And so we have to start from basics, and imagine the possibilities all over again. Raymond Williams tells us that 'It is the ability to raise a structure in imagination before erecting it in reality that marks out human activity from other kinds.'[3] So we should have more confidence in imagining, in describing and in testing out what might be possible and what we could achieve. We should not necessarily rely on the 'obvious', or on a master-plan. But any proposals should be predicated on an architecture of consumer control.

Is the consumer necessarily inadequate, *a priori*, in making personal judgements? I argue that this is not necessarily so. Granted, there is an information asymmetry – one which has been reinforced by NHS rationing and by Government deliberately restricting the flow of information in order to suppress demand. This denial of information to patients has proved inefficient, shown the structure to be vulnerable and unable to defend itself against its own weaknesses. However, we should recognise that much healthcare concerns lifestyle choice, in which the individual has the intimate and special information and self-knowledge about their own life. And if individuals join consumer co-operatives these will employ medical professionals in key management roles, where clinical expertise will link medical and personal knowledge, advise members, and deploy specialist skills on their behalf. Consumers will not live in the dark: services providing advice, information and counselling will proliferate, providing individuals with data and advocacy to help them make intelligent and informed choices.

The key is to place consumers in the position of spending a health credit as if it was their own money from an ordinary wage packet (as, in reality, it is, although they have been cut off from choice, true cost, and purchasing decisions by the State). The provider, too, will seek to appeal to a mass market peopled by individuals who can switch funding to preferred services.

Much more direct change will come from making sure the consumer has direct financial control than from any other proposed approach. Too often, in 'consultation', this means that service-users are co-opted into the defined processes of professionals – as Norma Raynes, Director of the Institute for Health and Social Care Research at the University of Salford, recently stressed. Or, in Lionel Trilling's words (from another and older context), they 'make a fine show of rushing out to meet the problems of modern life but their endowment was limited enough to keep them safe and platitudinous'.[4] And the roles of counsellors, advocates and lay assessors are ameliorative responses in the main to the consequences of State monopoly and the lack of individual empowerment.

It will be seen that this settles nothing, but merely initiates the problem. For it is insufficient to speak of freedom without enquiring into freedom's meaning or its uses. It hardly helps us at all to consider freedom as a horse to be ridden without noticing the nature of the animal. But if consumers are in charge, we will instead quickly see much innovation in a variety of better services, to provide creatively thoughtful service solutions tailored to the preferences of the financially-empowered individual. For the features which most people value – treatment mainly free at the point of use; care regardless of income; free Accident and Emergency service – can be more successfully provided if there is consumer empowerment and direct payment and incentive, inducement and encouragement. So, too, we can achieve more in preventive care and self-responsibility. All these features are characteristics, indeed, of social insurance systems. Money empowers all, including the silent, the unorganised, the discrete, the un-politicised patient who does not wish to join a pressure group or be an active, trained, citizen pre-occupied with healthcare structures and rationing in permanent 'consultation' with 'experts'. Existing providers, new investors and entrepreneurs will, too, be attracted to offer differentiated services, featuring different combinations of benefits valued by consumers.

Preference and acumen will soon combine, and consumer pressure will produce many new efficiencies as healthcare becomes customer-oriented. Government, too, as I argue below, will subsidise the poor as a morally legitimate claim upon the public purse and will police the system to ensure protection against abuse. In addition, risk adjustment will be integrated by law into the foundations of the system, to ensure that we do not see a system emerge where insurers attract the healthy and punish the sick. Indeed, by competitive insurance and Government risk adjustment the incentives will be to develop innovative treatments of the chronically ill in integrated and co-ordinated approaches which we notably lack now. Disorganised, poor care costs more than well co-ordinated quality services, for poor care and a lack of self-responsibility undermines individual health, and leads to costly illness, procedures, prescriptions and emergency care. In markets, too, the differences in quality between the best and the average narrow, and all legal products must be of adequate quality. In addition, consumer-driven quality care would release funding as it improved health status – either for new services, or for greater subsidy to the poor in purchasing care. Consumer-driven care, too, would cease to be focused on large general hospitals and the workplace of consultants who throw political clout. Instead, consumer co-operatives would insist on integrated care and diversity of delivery locations – for support in the home, for services in the community, in tertiary care facilities for access to specialist and complex care.

Action stations

To build understanding and support for change, we should take a number of conceptual steps.

First, we should set out the first principles of good care, and ask how these can be applied to the urgent necessities of improved care. This is a prerequisite, to give *unité d'action et d'ensemble*.

Secondly, we should offer explanations for the difficult realities that we see around us, by applying the insights of first principles to show why things are as they are, what individual events mean and why they persistently occur.

Thirdly, we should offer approaches to change which apply first principles and thus offer a credible and realistic agenda for change.

The fundamental task is to give a coherent account of first principles by which we can understand why and how things happen in the NHS, their meanings and the alternatives. In Matthew Arnold's words 'to see the object as it really is' – to sort out meaning from a vast multitude of facts awaiting and inviting comprehension. And to explain why putting consumers in charge will make the essential differences – to improve coverage and access, to enhance quality, to reduce costs and to integrate care over time – thus improving outcomes in long-term care and in the treatment of acute, chronic, mental and catastrophic illness. We must try to understand the organisational, economic and social, cultural and philosophical problems that we face. And why all attempts to improve quality, curb cost spirals and enhance self-responsibility have achieved little. Why, too, patients, doctors, nurses and hospitals are all so unhappy with the situation.

The identification of first principles – and the direct incentives which enable them to harmonise the interests of consumers and providers – is both a political and a moral necessity. We shall make no progress, we shall persuade no one and we shall build no political support unless we recognise these political facts of life. Since the most persuasive change is incremental change, this should be evolved and explained in terms of these principles. These both justify and enlarge understandings. They make visible both contradictions and alternatives. It is necessary to explain events in terms of a framework which makes principles explicit. This gradually builds understandings of why things are as they are, how they came about, and how they can be different. As Thomas Jefferson said, 'Fix reason firmly in her seat, and call to her tribunal every fact, every opinion'.

As we try to set out first principles, we quickly bump hard into value judgements – about the human condition, human nature and conduct. And so we should. For the problems of healthcare are not about *facts* alone. Nor can facts speak for themselves. As the economist Alfred Marshall said, controversy 'brings out the impossibility of learning anything from facts until they are examined and interpreted by reason'.[5]

So we need to reason out principles. We need to reason *from* principles. We need to do so quickly, too, since evidence from elsewhere shows that outcomes are consistently better where different approaches are taken to healthcare funding, purchasing and provision. We need, if we are to have this debate at all, to notice how three key roles have become confused, namely our interests as 'citizens' (or voters), our role as 'producers' (or voters again) and our demands as 'consumers' (subsumed into voting – which does not secure what is a necessarily personal, separable, intimate and individual service).

I believe that we can and must find answers to a whole series of interrelated questions to release a dynamic, cohesive and improving future for all, and within the traditions of mutual aid, co-operation and voluntary exchange. Here I urge that only individuals really know what matters to them – and that we should resist the blandishments of 'experts' and of 'emancipatory politics' which forces us to have what is 'good for us'. Instead we can set out the firm foundations and the specific devices by which we can really guarantee prompt access to optimal care for all, which the NHS has promised but has not consistently achieved. We can, too, make changes now which will improve, not worsen, the position of the unlucky, the disadvantaged and the poor who have done least well from the NHS – and which will give everyone, including them, access to sustained improvements. And if change is secured, Government (as rule maker) can be motivated to *sustain* the right rules, including maintaining the value of tax transfers to the poor – and thus convince the poor that they will not sooner or later come off worse in the new bargain. A new structure can change this position and at the same time prevent the poor from being marginalised further by changes in funding and access, so that tax revenues ensure cover for the poor, and for *their* power to have their individual preferences respected.

For the first time, they can have the power that the richer enjoy. Free choice – of doctor, of hospital – can be restored. The doctor–patient relationship rebuilt. Morale improved. And staff no longer feel at the behest of every political whim. Management will be freed of political control. It will be set clear objectives for performance by purchasers and by consumers. It will have the freedom to manage, and obtain the information necessary to do so and to measure performance. It will be accountable for quality, individual outcomes, and value for money – thus making a reality of the objects Foundation Hospitals seek. Everyone can win. Success will be rewarded (and failure penalised). Thus, Government will fuse ultimate national authority, immediate national responsibility, and the structure of re-assurance which will underpin local adaptive change, tempered by experience.

There is a search on for new forms of organisation and alternative models for ownership of industries currently in the public sector. The effort is to balance the State and subordinate centres of authority, between centralisation and localism, between compulsion and free choice, between greater freedom for some without markedly lesser freedom for others. There should be, too – in Lord Acton's words – 'the preservation of an inner sphere exempt from State power' in which, he believed, all liberty *in radice* consisted. Increasingly, the consideration focuses on mutualisation, and the 'public interest company' or 'social enterprise', to combine both the customer interest and the wider public interest.[6]

Here, we need to be alert about such apparently comforting words – such as 'mutualisation' – which are offered to break the log-jam between public and private. For example, does 'mutualisation' give the individual economic power, or merely 'a say' (or 'a greater say')? Mutualisation – or 'the local community properly and fairly represented' – is suddenly fashionable, and in some surprising circles. But if this merely means more 'active patients', politicised, and 'trained' to discuss planning choices in 'social enterprise', we make no progress. If it means the ability and freedom of the financially-empowered individual to choose between purchasing organisations which people willingly join, which are mutually owned, and in which no member stands in a more advantageous position than another in terms of voting rights, ownership or benefits, then we make genuine advances far beyond the NHS mutual promise of 'having a say'. I propose a new and entrepreneurial structure which will align direct payments and incentives, focus on outcomes which will be significantly defined by patients, and establish a clear framework of services accountable to patients. This is essential to any mutualisation.

And it is a structure which meets the claim that health is unsuited to competitive choices because provision is inherently monopolistic. It answers, too, the assertion that individual empowerment cannot be allowed since 'need' rather than ability to pay is the necessary moral emphasis.

There is a sense of epoch about these questions – a real feeling around us that major changes are coming rapidly, that we can see a loosened cliff giving way to seismic shifts, and that we can design market-based proposals to improve access, increase funding, enhance responsiveness to the individual and improve quality care. We can set in place real incentives, which improve personal concern for consequences.

A new framework of patient-guaranteed care

One of the greatest advocates of 'the people', Abraham Lincoln, accomplished his Gettysburg Address in 265 words. Few manage such brevity. And it is risky, too, to generalise about a system which 'delivers' some 12 million consultant episodes a year, another 12 million Accident and Emergency attendances, and some 250 million GP consultations. Yet my proposed reformed structure – which pivots on empowering both patients and general practitioners much more than is presently the case – will look like this (as concisely as I can manage):

1 patient-guaranteed care – a core of PGC, or pretty good care
2 patient fundholding – the essential financial structure, covering everyone
3 patient-guaranteed social insurance – the vital step empowering the individual with choices, spending the personal fund as a patient fundholder
4 patient-guaranteed care associations – where every individual would choose membership of a competing co-operative purchaser. These will be private associations mediating between the individual, the State and the producers of care. (Perhaps guaranteed patient care association would be a stronger formulation?)
5 patient-guaranteed care providers – a diversity of registered providers
6 Government as rule maker – to guarantee the structure and to maintain the pool of risk inherent in health services with universal access
7 open information – to inform the consumer and support evaluations by them and their purchasers
8 direct incentives for preventive care
9 every opportunity for the individual to top up spending
10 a presumption within the system against the 'problematisation' of normality, and that the biomedical model will be seriously queried
11 the whole functioning through effective direct incentives and legally enforce-able contract arrangements, rather than as services received as 'acts of grace'
12 the structure funded in the main by general taxation – the middle class paying for the less well off.

The role of the individual should be to be in charge of their own life and their own care. Thus they will select an insurer and a care plan with a purchasing co-operative (representing collective action without collectiv*ism*), to negotiate choices and to offer individuals an opportunity to provide additional supplementary funding. They should also take personal preventive care seriously. The State is often perceived to be the problem, but this is only a half truth. The patient is a problem, too, especially when we look at preventive care – because we are not permitted to be in charge of our lives, and because the incentives to think and act more with regard to our healthcare are subdued by the State.

The benefits of greater individual responsibility for preventive care would be huge, not least in terms of funding for services and staff presently denied. The Wanless Report estimated that high levels of individual engagement could deliver savings by 2020 of £30 billion – equivalent to half of the existing NHS budget. For each £100 spent on encouraging self-care, some £150 of benefits can be returned. Varying estimates suggest that 60–75% of healthcare costs are now associated with people with chronic conditions – and many of these costly medical conditions are preventable, or can be postponed, by effective disease management. Notably, by co-ordinated interventions, often by healthcare professionals allied to doctors. And it is clear, too, that a sense of self-worth, of control over one's life, of being able to shape and express personal preference and of being financially empowered to do so, is a crucial element in well-being.

The basic source of good individual health is the individual. How we live. We need to narrow the role of the State as we enlarge the role of the individual. More individual choice, of course. But more individual concern with preventive care, more concern with consequences, and more incentives to be so concerned. Under my patient-guaranteed care plan there would be direct incentives for the individual to agree a longer-term contract with an insurer, by which they negotiate preventive care gains and receive bonus benefits as a result – including gains which they truly value, depending on their interests (e.g. holiday vouchers, tickets to concerts, to Arsenal or to Wimbledon, bought by the insurer for achieving an improvement, for example, in blood pressure). Thus a well-person incentive would impact directly on preventive care, where gains have proved so elusive under the NHS. In the USA, for example, enrolees who follow Destiny Health's guidelines by participating in smoking cessation or weight loss programmes earn additional benefits such as higher interest levels on their personal medical funds, waivers of plan premiums, air-miles and hotel discounts.[7]

The role of Government should be to guarantee core care, to fund it by taxation, and to ensure individual financial leverage, choice and competition. It should withdraw from its 'triple monopoly' of funding, purchasing and providing, retaining the key role of guaranteeing funds by taxation but otherwise leaving well alone. It would ensure the provision of 'public goods' by efficient providers. Government should, too, ensure that real prices and complete price transparency are characteristic of the fullest information which they ensure is available, so that people make informed decisions between purchasing and provider organisations. Here the information which people most want must be published. This concerns what I have called the 'my daughter' test – where would a doctor send *his* daughter? People want to know about the performance of specific doctors, teams and units within hospitals. This information is not available to users, although it is known informally by many doctors. If a market is to function properly, there must be systematic, up-to-date disclosure of such knowledge, instead of generalised star ratings concerned merely with processes and volume measures. If consumers are in charge, information services will evolve, offering standardised ratings which reflect quality, consumer reporting on issues which matter to them (including the experiences of care) and comparative analysis. Information will be necessary to help consumers choose a co-operative purchaser and an insurer, and to accept recommendations from their purchaser concerning specific services and doctors. This will include guidance on specific medical conditions, and sources of detailed advice.

The role of providers should be to set their own prices, specify their quality and benefits, and then seek willing purchasers (members joining co-operatives) who have choices. These purchasing organisations will be like the old Friendly Societies (or Public Interest Companies, as they are sometimes now retitled). These arose in the heartland of an old, self-organising, labour tradition. If we want providers to turn outwards, to change systems, productivity and personnel management, and to focus on consumers, we must require them to seek revenues from individuals or their co-operatives which have a genuine choice and can go round the corner to another provider if they wish, and take their money with them. One result will be a wider choice of providers, including the correction of fragmented (and thus costly and ineffective) care by new, integrated, multidisciplinary provision specialising in specific diseases (such as diabetes) and improved quality.

The role of insurers will be to offer consumers information about choice, services and options. Insurance will cover the guaranteed care package – which will protect every individual from catastrophic and costly medical events. It will also offer other voluntary options. The individual will be enabled to negotiate a specific package of care which suits their requirements, and to customise care. They will also have an incentive to make trade-offs, for example by accepting a higher 'excess' they might secure greater benefits or pay a lower premium with their 'NHS credit' and carry forward the difference into a long-term elderly care plan.

To make the most effective use of money, every individual could be permitted to organise in voluntary co-operatives which do the actual purchasing. In a competitive environment, these would secure value for money for everyone, including the poor (who receive tax transfers with which to buy policies), good standards of care, and represent the patient as a strong and empowered customer. This would recover an important aspect of our traditions, for voluntary bodies, mutual-aid co-operatives and other associations were enormous – not universal – mutual bodies of working men, engaged (both in theory and in practice) in collective self-help (but without collect*ivism*). To recover this ambient (and still waiting) tradition, it would ultimately be the customer who made the decision as to whether a service was good value.

We can hope, indeed, for what Herzlinger has urged:

> *health care providers responding to consumer demands by pursuing three dramatic innovations:* focused factories *of providers that work together to better treat specific diseases or patient groups,* integrated information *records that consolidate*

currently dispersed patient information, and personalised medical technologies
that enable treatments to be designed for individuals. (italics in original)[7]

Consumers in charge of their NHS fund will choose a consumer-purchasing
co-operative that is able to secure specialised, integrated, comprehensive care
for their particular condition, and the incentive will be for providers to offer
integrated care. Integrated patient information will be necessary, and again direct
payment and direct incentives to achieve this apparent impossibility among
fragmented care services will be necessarily and promptly effective. Integrated
records will be essential when co-operatives make purchasing choices, and to
achieve quality outcomes these will also be necessary for consumers to select an
insurer and a consumer co-operative.

I do not suggest that the plan I outline in this book is a fully worked out
structure. Indeed, it is offered more by way of an ideal type – an institutional
framework at which to aim – a prologue with the intention of achieving a
consumer-driven system. There is clearly work to be done to achieve strategic
purposes, notably by economists. I shall examine the detail of thinking this
through operationally in my two linked chapters on 'Getting it done' (pages
177–214). To achieve these things we need to frame institutional foundations which will encourage new healthcare providers to respond directly to competition, to ensure individual patient control and choice, to drive down costs
(in part by reducing much waste), and by enhancing quality in many respects,
including fully integrating the comprehensive care of complex diseases and
diversifying the locations of care.

Some suggest that individuals are not capable of exercising choices. Certainly,
there is an information asymmetry in the system. But consumer ignorance
is neither inevitable nor a priori. It is a result of a rationing structure (and of a
wider educational failing) which necessarily suppresses knowledge in order to
curtail demand. However, with the individual financially empowered, there will
be devices to enable us all to express our common motivation to improve our
health and to educate ourselves about our choices.

A key question is how service-users (or consumers) can effectively express
preferences.

How consumers express a preference

There are two ways by which consumers express preferences in ordinary life – by
voting and by spending; as voters, in elections, and as consumers, when holding
money. I argue that it is only direct consumer control which can reform healthcare. Voting and shopping are different *in kind* – one is a very indirect action, the
other very direct. One is diffuse and generalised, the other specific and particu-
larised. One is disconnected from direct results, the other very directly connected.
One disempowers the individual – by submerging minorities beneath majorities
– the other empowers individuals in concert – by empowering the personal voice
within a purchasing co-operative, without detracting from social solidarity.

I believe the key to successful, cost-effective reform is to put consumers in charge both of themselves and of choosing a purchaser. We need to ask how to do it; why do it; how to convince people that they should want to do it. We can see movement, as I discuss, in giving users direct cash payments. I believe this is the beginning of patient fundholding, or direct cash control. To generalise this to the NHS as a whole is a huge but essential challenge. The project is harder than it might look, for all sorts of cultural and political reasons. But we need to begin with first principles which people recognise, which they endorse, by which they justify their actions, and which they identify as appropriate incentives for agreeing to change in approaches, systems, structures and *personal* responsibilities.

The pivotal point about how people express a choice is this – there is a fundamental distinction between being able *to command a specific service* (by spending money or calling upon social insurance) and being able to *discipline a system* (by occasional voting, or taking part in planning consultations). Having a say in *how a system is run* is different to having a say about *a personal service* supplied when you want it, when prices are quoted, and when cash (or a voucher/'NHS credit') is to hand. Having the option of moving your account to a preferred provider is more powerful than an occasional vote, which is itself lost in the big bundle of election questions and answers. It was HG Wells who noted that one of the last English illusions is that one class is capable of properly speaking for another, and that 'free political institutions do not guarantee the well-being of the toiling class'.

Power is its own currency. And cash is the most concentrated form of power. Real choice, too, is both a social and a *moral* experience. It turns on free will, the capacity to choose – which is *learned* – and the expectation to do so. The processes of NHS 'consultation' subsume the particularities of individual lives without empowering them. This undermines the participation of the individual in their own life. It reduces the role of the person. It denigrates individuality and freedom, in favour of decisions dependent on 'general causes'. The process takes away from the people themselves the faculty of modifying their own lot and instead asks them to rely on the expertise of others, or an inflexible providence, or on a determinist and blind fatality. Crucially, the processes undermine free will (and thus self-responsibility which is acknowledged to be at the heart of health status). This belittles the will, ideas, and actions of free individuals.

There is, too, another absolutely bedrock distinction to be made – between 'needs' (determined, defined, delivered by 'experts') and 'wants' (which come 'from within' the individual). In the past, this distinction was reflected in a key organisational distinction between working-class self-organisation and mutual aid on the one hand and a 'Webbian' management from above by a professional elite on the other. Unfortunately, the founding of the NHS in 1948 suffocated the first model (of voluntary and mutual aid) and substituted the second (of elite management which 'knows best'). This structure remains a determined barrier to all attempts at reform. It represents what TE Lawrence – in *The Seven Pillars of Wisdom* – called 'the vicarious policemanship which is the strongest emotion of an Englishman towards another man's muddle'. This key difficulty is the subject of my chapter on 'needs' and 'wants' (*see* pages 129–36). It is indeed the backbone theme and constant explanatory reference point of the whole book.

For however 'consultation' may be sensitised or 'improved', we can make no fundamental progress under the flag of 'needs'. For here, to borrow from Dennis Severs' book on Spitalfields (which deals with 'the true comic conflict of Reason with Passion'), 'whenever we have approached the centre of any subject, we are somehow – always kept apart. We stand in the cold draught of a pause.'[8]

Concerning consultation (and de-centralisation), we should sort illusion and control from the offer of influence, if we are to see the realities that many patients experience. In a market – by contrast with voting – it is often good enough to voice a question in order to get an answer. And if enough do so, it is acted upon. In NHS consultations it is difficult to know – even if you are an activist – whether a question has been acted upon, clearly and surely. And if it has, will it be allowed to slip back when you look away? A customer is more easily aware of change, as the signals are explicit on both sides of the lines. And if 'conscious competent behaviour' is one key element of learning, this too is more obviously secured by a market. Pressure groups, too, which repeat messages find that this itself ensures that they are often not heard, even when they believe that they have been consulted. This is the problem of being characterised as 'the one that *always* goes on about *that*'.[9]

In a market, there is always a frontier, and it shifts constantly in response to consumer preferences. Without a market, too, it is very difficult in consultations to deal with 'the unsaid' – the statements which people dare not make, and the descriptions of their experiences which they find hard to formulate or of which they are not fully conscious. Yet good communication is an essential element and a prerequisite of a market, which is about listening best as well as knowing best – about hearing as well as talking, about empowering the silent as well as the activist. Tacit assumptions, the unsaid, the statements in the spaces between the words, are all fundamental. But these are difficult to capture in 'consultation', whereas they find ready if silent expression through prices. A response to a priced service is easier for us all to rely upon. It is, too, a more individually empowering alternative to the consultation in which a patient engages when management and professionals too often decide the important things – and indeed what *are* the important things. The consultative process in the NHS, too, shows that many problems go round in circles, but are never resolved. The problem of mixed wards is but one example. We cannot rely either on officials who may or may not allow things to happen after an election has passed. For even if I vote to ensure that other people pay the tax, I do not necessarily secure the service, or the control that consumers enjoy. We should notice, *after the vote*, who it is who are in the positions of power. Who calls the shots? Who exercises primary control? Just as key predators in nature exercise an overwhelmingly important influence over entire communities, we should see what is made possible and what made very difficult by the big beasts. I shall explore this further below, in discussing what Milton Friedman has called 'the iron triangle' of politicians, managers and professionals, and their success in wielding sufficient political power to protect their interests compared with that of the scattered and unorganised patient. Yet, as Umberto Eco reminds us, *The Three Musketeers* is the tale of the fourth.[10] In most debates and 'consultations' it is the professionals who determine outcomes, in what Professor Elie Kedourie called 'their equivocal transactions' with civil servants and politicians.[11]

In elections, as in opinion polls, people, too, inevitably give much more weight to their demands if they do not have to consider the prices – which is the lesson of the unpriced opinion poll. And when a decision is made separately by an individual in a market – including deciding to which co-operative to subscribe – the cumulative effects are more carefully considered by the individual than when voting on a bundle of issues. For in an election, the cumulative social and economic effects, too, tend neither to be fully recognised nor taken into account. Here, too, at an election it is easier to vote other people's money than to decide to spend your own on a priced choice. It is individually painless in terms of cost (if unproductive in terms of concrete personal service) to be in favour of free services, too, and to vote for them. We can see, too, that in past decades there has been considerable demand for the reform of failing public services – that is, reform *for everyone else*, whilst many have viewed their *own* area of professional activity as a special case deserving of exemption.

In addition to an occasional vote, the service user is offered a re-emphasis on 'consultation'. This should be understood as a form of technocratic control. For the idea of more 'participatory democracy' substitutes group decision making (as urged by politicians leading all three major parties) for individual choices and individual self-responsibility. It insists on public decision making about private issues. And these consolations we are offered concern 'the plan'. They do not support individual, decentralised trial and error, responsibility and self-reliance. And they contradict the first premise of democracy, that the individual has the capability of interpreting the world, and choosing a course of action.

The substitution of a political choice for individual preference to secure a service leaves Government in great difficulty, too, in settling upon what to spend and what to buy. It has to try to define an 'adequate' service, and to find the 'right' amount to spend. It does so without prices, which otherwise deal with the challenge of balancing demand with resources. Consultation wrestles with several intractable (and often heartbreaking) difficulties – how to 'fairly' share out a rationed pot between competing (vocal, political, skilled) pressure groups; how to ration between one urgent case and another when both patients have capacity to benefit; how to discriminate, say, between cancer care and elderly care; why and how to deny a cancer patient an effective but expensive drug but to provide a renal patient with dialysis, or vice versa; how to define what healthcare, and in what quantity, the individual should receive; how to determine the 'right' amount of money that should be available and spent, and on whom.

Decentralisation: a diversion?

Then there is decentralisation (and its fashionable companion, mutualisation). It is insufficient to decentralise to a localised group. This gives no economic power to the individual, and it does not ensure consumer-driven choice. Although it seems to draw on the benefits of shifting decisions from the centre, it does not endorse personal choice and responsibility. A shift from central agencies and experts to the public groupings of localities demands the politicisation of the patient without any gain in personal power in securing a specific service. For instead of making a cost-conscious choice as a purchaser when the service is wanted, the potential or actual patient must devote time to planning, meetings and specialised issues in advance of any requirement for the service itself. They – probably seeking to call from within themselves tacit knowledge and preferences, often in a hypothetical situation – must learn to offer 'good reasons' for preferences, or reasons which will be regarded as suitable by the 'experts', who enjoy 'occupational prestige', and who seek to train people to see 'problems' from the management's point of view.

No satisfactory reform will be achieved by more tinkering and twiddling in the margins – with some supply-side adjustment and some notional empowerment of the individual. Radical, systemic change is both inevitable and desirable. The alternative (to use Evelyn Waugh's words) is 'cumulative futility'. The necessary amendments will not come if we confine ourselves to what Simon Jenkins has recently called 'a fidget of inchoate reform' under governments of both main parties.[12] Decentralisation without individual economic control is a fidget, not a step-change.

Foundation Hospitals

Here, the innovation of Foundation Hospitals now stands as a meeting place for all the forces at work on the imagination and for the necessity of innovation. Foundation Hospitals have been offered as a way to offer empowerment to the local community, to call managements to account, to generate participation of patients in decision making 'as citizens' and to get them 'involved' in the system. They are said, too, to be a means of introducing choice and diversity – but without (in Mr Milburn's words) 'right wing solutions'.

However, we should not let the vociferous opposition to Foundation Hospitals from 'old Labour' mislead us into thinking that the idea in its present form is more radical than it actually is. For, in the continued denial of individual economic power, the proposal is still deficient. It is, too, overly concerned with stability and order, with continuity and tradition, rather than with real progress and change in terms of consumer choice and individual empowerment. To this extent the policy can be seen as a profoundly conservative policy. Its difficulties arise not from what it proposes but from what it dare not yet propose.

However, Mr Milburn surely understands that you can only fight one political culture with another. The policy is a device to stress the necessity of designing services round the patient journey, and to unleash innovation, entrepreneurship and rewards for good service. It is, too, a device for managing the risk of getting greater autonomy into the system. But the real risk is that too little autonomy will be offered. Nevertheless, the Foundation Hospital will do more to dramatise and reveal the contradictions in the system. Notably, that you cannot make a State monopoly consumer-led unless you give the consumers the actual individual economic powers; that mutuality is no substitute for monopoly unless individuals are financially empowered; that there remains a key distinction between disciplining a system by occasional voting and commanding a personal service by expressing an empowered preference. The Conservative attempt to run a quasi-market revealed the contradiction between a bureaucratic approach to the allocation of resources and a market-led approach. The conflict could not be reconciled, and so – in the interests of political security – NHS Trusts were denied the fundamental freedoms to manage, and purchasers the powers to contract for quality. Service users had no economic power and no individual freedom to migrate to a preferred provider. A tradition of refusing to seriously examine the economic issues and the sources of genuine user empowerment has continued, notably in the Wanless Report.[13]

Foundation Hospitals offer NHS Trusts more management freedoms (for example, on the crucial issue of pay bargaining) and they offer the individual more involvement, more voting, more opportunities – but as 'stakeholders'. They offer, indeed, everything *but what you really want*, which is control over a personal fund to buy guaranteed individual care when and where you want it, and from whom you want it. The irreconcilable conflicts between real personal choice and a system which excludes individual financial empowerment will become more obvious as the alternatives continue to fail. Mr Milburn has shown himself bright and sensitive, quick-footed and politically nimble. He must know that these contradictions will become increasingly obvious, and be aware that this in itself is a necessary increment towards real reform, of advance via frustration. Meanwhile, Foundation Hospitals will remain block-funded, and thus protected from consumer preferences. There will be 12 initially, and they remain the subject of fundamental dispute between the Secretary of State for Health and the Chancellor of the Exchequer, who wishes to control costs within an apparently unified national structure.

In a sense, Mr Milburn has developed Foundation Hospitals as an attitude as much as a policy. This seems to follow on from his appreciation that extra spending alone cannot deliver sufficient improvement in the NHS. It is the approach that Foundation Hospitals represent – weakening Whitehall controls – which matters, and where it can lead. As the ideas are presently stated there is no freedom for the individual to take their NHS fund to a preferred purchaser. So it remains difficult to see what it means to say people will own the hospital, or share power with managers and professionals. It is difficult to see how consumers can persuade them to allow it (whatever it might mean). And it is hard to see what the incentives would be for managers to do so. A board of differing stakeholders somehow 'representing' (and 'balancing') 'interests' will not do to empower choices by individuals. It is problematic to imagine how boards of this kind – and those of Foundation Hospitals – can be governed by 'elected patients and staff', how decisions by local communities about priorities can be made, and why the project is more appealing to the voter than voting in local government, where the response is generally bleakly poor. And it is hard to see how such boards might function coherently, and where power will truly lie. Certainly, non-executive members of NHS Trusts (or, indeed, of national, bureaucratic, cumbersome and costly regulatory bodies) have found it an elusive struggle to get staff to 'represent' users and to make the user's voice more effective, to achieve meaningful leadership on behalf of user power.

Indeed, inspection – in my view necessarily, ineffectively and expensively – has substituted for consumer power. The lay voice, too, is always too weak, in the absence of individual choice backed up by the power to wield money or a voucher – both at the national and at the local level. This is so, *even if* lay-assessors are involved, *even if* users 'open up' more to them than to inspectors of services, *even if* this 'paints a truer picture of the real strengths and faults of a service', *even if* they seek to offer imagination and not merely administration. The key discipline of executive action (and, incidentally, the facilitator of staff empowerment and higher morale) is, too, not one of constitutional balance. It is instead when customers can leave, go to another purchaser or provider offering better, more convenient, cheaper, or more diverse services.

The historian Lynn White Jr said that 'history is a bag of tricks which the dead have played on historians'.[14] Yet just as historians seek to discover the 'truth' about the past – not least from 'the unlettered portions of the past' where 'the peasant was the last to find his voice' – we need to try to discover the truth about the present. And so, in assessing Foundation Hospitals, we need to try to make sense of the 'NHS debate', or rather the debate about the future of English health and social care. To assess the particular in the context of the whole. And so I begin by identifying first principles which I believe everyone will recognise. And by which I believe healthcare (including how we see ourselves, and how seriously we take our responsibilities for ourselves and for others) can be successfully reformed. By these changes, too, many other aspects of our lives can be bettered, so that we live in a society of liberty. Meanwhile we continue to be showered by the falling leaves of the cultural, political and empirical inheritance of the NHS. Much that was only recently accepted as permanent has been lately subjected to what Marx called 'the gnawing of the mice'. Notably, the moral particularism which assured NHS superiority as a system. And the NHS is itself a peephole into the cultural assumptions of its founding period, and into the rather different cultural changes we see all around us and which are changing the context and consideration of the NHS itself. What we have inherited rests on cultural judgements about values, about what matters, about what has been taken for granted as to what and who belongs where. These judgements concern how we should each live our lives, with what competence we can be trusted, and what can count as private space. Foundation Hospitals focus this debate.

The contrast between dynamism and stasism

Meanwhile, we face a surprisingly fractured landscape where new possibilities are suddenly contested. We are seeing, too, the revival of interest in old approaches to structures – notably in voluntarism and mutual aid, and in non-profit institutions – to do what has been thought of as public work. This is offering a new context in which to think about ways to increase cash, capacity, communication, caring, competition, access and quality. It has, too, revived consideration of the principle of latency – or to what extent the individual has within them the capacity to exercise meaningful choices for themselves, and how this could be released and supported for individual and general benefits.

Here we should revisit Lord Beveridge, one of the architects of the NHS. He is more quoted than read on the proper relations between public and private interests. But his ideas present one of several competing modes of cultural and political authority. They offer a particular way to think about how we belong – to ourselves, to one another and in society. They do, too, offer a specific narrative of working-class history, and they say a good deal about the England we might have had if a different step had been taken in 1948, avoiding NHS monopoly. For one of the objectives is to discover – to use some words of Lord Beveridge – 'the duties of the State, that is the organised community, and the individual, in social advance'.[15]

To find answers which enable the duties of the State and those of the individual to be successfully expressed and interrelated, I emphasise dynamist initiatives in place of statist controls and elitist decision making. As an early English co-operative spokesman said, 'It is marvellous how many persons are desirous of controlling the affairs we ought to control ourselves.'[16] Dynamism implies just such personal responsibility, and in just that 'social world' of working-class self-organisation, educational groupings, friendly societies, trade unions and co-operative bodies whose creativity, size, imagination and knowledge characterised British experience prior to the Welfare State. However, this substituted dynamism for bureaucratic collectivism, and control from above for collective action. This, as Professor Stephen Yeo has demonstrated, was a *culture* in itself, and was seen as such at the time. JM Baernreither published a study, *English Associations of Working Men* (1889), in which he saw England as a 'gigantic theatre of associated life'.[17] Yeo has argued that this was a working-class practice, and not just 'socialist theory'. Indeed, observably it was often not socialist at all, but *individualist in its impulse* even if collective in its gathering of individuals together in mutual aid. Its recovery is an essential of ceasing to knit with water, in shifting the deck chairs in which planners find comfort but where users discover no choices and have no outlet for self-organisation and self-responsibility.

Dynamism relies on the twin concepts of state of the art and of innovations to come – the realisation that wonders do truly never cease. Stasism implies the concept of control from above, and by a professional class on behalf of others. It has continuity *whichever* political party is in power. The machinery persists unchanged, save at the margin. It has, for example, in the NHS been more like the barrel organ, with a pre-set tune produced by turning a handle, than like the older world of mutual aid which saw people making their own music.

There is a long tradition of debate about these choices, but it is not yet well understood or even discussed by that closed world which calls itself 'the NHS policy community'. Indeed, it is ignored – for example, by such stasist documents as The King's Fund's *The Future of the NHS: a framework for debate* and other pertinent Government and Audit Commission documents.[18] However, it is a central debate both between the theoretical base of the centraliser position and what we could broadly call libertarians, as it is too among some intellectuals *within the Labour movement itself* – that is, between the advocates of self-organisation and co-operation in consumer control on the one hand, and those who articulate ideas about state control, state socialism and collectivism on the other. In 1900, one spokesman for a policy of mutual aid, co-operation and self-organisation (or *workers' socialism*, as it was then described) contrasted this approach with a *state* socialism in which 'the country was to be transformed into a vast bureaucracy'.[19] I explore this important tension – and its implications for NHS reform – further in my chapter on 'needs' and 'wants' (*see* pages 129–36). However, it is important to offer an outline here to inform the discussion.

The foundation of the NHS in 1948 was the culmination of a process which began with national insurance legislation in 1911, which subordinated Friendly Societies both to the state and to commercial competitors. This represented the triumph of a bureaucratic state socialism, content to function within an administrative system. It marginalised both a 'workers' socialism' of mutual aid and cooperation – the world of working people's self-organisation and co-operation – as well as the impulses of individualism and self-responsibility. As Yeo says, for Fabians, the State was no shy, neutral, hidden thing. It subsumed 'the community'. The State was to be personified by collectivist experts, trained through institutions such as the London School of Economics. Its construction was to constitute a break, a new civilisation run by a new cadre of professionals. The NHS replaced a culture of anti-statist but still collective capacity for self-control, self-government and forward-looking saving and provision in co-operative endeavour.[20] These working people's organisations tended to be anti-State and even, as part of the same package, anti-Socialist. Above all, they stood for federated association as the instrument but also as the achievement of a fully social life.[21]

It was not inevitable or 'obvious' that this world would and should give way to the NHS. And we have indeed been the loser both by what did occur and by what did not happen but which might have evolved if the culture of independence had been sustained. This might have been done – and could be done now – by using tax transfers to enhance purchasing power for the poor. As Yeo has said – although arguing for a differently balanced solution, in 'class' terms, which I do not – 'The task, as always, is to make space between what has been and is, and what could be: or to use what has been, as a resource for making a different future.'[22]

This analysis offers an account of why social problems inevitably arise in the specific statist system under review – the NHS system of triple monopoly of payment, purchase and provision, directed from 'above'. It focuses particular attention on 'the problem of agency' – of who does what on our behalf, and with which justifications. And it seeks to recover lost potentials.

The poor and the class gulf in the NHS

When Mr Milburn announced (in January 2001) the first ever health inequality targets, concentrating on reducing infant mortality rates and premature adult deaths in the poorest parts of England, he drew attention to the class gulf in the NHS and its results. He has subsequently spoken of 40 years of irregularity in health provision. We are indeed a long way from the 'universal republic' of which Richard Cobden once dreamed, and which the NHS promised. Mr Milburn has also said more recently that 'standards of public service – schools, hospitals, policing – are often lowest where communities are poorest'.[23] And the data show that for all specified conditions – stroke, lung cancer, coronary heart disease, accidents, poisoning, violence and suicide – mortality for those in the lowest class (5, unskilled) is nearly three times the rate for those in the highest class (1, professional). The unskilled are nearly five times as likely to die from lung cancer as those in the highest social class. Lung cancer accounts for 22% of cancer deaths. Those in the bottom two social classes have more than a 60% greater chance of dying between the age of 35 and 64 years than people in the top two classes.

Of course, this is not all down to the failings of the NHS. A significant part of it is due to socio-economic differentials and lifestyles – for example, smoking or not. But the wide inequalities in health persist consistently over time. And this has not changed significantly in the lifetime of the NHS, despite the relative changes in the quality of life *for everyone* in the past half century. There is continuing evidence of a marked social-class inequality in people who die from cancer, particularly those cancers related to smoking. Indeed, even though death rates have fallen in the last 20 years, the differential in rates between social classes has widened. I suggest that to some extent (we have no well-grounded measurement) the social skills of the higher classes enable them to access services more effectively, and that this – together with attitudes towards the less able – has impacted on health outcomes.

The system must change so that this stops, and so that the poor can buy for themselves what the middle class expects to get. Governments usually think that the key to change is reorganisation. But the more certain answer is to move individuals up the socio-economic distribution, as the overall socio-economic status (and hence health) of the community improves. This means market-driven care in which the poor both improve their status and have the buying power of the middle class, with targeted tax transfers with which to pay social insurance premiums.[24]

The 'co-rrob-orative evidence' from Europe proves the point. In each of these differing countries, patients with market choices are significantly better served. In a modern democratic society the poorest, the disadvantaged, the unemployed, the pensioned elderly, the mentally ill, and the acute and chronic sufferers from disease should all have prompt access to the highest standards in the same way as the articulate middle class. This is not the case in the UK today. Rather, the contrary is generally true. We do not attain either the levels of outcome or the equality of access that are routinely and swiftly achieved in France and in Germany (which has absorbed the burden of recovering civil society and economic reform in the former Soviet bloc East Germany), in The Netherlands and elsewhere. Yet medical knowledge and methods are shared in common with the UK. So what is the basis for these differences? Rapid access for all to high-quality care is also routinely achieved in the Swiss system, which in my view is the best combination which can be a model for the NHS. In Dr Heinz Redwood's view, too, it 'is probably the clearest signpost to a compromise between solidarity, public sector control, and market forces'. This blend runs with the grain of New Labour's interest in asset building for the poor, and in its shift away from untargeted equal benefits for all.

In European approaches there is, too, an important link – because of direct incentives and the financial structure – between individual behaviour and consequences. In France and Germany (although there is less competition in Germany than in France) standards seem higher, if the Organisation for Economic Co-operation and Development (OECD) is to be believed. There is equality of access. Everyone is covered. Treatment is prompt. Costs are generally lower than ours. Incentives function directly. There is solidarity, cohesion, differentiation and ethical competition, where individuals and their co-operatives make judgements about the reputation of providers for quality care or for unsatisfactory performance. Of course, people do many things from non-financial motives. As Paolo (Commissario Brunetti's wife, and a close student of Henry James) says, 'Different goals drive different people to different lengths. Or perhaps people are driven by different goals. At any rate, I think people will do more if they are after something they view as a manifestation of money than if they view it as a manifestation of beauty.' This is not intended to be cynical, but merely realistic.[25]

We need to enable the working class to come back into the full market for healthcare, rather than to go on with the idea that it is markets which have damaged their care, or that markets are unsuitable for health and social care. The opposite is the case. Indeed, Government must ensure genuine competition and transparency in order to make choices a reality to the individual, and to make genuine differences between people actually count as they make their own choices. In Europe, much better access, higher quality, improved lives and longevity have all been positively and creatively influenced by consumer choice in a market. There is individual autonomy and bargaining power, competition and investment, and transparency of information. And the permanent necessity of insurers, purchasing co-operatives and providers to satisfy consumers in order to win support, markets and revenues. Having to seek revenues and satisfy service users has a startling effect. So, alas, does not having to do so. A true crisis of consumer confidence in a market forces you to deal with it. But nationalised services in permanent crisis can sustain themselves by receiving budgets from above over many years, as we have seen.[26]

Social insurance systems in Europe show that the poorest are treated immeasurably better, with legally guaranteed entitlements to fuller health coverage. Good health, too, is recognised as one of the rewards of economic and social power, of education and understanding, and of fortunate birth. I believe the most effective and efficient mechanisms for achieving routine access to good care for all are market devices, where direct incentives function, and by which we ensure that the poor have the buying power of the middle class. It is the absence of markets, rather than their failure, which has prevented modern development in healthcare and access to good services by the poor in the UK. The NHS has been a middle-class organisation from which the middle class have derived the greatest benefit. The best doctors, too, have tended to work in privileged areas.[27]

Incentive is an essential ingredient to achieve the optimal use of the scarcest resources of human capital, skills and cultivated human potentials. These are the most important qualitative elements of provision. To release these successfully, the regulated market environment is one that must be realised first if progress is to be made in improving healthcare. The market pre-conditions must be constructed before the required improvements can happen. But it is – to borrow a phrase from the historian WG Hoskins – 'the acid fingers of the twentieth century' which have taken away markets and mutual aid when the NHS abrogated the responsibilities of the individual customer.[28]

The *processes* I investigate will, I suggest, increase opportunity, access and better outcomes – which should be significantly defined by the recipients of services. I would like to see spending on healthcare expanded. But not by transferring resource from the efficient private sector of the economy to a State sector which is the opposite. We need much improved access to good care – certainly much better, generally, than the NHS usually offers – for all. I seek to square private and public goods, notably by releasing genuine direct incentives. I would maintain the tax base, but enable individuals to control a personal fund which can only be spent on healthcare. I am an optimist about change, which is tricky but not impossible. We are, after all, a nation of native flair and resourcefulness, of which it has been said often that 'we are capable of doing almost anything'.[29]

A society of liberty

The absolutely fundamental principle is a liberal society. A society of liberty and independent fulfilment is significantly supported and expressed by ensuring that everyone has routine and reliable access to good-quality healthcare. This offers a choice between two different visions of life: a society of individual and self-responsible liberty, or one of hierarchical control.

- A society of liberty and independent fulfilment is significantly supported – and expressed – by ensuring that everyone has routine and reliable access to good-quality health and social care.
- A society of liberty should expect people to act for themselves, to be responsible for consequences, and to be empowered to be responsible for them by being able to make genuine and attainable choices.
- A society of liberty should expect every person – in and through voluntary association – to govern themselves.
- A society of liberty and self-responsibility itself offers order, in contrast with the order of hierarchical control, with welfarism, with politicised equality and with a society of dependency.
- A society of liberty encourages people not to ask why doesn't Government do something (for example, about obesity), but to ask why I or we don't do something. An early analyst of the NHS, Dr DS Lees, said that 'The major aim of the liberal is to leave the ethical problem for the individual to wrestle with.'[30] The issue is not that we must try to make Ministers and Whitehall more accountable, but to ask why decisions which are so personal are being made by Whitehall at all.

No one system

This book is optimistic about change. It urges that we should not seek to replace one 'system' with another. It does not seek to offer yet another holistic 'transformation', or a clutch of 'solutions' to 'problems'. Instead, it asks for individuals to be able to make their own decisions. It constructs *an approach* to individual possibilities. Unavoidably perhaps, I use the word 'system' as a shorthand. This is not because I believe that we can, should or even possibly could have a single manageable world which fits all. I adopt the shorthand, instead, in the sense of constructing an approach which will permit a plurality of decisions by individuals about their care and its coherence *to them*. It is necessary to offer some outline of formal institutions and constructions, but this is not the chief preoccupation. Instead, we should seek a structure which permits constant adjustment and exchanges, with the fullest expression of the civilised individuality of all, benefiting from experiences in making decisions about life and health.

Insofar as a new structure is proposed – and there can be no credibility in argument for change without at least a firm outline with which to begin the process of adjustment – this is intended to be so structured as to evolve and adapt in response to consumer wishes. As Timothy Fuller said (of Michael Oakeshott's work), 'What he meant was that each generation must do the best it can with the resources it has in responding to circumstances it did not choose but cannot avoid.'[31]

This view outlaws once-and-for-all solutions. It bars reducing the meaning of life to political action. It shows that we should not seek the closure of choices or the collapse of possibilities into a single 'system'. It encourages an approach to differences – where patients hold the initiative – within a moral world of reassurance about the availability of services for all. Instead of *the* system, we should seek a permissive structure, with individual empowerment intended not merely to instrumentally acquire power over one particular approach. Instead, empowerment should enable the individual to explore the complexity of their own self, in a readiness to cope with life's risks and contingencies, and to express their response by making choices which the approach (or adaptive structure) enables them to make effective. This is an attitude of mind much influenced by Oakeshott's ideas, notably in his *Rationalism in Politics*.[32]

I suggest that less government will lead to more effective self-reliance and better caring for others, through initiatives in civil association. Noel O'Sullivan summarises Oakeshott's concept of the State, which this reflects. Thus:

> *a formal association of citizens united, not by a common purpose to be imposed by managerial government, but by mutual obligation of a civil authority which never constrains liberty because, unlike managerial government, it imposes no plan or purpose: what it does is to make laws which do not specify actions or purposes, but only lay down non-instrumental conditions to be observed by citizens in the course of pursuing whatever ends or purposes they may choose for themselves.*[33]

When we begin to think about issues in this frame of mind, we are immediately confronted by many powerful 'givens'. As we try to widen the angle of our vision, it is striking that the NHS, despite its many deficits and denials, remains an enormously powerful 'brand', to which there remains a deep culturally embedded loyalty. The challenge is to genuinely deliver its intentions of good healthcare for all, but by Government withdrawing to the battlements, making general rules but not making managerial decisions. It should fulfil this role without imposing equality as a political value by depressing quality and access, curtailing individual choice and hindering the evolution of direct incentives for responsibility. These challenges raise fundamental challenges at the level of what we mean by 'democracy' and 'choice' and 'responsibility' and the role of 'the State'.

Incentive, choice, competition, professionalism and direct patient responsibility are all key elements in these considerations. So, too, is social cohesion and solidarity. Overall, on funding, I believe that we should maintain the basis of the services by general taxation, with the poor and the disadvantaged being paid for by the younger and the richer. But that this 'NHS credit' should be used to buy a social insurance, which Lord Beveridge regarded as necessarily compulsory, and the method by which men would stand together with their fellows.[34]

The individual will use the 'NHS credit' to subscribe to a co-operative, mutual-aid purchaser of care, recognising that by this means they can express their wishes, and whose development they can influence. This will be constructed on mutual, local, autonomous, self-governing lines, with minimal Government interference. Consumers will be subscribing *members* whose funds will be used to purchase care and distribute benefits to individuals. And by this means – combined with tax transfers – the unequal social arrangements structured from above by the State, which have seen the poor do least well under the NHS, can be corrected. This, too, without dragging others down.[35]

Questions to resolve

I offer an approach which starts with the insistence on patient-*guaranteed* care for all – with a core of certain, specific, legally guaranteed services, and on the patient as the fundholder. This approach is helpful in considering – indeed, even in noticing – key choices. These are questions which we ask ourselves every day, and which are the underlying realities of all discussion about the source of the difficulties of the NHS. As Yeo has shown, they concern:

- how to combine equity and economy
- how to connect locality and nation, and thus to integrate local autonomy and accessibility with control – preferably from below, with much more personal responsibility for behaviour and consequences, and for decisions and results
- how to combine the contradictory imperatives of local autonomy/accessibility with central financial and political strength
- how to universalise services while maintaining local sensitivities and control
- how to maintain the morale and skills of professionalism in medicine, but with transparency and accountability

- how to bring together large numbers of financially empowered subscribers in a
  co-operative healthcare-purchasing organisation without the individual being
  submerged in the mass – being 'deskilled' by the 'representation' of an agent,
  whether they be a doctor, a manager, a pressure group, an official, a health
  authority or a primary care trust
- how to delegate authority upwards, while enabling the subscribing members
  both to mandate and to recall powers
- how to control costs but achieve quality – how to ensure access without restricting capacity and without encouraging irresponsible 'demand', which overwhelms
  the present NHS
- how to reduce the medicalisation of our lives, to the greater benefit of self-
  reliance and self-expression.

'Ordinary' people in mutual-aid organisations sought to find answers to these
questions which worked for them in their own lives. The replacement of this approach by State institutions has often provoked apathy and disillusion, as people
have found themselves managed by 'social administration', with professionals
distributing rationed benefits.[36] However, there is no irreconcilable conflict
between democracy and order, between freedom and organisation, and between
populace and State, as I show.

The problems of healthcare are thus cultural, economic, personal and organisational. They are moral questions, as well as being matters of law and regulation.
They are, too, inherently complex. No answer is without its cost in trade-offs. We
have to make choices for ourselves about questions, answers, problems and solutions. The emphasis here is on the civil association described by Oakeshott, by
contrast with intrusive, goal-directed, ideologically derived, managerial government. To permit the approach I outline to evolve – which is generally characterised as 'dynamist' as opposed to 'statism' – Government will be the umpire. It will
administer neutral rules of behaviour, permitting many choices to be co-possible.
Within this framework of rules, individuals will themselves 'get it done', pursuing
their own goals. And thus the social order will be one of enduring adjustments
and exchanges – adaptive, dynamic, mutually respecting. There will be no overall
master-plan, no one 'system', no ideologically driven approach, save that Government will foster a situation where individuals can exist at civilised levels.

In summary, so far …

One key problem is the medicalisation of our lives. Here we should consider
more carefully when we think medicine can do good and when it might do harm.
It means the individual choosing between opportunity costs, too – choices both
between one *kind* of treatment rather than another, one *course* of treatment and
another, and between medicine or other non-medical investments (like a holiday,
which may often do more good).

This is a debate about how we can benefit from our own knowledge, in our own
lives. One condition of doing so successfully is a system of limited government

which encourages those devices which we know increase *economic* freedom. This implies particular ideas of how such services as healthcare should be governed in localities, and how they should and can respond to individually and financially empowered individuals. Notably, too, that ultimately – and no matter what advice they get – individuals must seek for guidance for decisions *from within themselves*. To make their decisions about specific services stick they must be able to deploy specific devices. There is none more compelling than money. Advice and advocacy are others, but they are supporters of the crest, not its alternative. And a Patient Guaranteed Care Association, or consumer co-operative, would put in place all the advocacy services which user groups (such as those in mental health) seek, without the need for a homogeneous national and professionalised advocacy service (and thus, a new vested interest). Patients would achieve local advocacy, which would be non-judgemental, independent of the provider, and which would compellingly express the user's voice to providers. The PGCA would be a power base with a clear sense of consumer direction. It would be a genuine co-operative association, a community of purpose of willing members, and not merely a gregarious gathering like many 'communities' sharing a local NHS facility or a local Council. This is the distinction between crowd and community, between control and cohesion, between phrase and fact.

In my proposals, the consumer will instead again have these older, effective choices of insurer, and of purchasing co-operative, and thus of provider. This is the case in social insurance approaches, where spending levels (and thus capacity) tend to be higher than in structures restricted to tax income, and where satisfaction rates are higher, too.[37] Direct incentives would urge providers to offer high standards of care. My proposed co-operative buying organisations (patient-guaranteed care associations) would filter out poor providers by switching funds away from their services. They would also actually make use of the mass of data which the NHS collects but does not use. The financial structure, too, would balance expectations and resources. In civil society these bodies would be guided by the civilising values of custom, tradition and compromise. The habit of reasonableness and of trust would be embodied in legal arrangements which promote and protect these civic virtues and their individual results. This is collective action, but without collectiv*ism*. It is social solidarity without solecism. It is unanimity without conformity. And it is, too, an effective form of proportional representation. For people in every income category would have equal power in the market.

This dynamist alternative offers a demonstrable healthcare benefit from choice and competition in place of statism. It is democratic, for it is derived directly from the specific democracy of the marketplace – in which the poor, who do least well from the NHS, would be financially empowered through tax transfers. This is to speak of consumerism rather than of control from above. And it offers a living example of how progress really occurs. It shows, too, that the issue concerning markets is not how to protect people *from* them, but how to get everybody *into them* as effective and empowered players. As we consider these possibilities we come across problems concerning price and profit, information, and advocacy. I address these. Yet price is the only way we know to successfully balance demand and resources, and to relate the immediate demand to the ultimate end. And the issue concerning profit (or 'surplus' – or in New Labour terms, a 'community dividend') is not that it is immoral, but how it is used to increase investment, support constructive change, improve services, innovate and adapt.

Consumers outnumber everyone else. And change can only come when consumers think of themselves *as consumers*, rather than as voters, or citizens, or producers, or spectators, or the passive and fortunate recipients of services provided from above by experts. Patients and patients alone have the very direct and personal experience of what services do *to* and *for* them. This is something which voters do not have *as voters*. It is something which purchasers and providers do not have in discharging their roles. And which professionals, politicians and managers do not have, however empathetic they may seek to become.

The intellectual origins of the NHS

The NHS tells us about our 'needs', and either provides for them or puts us on a waiting list. It does not empower our 'wants'. In order to understand the misleading 'needs analysis' of the NHS, which disempowers the individual, I examine the origins of the collectivist identification of our 'needs'. Here, *both* working-class autonomous, prudential, federated self-organisation (Friendly Societies, &c.) and early twentieth-century working-class political aspirations (and collaborative culture) were replaced by a new cadre of professional 'social scientists' (the archetypes were Beatrice and Sidney Webb) who captured both the Labour Party itself and the welfare systems it erected:

> *The whole group of which they were archetypical has an elective affinity with socialism as planning, as scientific theory…. They proposed a disembodied knowledge, value free, a science which was in fact their own ideology.*[38]

However, the Webbs had recognised in the conclusion to their *History of Trade Unionism* that 'the trade unions offer the century-long experience of a thousand self-governing working-class communities', including proving capable of producing a leadership largely independent of middle-class intellectuals.[39] The historical development which the Webbs sponsored and for which they were the intellectual touchstone, pivoted on the substitution by 'the State' of working-class co-operation, de-emphasising the role of the organisation of 'ordinary' people as both consumers and producers, and instead focusing on their role as producers for whom consumption decisions would be made by others. Sidney Webb carried his political ideas into the most intimate quarters. He spoke of marriage as 'the ultimate committee'. Beatrice Webb said that in marriage the man should take the important decisions, but she added that she would determine which were which![40]

The alternative view had offered a critique of 'the State' which was suspicious of direction from above by 'experts' who 'know' our interests better than we do ourselves:

> *Active agency by the state-as-subject would turn the people into objects rather than the subjects of the social sentence they should properly be. The project was,*

in good part, about agency. *How changes happened from working people's point of view was a big part of what changes were.*[41]

Yeo argues that there were choices made in favour of State action, which replaced working-class mutual organisations, actual and potential collaborative endeavours. And, indeed, in 1948 with the establishment of the NHS and earlier welfare measures (notably the National Insurance Act, 1911) – this has hidden from view alternative definitions of what co-operation could mean (and of what 'socialism' might have meant and become). I re-iterate this history to suggest that we pay attention to the words 'needs' and 'wants', which are distinctly not interchangeable. I also examine their history, insofar as the Webbian origins of the elitist attitudes captured in 'needs' help us to consider choices now. It is necessary to unpack this dangerous word 'need', and be wary of it. 'Need' is a top-down concept. It is, too, an imprecise one, and it excludes more than it includes. It contrasts with and contradicts the idea of 'wants', or personal preference. It is open to subjective interpretations – and it is convenient for political, ethical and administrative judgements. But the objects and the emotions of the 'decision maker' are not necessarily those of the patient, explicit or tacit. The language of 'needs' – to which the majority of NHS managers and centralising institutes like the King's Fund cling keenly – is part of the armoury of centralised rationing, bureaucratic allocation and control.[42] Consumer 'wants' as a concept is only coherent, too, if it is expressed as a willingness to devote personal resource – which is not just money – to an objective. It is this self-reliant approach in the wider economy which produces a fabric of individual transactions and transfers which is reasonable, legitimate, negotiated and constantly evolving.

The real question is put by Misselbrook:

> *So what is healthcare* for? *However advanced our treatment of disease may be, we can never banish illness. At the very least medicine must recognise and deal with both disease and illness, and the disability that may stem from either. Healthcare exists for the benefit of the patient. Healthcare must therefore include both processes and outcomes that are valid primarily in the world of the patient, not primarily in the world of the doctor [or of the government, or its 'agencies' deciding 'needs' on our behalf – JS].*[43]

So there are many 'shoulds'. We should remove Government into the background. We should motivate and value professionals. We should empower patients. We should increase the accountability of both. The opportunity for cultural change is evident. There has already been a significant shift in mood and meaning in public discourse – led in the main by the media – about the future of our healthcare. But this remains too much focused on instrumentalities – on which funding system will do more, on which structures will improve quality, on which investments make most sense (for whom). Yet a new tone of openness – and of seeking other paths – is more inviting to the discussion of alternatives. But it must be focused on cultural changes which truly recognise the foundations of liberty, autonomy and choice. And which are expressed in terms of the individual's world being at the centre of decision making. The imperative is neither to maintain the near-exclusive grip of the biomedical paradigm nor to continue with Government's managerial approach to healthcare. Instead, we need co-operative, mutual organisations of patients (we could adopt the Government's own language, of community interest companies) which will place the patient's perspective – whatever that might be – at the centre. Current debates are indeed enabling new ideas to be seriously considered as legitimate. These include many which until very recently have been ignored or only discussed by 'outsiders'. But few of the ideas listed above are yet a full part of the debate.

Misselbrook emphasises that if we insist on belief in a multi-dimensional model of health – which includes the biomedical, social, psychological, anthropological and spiritual dimensions as genuine partners – then we swim against the political stream. So be it, for we should. For, as he shows, the current NHS reforms are 'staunchly biomedical and managerial in their gaze'. The drive for evidence-based medicine is chiefly biological. The proclaimed concern with patient 'needs' is formulated around a model of the 'expert knowing best'. There is still no genuine stretching out to understand *individual preferences* and to empower them. Patients are regarded as just one of the many 'interests' in the picture, rather than the reason for the existence of all others. The NHS still buys in bulk, and for 'populations' – incidentally overlooking the fact that in nature (as John Stewart Collis reminds us) the size of a thing bears no relation to its significance or its complexity. We cannot see the human sperm, for example, from which we all commence, unless we magnify it 160 times.[44] The State (and its agencies and officials) has remained in control, despite a rhetoric that suggested co-ordinating voluntary and State endeavour (Beveridge's emphasis) and advancing the claim of democratic decision making.

The present work, like Misselbrook's, is an attempt to identify how patients' wishes might be empowered, and how a truly patient-friendly approach could evolve. It seeks a risk-accepting society, where we do not expect every problem to have a packaged solution. And where 'health' is not a state of permanent introspection and of 'needs' analysis – but instead one of coping in self-reliance if possible with the challenges of being human. It seeks the recovery of willing collaboration, but with the role of the 'expert' advisory, not exemplary, and it offers the argument that, by willingly collaborating in mutual purchasing organisations, the individually empowered patient can benefit from capital itself and from the benefits it delivers. Without this emphasis on a reconciliation of consumerism and care we shall remain in the position of Glendower in Shakespeare's play, unable to achieve self-responsibility, on which whole worlds turn. 'I can call spirits from the vasty deep,' said Glendower to Hotspur. 'But will they come when you do call them?' asked the latter.

Favours to the middle class

The present NHS system favours the middle class, and those interests equipped for its particular kind of localised and specialised governance. For this system rewards those with the patience to endure endless meetings, and who have the connections and the experience, the articulateness and the social command which has always favoured the favoured. This is an attractive model – even though it creates a beggar-my-neighbour problem, and among local neighbours, too – to self-appointed activists, who can veto other people's choices and their potential experiments with preferred services. It recommends itself to centralising charities like the King's Fund, which would hold on to hierarchy as the path to an egalitarian politics. But as Postrel says:

> *Whatever its form, technocratic governance by its very nature slows dynamic processes. It transfers to deliberate, centralised authorities decisions that would otherwise be made nimbly, through competition and feedback in dispersed, evolving markets, not only for goods and services but also for ideas. Technocrats therefore supply the machinery that reactionaries need to work their will.*[45]

Yet healthcare is by its nature necessarily personal, intimate, specific to the individual, separable, uniquely timely in its character and reliant on access to appropriate services as well as on self-responsibility and preventive care.

This is why personal leverage and its potential in an evolving and responsive market to secure a specific service is fundamental. The centraliser's model – under the apparently neutral and scientific or merely technical decision-making process – determines 'need', 'efficiency' and its risk–benefit calculations by experts. This takes away the judgements essential to the individual in living their life, notably the assessment of risks (with which we all co-exist) and what the individual is prepared to live with. It emphasises universal access – but it does not have the capacity to provide it – while diminishing the potential for variety, service innovation and choices. This is not only a question of not having the funds. It does not have faith in the potentials of competition, choice and variety. And it fails to offer staff direct incentives to serve patients. It denies potential providers evolving opportunities and freer access to revenues controlled by patients or by their co-operatives. Without these essential echoes, however, such chimes which promise change are a chimera.

Changing a million minds

The NHS employs more than a million people. It does so in a system where there is no reward for good performance, and little definition of what that might be. Economic realities, too, suggest that poor performance takes over when good performance is not recognised. And so to reform a huge and diverse institution like the NHS demands huge, devolved, driving (even enraged) energy *from literally hundreds of thousands of people*, many of whom remain reluctant to change, many of whom have deliberately elected to work in a non-competitive environment, and who have found no penalty in their lives from attitudes and behaviours which have marginalised the individual patient's feelings. They presently have no incentives to change. But the reform of the NHS demands huge, driving energy, and it is not a piecemeal task. It demands that most difficult of conjuring tricks, a change of *thought*. The revolution required is not a job which can be done by centralised exhortation, targets and moral campaigns alone. It will take the impact of competitive razors, with the cutting edge of crispy notes. It cannot be done without the likelihood of greater reward for successes, and of definite censure for failures[46] – the prompts for the individual to translate policy into *personal* action. And to refer what they do each day to specific first principles, notably the enlargement of free choice and responsibility.

While hundreds of thousands of public employees believe in State intervention, the hamster will continue to run in its wheel. In the activist State, in 'needs'-led analysis, the change will not come. It is necessary, too, for employees to realise *for themselves* that much of which they complain – more guidelines, strategic targets, priorities, monitoring, bureaucracy – is an integral part of central direction, which they wish to protect while at the same time expecting to be otherwise left alone to get on with the job. They are no less the victim. The lack of employee autonomy is inextricably linked with the lack of patient autonomy. The central control of the employee reflects the central control of the patient. People working in the NHS tend to see developments as a responsibility of the *organisation*, rather than of theirs. Yet a change in this attitude is essential if they are to respond to customers. Many, too, may work very hard but they do not necessarily *contribute* to making a difference – there is no market test in place; there are no real budgets. Moreover, the customers do not establish the culture of the organisation. The service is seen from within as one of control, not of service to the customer in which there is a continuous market process of adjustment, transparency and reinforcement of strengths. There is no expectation of helping the informed user to make decisions. In a competitive environment, people make their living giving service and then sending people invoices; in the NHS, people make their living controlling enforced scarcity and then sending people minutes. It has, too, proved very difficult to change a culture of dependency once it is in place. Yet this must occur if consumer preference is to be the canon of valuation, dominate the system, and move its springs.

Rewards are deserved, too, for helping others. For just as individuals should bear the costs of their choices, so too individuals should gain some of the bouquets and prizes of success. For it is individuals who respond to incentives, not institutions or systems which react and which acknowledge ineluctable pressures. It is to the individual on both sides of the service desk to whom attention should be paid. This is the iron chain of necessity.

This especially highlights cultural change. Here, let my voice slip into **bold type**, and the tone into *italic*: **cultural change is not merely an aspect of the challenge. It is *the* challenge**. For, in the final analysis, any organisation is no more than the collective capacity of its employees to create value which is recognised by and which will be paid for by its customers. All the talk of strategies, of vision, of management, of reforms are facilitators to this end. And the culture must be connected by everyone working in the organisation in their own lives and at every level to what they do, why they do it, and how they do it on Monday morning. Everyone and every action must be directly and clearly connected to what the enterprise itself is all about – good outcomes which satisfy the consumer. Yet to change the attitudes and behaviours of hundreds of thousands of people is one of the hardest of all hard tasks. It is constantly under-estimated. Speeches, statements of intent, solemn and binding undertakings, strategies and White Papers – none of them do it. We should recognise that it is a mix of money and management in a different kind of culture which delivers both social solidarity and good care which does the job, if it can be done at all.

Direct incentive is essential to change attitudes and behaviours towards consumers by individual employees and to change attitudes of consumers to their own selves, as well as to maximise the benefits from investments made by the public, and by independent decision makers. Otherwise, it looks unlikely that Santa will get the letter – or that people will see the freight train coming. Words will continue to be produced, documents circulated, but this does not mean that anything real has to happen. And without direct incentives people will continue to deal with appearances rather than with reality. They will not shift to see reality through a different lens, nor make the necessary leap of imagination to focus on the empowered consumer. They will continue to apply a political template to reality, struggle to fit events into a political theory (which gives managers power and status), and largely ignore information that doesn't match up with preconceptions.[46]

In bureaucracies, the rule is 'protect yourself as number one'. In markets, the rule is satisfy the consumer. The former offers delay, obfuscation, and obstruction when a policy is disapproved. The latter leaves no space for those charms. In a State monopoly service you are notified when your number comes up. In markets, the failing system sees that it is its number which is up. Good care is made up of many small things, rooted, too, in positive and concerned attitudes as well as in professional skills. And it is only an essential cultural shift which encourages the individual to focus on the particular in their own work and the patient's perspective which can help create the conditions for change. For the necessity is for the consumer and for management to invite itself and the workforce, too, to make the changes. For each employee must take *personal* responsibility for the change, and for the outcome. They must seek possibilities and opportunities, instead of fear, danger and threat. They must both want to make a difference and believe that they are capable of it, might even enjoy it, will be rewarded for it in many different ways, and that patients will want it and benefit from it.

Expectations and elections

If we accept this analysis and the importance of incentive – and of price and markets – we gain access to a powerful body of theory and analysis which can help us understand the nature of the challenges, and find solutions. These ideas need no longer be the wandering banditti of the right. Indeed, they can help us answer the question of how we can pass most swiftly – and in social solidarity – from point to point. If we accept that people differ greatly in the emphasis they place on particular values – and the kind of life they wish to live – we should seek ways to enable these alternatives to be expressed, prompted by incentives. This is what free choice and cost-consciousness mean. This carries implications, of course, concerning costing choices. But we should try to encourage the evolution of a diverse structure, with a diversity of excellencies and opportunities. With each structure and each individual benefiting from living with others – being mutually supportive and complementing one another. This cannot be done from 79 Whitehall, as Mr Milburn has seen.

Meanwhile, in the absence of proper structures of incentive we should, in particular, listen out carefully when we hear *patient empowerment* and *public participation* treated *as if they are the same thing*, and offered as a package to ensure patient empowerment.[47]

For this combination of ideas is itself a substitute for individual leverage over a specific service. It usually confuses, too, 'needs' (where 'experts' make decisions on our behalf) and 'wants' (which empowered consumers express when faced with costed alternatives). In this debate, how centrally the discussion of patient empowerment is situated tells us much about assumptions. And the confusion between empowerment and participation shows whose authority matters, who has power and who has none. And so what is the message of 'consultation' for patients? Do not ask to whom the bell calls, patients, it harkens not to thee. As I have argued, all healthcare is by its nature *necessarily* personal, intimate, specific to the individual, separable and uniquely timely in its character. This dramatises a key point – that the option of being enabled to discipline a system by an occasional vote is not the same as an individual commanding a personal service when, where and from whom they want it. So, too, offers of greater local accountability of service providers are both the personal and the national problem writ small. They are not an answer to the problems of personal command over appropriate individual care. This is not secured by the individual from bringing 'accountability for public spending closer to its consumers through the agencies of local democracy.'

As we consider how to set in place real devices which will leverage changes, we should recognise that in terms of social solidarity, what might be called the stock of images from the past continues to assert pressure. As William Faulkner said, 'The past isn't dead. It isn't even past.' We do need to recognise that the past is drawn into the present, and that the present is restricted by the past. Curiously, too, for many and despite its evident difficulties, the NHS remains both a comfort and yet severely controlling. Large-scale cultural changes are requiring both patients and politicians to look afresh at how this comfort can be maintained, while we escape from the difficulties. This concerns how healthcare can best be funded, purchased and provided in a structure of self-responsibility.

I do not envisage change in healthcare alone, for this is never independent of education and many other social factors. Reform of a healthcare system alone cannot change the culture. For this we need root and branch change in education, and in the cultural context of politics where we press politicians to enable our healthcare to be safe in *our* hands. I do not believe that the health sector alone can change the culture. I assume simultaneous reform in education and in many other social policies.

Politicians take their hands away from electrified wires. And the charge in the wire is increasing as new understandings about choices and other overseas approaches are developing. The context within which politicians function is shifting radically. I do not see the issue in terms of the survival or renewal of one political party rather than another, one Prime Minister or a successor rather than another – although it may turn out that the electoral threat to the survival of the Labour Party may lead it, surprisingly, towards a market-driven solution. As Francis Bacon says, 'Frost burns'. Here the unparalleled political capital the Prime Minister has twice accumulated offered a clear opportunity to make the necessary radical changes. The electoral consequences of failing to achieve cultural and contextual change are themselves creating new opportunities. Perplexity and some panic may combine to encourage the reappraisal of what we have, why it is as it is, and what else we might evolve from the present malaise. The great persuader is personal experience. Of course, habit and custom exercise great power over the minds of men. Yet everyday experiences are changing the respect people bestow on the failing structure. The hour may be late. The situation is more difficult than it need have been. But the opportunity remains, even if it is now taken up on the electoral cliff edge.

Mrs Thatcher once spoke of the health service being 'safe in our hands'. But the role of politicians should *not* be to offer us a health service safe in their hands, unless by this they mean that they intend to pass power back to the people. Their role should instead be to respond to the much changed (and still changing) context of debate and understanding and to withdraw to the ramparts of minimum regulation. There they should legally guarantee a coherent core package of services, focused on serious and long-term diseases such as cancer, and others for which there are effective treatments. These should be made routinely and swiftly accessible to all. And there should be an appropriate and diverse funding structure which will be more robust than the present tax system, with its severe political limitations.

Leadership matters on these issues, and on the others I have outlined. How to persuade people? Experience educates. So, too, does the explicit reminder of first principles when these are called upon in explaining current events. The clear focus, sheer zest, determination, courage, and refusal to capitulate to vested-interests and to 'old Labour' – seen in the campaign to liberate Iraq – now needs to be focused by Mr Blair on health reform and genuine, financially-empowered choice.

Henry Fairlie wrote persuasively about another important factor, which is expectations. He wrote:

> There is a place for the arousal of expectation in politics; without it, man would hardly have progressed. Politics is not only the art of the possible, which is too often a thoughtless commonplace in small minds; but neither is it the art of the impossible.... Politics can be made the art of the necessary. A people can be nourished to believe that there are necessary things to be done, which they have overlooked, and that they have the necessary capacity to do them. That was the art preached by Franklin Roosevelt, the greatest political leader of this [twentieth] century ... that the necessary can be accomplished.[48]

In addition, if disenchantment spreads, if new investment fails to deliver improvement in services, politicians will necessarily respond.

Repetition, too, is essential to help secure change by explaining the meaning of events, discovering the meaning of meaning. And, as Raymond Williams says, 'the problem of meanings seems … inextricably bound up with the problems [they are] being used to discuss'.[49] To offer new policies, having carefully and constantly prepared public understanding of the required new framework of funding and provision, and the moral, practical and principled basis for systemic change. Thus events can be explained as they arise, in terms of first principles, and people can be helped to understand why difficulties arise and what they mean. John Manning, the literary scholar, has reminded us too that new ideas need to be reinforced by copious and various repetition: 'Knowledge was, after all, a process of remembering, recollecting, recuperating, and reminding.'[50] Or, ex *nugis seriea* – from trifles, serious matters. This makes quite literally biblical sense, for as the seventeenth-century cleric John Lightfoot remarked, 'It was the course of Nehemiah when he was reforming that he caused not the law only to be read and the sense given, but also caused the people "to understand the reading".'[51] This is Mr Blair's opportunity.

The sea change in sentiment

Speaking up against the NHS monopoly no longer seems like challenging the earth's orbit. Context and politics have changed radically and rapidly. The old landmarks remain, but are being seen by different eyes. What was seen as a mystical institution is now seen as a mechanical construction made and unmade by men. We are in the middle of a revolution, and patients are moving beyond their previously allotted parts. Politics has a leading part to play, not least in stepping aside. But proposals for reform do not rely on politics, nor are they determinist like the ticking of a clock. They rely on self-responsibility. However, there is the contradiction that more politics and political direction in healthcare are not the answer, but change can only come about through politics itself. One of the most constructive ways to enable necessary change is for politicians to continue to introduce incremental, educative change. Mr Milburn has taken some important steps on direct cash payments. I suggest that the gradual widening of direct cash payment can do much to encourage understanding about the basis of successful, incremental development towards a consumer-led, market-led system. Here the three key pressure points are Mr Milburn's introduction of choice for cardiac patients and the innovation of direct cash payment for aspects of social care – some £9 million is to be given to older people's organisations and other voluntary bodies, 'to make a reality of direct payments' – and the revolution in optical services during the past 20 years which offers a successful British model for NHS change as a whole.

Free; strengthen; require

Good health is recognised as one of the rewards of economic and social power, education and understanding. We must do three things together – first, free the individual; second, strengthen the individual; third, require (and encourage by education, information and incentive) that s/he is a responsible and participating person. For the purpose of healthcare, as of all social arrangements, should be to enhance the individual life, and to encourage human lives to be lived humanely and responsibly, with freedom to discover ourselves and learn to choose. It is not for 'experts' to define for any individual the purpose and meaning of a life. And we should each contribute to the evolution of the social conditions in which the individual can find his or her own purposes and meaning in their *own* lives.

GM Young said in his *Victorian England, Portrait of An Age* that the natural end of every refuted dogma need not be another dogma.[52] I am exceptionally conscious, too, that much further work remains to be done – both of a theoretical nature and of a practical navigation. This latter concerns number crunching and developments in the organisational framework. Much of this amendment, correction and addition can only occur as we realise and observe adaptive processes in action. Here, we should value surprises – and recognise (as Michael Crichton has stressed) that some random behaviour is necessary for innovation and creative change. For, if someone does not have the vision and the courage to strike out in new directions no progress happens. Ever.[53] And we should cherish the fact that in an evolving, dynamist system the work must always and necessarily be unfinished and incomplete.

There are few short cuts to what WL Burn called 'the fancied good of humanity' or to individual self-responsibility (caring for yourself; caring for those close to you) and good care for all. As he points out, 'while our own age can face specific emergencies with equal courage [as did our Victorian predecessors] it does not face life as a whole with the same resolution'. And: 'One of the cardinal differences between the mid-Victorians and ourselves lies not in their optimism and our pessimism but in the much greater faith they had in the power of the human will.'[54] However, as Burn suggests, we are not necessarily the helpless playthings and products of our circumstances alone. We have our own part to play, not least in our health. This does not mean that individualism implies a solitary life. Nor, in Balzac's words, is this 'solidified selfishness'. It may and does go along with many forms of mutual dependence. And, ultimately (in the words of the early co-operative leader JTW Mitchell): 'Not only must we bear our own burdens but each other's burdens.'[55] The objective is not to re-Victorianise society, but to actually deliver the access to quality services which the NHS promised to us all.

The older presumption was that the individual was more likely to provide successfully for their own welfare. And better than Government could provide for them. The idea was, too, that the common welfare is best likely to be promoted by individuals promoting their own private interest intelligently and in co-operation with others, by dint of contract. As Henry Sidgwick observed in his *Elements of Politics* (1891) – 'the main link by which the complex system of co-operation which characterises a modern civilised society is knit together'. And so, perhaps the key messages of the present book are to raise suspicions about final answers, to diminish both faith in and expectation of 'Government', to replace 'representative agencies' by personal self-reliance, and to urge every patient and professional to ask their *own* questions and to take responsibility for their own actions and the consequences. To do these things, too, with a conscience about others – each self being a social self. To resist the inefficiencies of Government, which withdraws projects from the spontaneous efforts of individuals or voluntary groups otherwise capable of organising for their provision, increases the complexity of enterprises, puts them beyond the comprehension and the reach of individuals, and undermines the moral alternative. Most notably, it undermines self-responsibility (and self-restraint), individual character, moral capacity, duty, and willpower.

We are considering perplexing issues which demand a seriousness about public affairs that go beyond party and politics in the day-to-day sense. This is to urge a seriousness about ideas and about practical philosophy that is far from academic. It forwards moral issues which are teasing and taut. It sees universals in public affairs, and not merely particulars. It underlines principles, and (as Gertrude Himmelfarb has emphasised in another context) not merely self-serving interests. In each, we need to discover our own guides. Above all, as Himmelfarb has stressed, this is all a challenge to what Lionel Trilling called 'the moral imagination'.[56]

'Painting,' Constable once said, 'is a science of which pictures are the experiments.' Healthcare, in these terms, is an experiment by each and every sovereign individual in which self-responsible and moral decisions about the unavoidably risky unknown must be taken by everyone. Selection and choice are inevitable. Trade-offs must be made. Mill urged that ultimately 'the question of government ought to be decided by the governed'. Is it not then best, perhaps, for decisions about *your* body to be made by *you*?

There are a number of issues to which I would have given more attention if space had allowed. These include such perennial topics as whether 'consumer ignorance' necessarily disables choice; the limits of liberty which the recent MMR debate illustrates (by contrast with the decision concerning Miss B and her right to make a decision about her own treatment); whether healthcare is different from other personal purchases; whether choice is a licence for unbridled self; how Accident and Emergency services can be placed in a market context; and whether, and how, doctors can make partnerships with patients work well. However, I do explore these questions in detail in my book of essays, *'Coming, Ready or Not!' Politics and the Future of Health Care. The Potential of Consumer Power to Renovate Health Care*.[57]

Notes

1 Comment by Ed Murrow, cited by Keegan J (2002) *Churchill*. Weidenfeld & Nicholson, London, p.133.
2 Herzlinger RE (2002) Let's put consumers in charge of health care. *Harvard Bus Rev.* 44–55. I am grateful to Doug Perkins for drawing my attention to this article, which enabled me to add these references after completing my text.
3 Williams R (1979) *Politics and Letters. Interviews with New Left Review*. New Left Books, London.
4 Cited in Valios N (2002) Voice of experience. *Community Care*. **28 November–4 December**; Trilling L (1936) (Unwin University Books edition, London (1963) p.149).
5 Cited by Kemp A (1964) The mixed US system. In: *Monopoly or Choice in Health Services?* Institute of Economic Affairs, London, p.48.

6 See Burn WL (1964) *The Age of Equipoise. A study of the mid-Victorian generation* G Allen & Unwin, London on *laisser-faire*, p.287 and on Lord Acton, p.330. For a study of some of the present possibilities of mutuality – but generally with an over-politicised stress on 'participation' and little if any stress on individual budgetary-control – see R Lea, E Mayo, *The Mutual Health Service. How to decentralise the NHS* (Institute of Directors/New Economics Foundation, London, November 2002). See also *Social Enterprise: a strategy for success* (Department of Trade and Industry, London, July 2002) which documents competitive membership co-operatives and adaptive experiment and initiative in many fields. G Day, *Management, Mutuality and Risk: better ways to run the National Health Service* (Institute of Directors Research Paper, London, October 2000) surveys successful user-owned consumer co-operatives in healthcare in many countries. On public interest companies and co-operative experimentation, see P Corrigan, J Steele, G Parstons, *The Case For The Public Interest Company. A new form of enterprise for public service delivery* (Public Management Foundation, London, 2001); E Mayo, H Moore, *The Mutual State. How local communities can run public services* (New Economics Foundation, London, 2001); E Mayo, H Moore (eds) *Building The Mutual State* (NEF, London, 2002); J Birchall (ed.) *The New Mutualism in Public Policy* (Routledge, London, 2001); A Westall, *Value-led Market-Driven Social Enterprise Solutions to Public Policy Goods* (Institute for Public Policy Research, London, 2001); Blears H, Mills C and Hunt P, *Making Healthcare Mutual. A publicly funded, locally accountable NHS* (Mutuo, London, 2002).

7 Herzlinger RE, op. cit.

8 Severs D (2001) *18 Folgate Street. The tale of a house in Spitalfields.* Chatto & Windus, London, p.240.

9 I owe this observation to Robin Douglas of the Office of Public Management, London.

10 Eco U (1985) (trans. W Weaver) *Reflections on the Name of The Rose.* Martin Secker & Warburg, London, p.54.

11 Kedourie E (1993) A colleague's view. In: J Norman (ed.) *The Achievement of Michael Oakeshott.* G Duckworth, London, p.98.

12 Jenkins S (2002) Come back BR and the NHS – all is forgiven. *The Times.* **16 January**.

13 Wanless Report (2002) *Securing our Future Health. Taking a long-term view. Review of the trends affecting the health service in the UK.* HM Treasury Health Tender Teams, London.

14 White L Jr (1962) *Medieval Technology and Social Change.* Oxford University Press, Oxford, p.vii.

15 Beveridge WH (1948) *Voluntary Action. A report on methods of social advance.* G Allen & Unwin, London, p.7; also see WH Beveridge and AF Wells (eds) *The Evidence for Voluntary Action* (G Allen & Unwin, London, 1949). WL Burn (in *The Age of Equipoise*) has shown that it is highly unsafe to look back at the Victorians in the search for a holistic anti-collectivist model. For not every action by the State is necessarily anti-individualist nor every action by an individual anti-collectivist. The State has undertaken large-scale clearing actions designed not for collectivist purposes – Mrs Thatcher's programme, most recently – but in order to give individual energies fuller scope. And these energies, even if expressed in a *laisser-faire* spirit, rely upon the machinery of the State for their effectiveness. It is the State which enforces contracts, for example. And we seek a blend of interventionism by the State and the mutual assistance of individual energies, whilst insisting upon a greatly more residual and a significantly reduced tax-based financing role for the State. The arbitration between the State and

the individual – and between conflicting claims in the distribution of scarce resources – should itself be one of adaptive change.

16 Hall L, *Root Remedies and Free Socialism Versus Collectivist Quackery and Glorified Pauperism.* I have mislaid publication details of this 19th century pamphlet.

17 Baernreither JM (1889) *English Associations of Working Men.* Swan Sonnenschein, London.

18 King's Fund (2002) *The Future of the NHS. A framework for debate. Discussion paper.* King's Fund, London. There is no hint of such tensions and choices in the Department of Health's *Shifting the Balance of Power Within the NHS* (Department of Health, London, July 2001), or in F Campbell, *Health and the New Political Structures in Local Government* (Democratic Health Network, London, 2001), nor is it visible in such Audit Commission publications as *We Hold These Truths to be Self-Evident. Essential principles to guide political restructuring* (Audit Commission, London, 2001), *To Whom Much is Given: new ways of working for councillors following political restructuring* (Audit Commission, London, 2001) and *A Healthy Outlook. Local authority overview and scrutiny of health* (Audit Commission, London, 2001).

19 Yeo quotes a South Wales miner (born in 1919), saying 'The Labour Party has always talked about what it will do for you; never what you can do for yourself, and that's where it has made its mistake.' Yeo, in C Levy (ed.) *Socialism and the Intelligentsia, 1880–1914* (Routledge & Kegan Paul, London, 1987, p.247). For Yeo, 'this is a tragic case of arrested development, losing us the predominantly delegatory culture of English associations of working people'. Again, the strongest statement of this has been from the left of centre, rather than from the right. Thus Mike Hales wrote of the 'systematic undermining of commendations of autonomous working-class practice, sabotage of working-class cultures, even identity'. M Hales, *Living Thinkwork. Where do labour processes come from?* (CSE Books, London, 1980, p.110). I owe the reference to Yeo, in Levy (ed.) op. cit., p.226.

20 Webb B (1979) *My Apprenticeship.* Cambridge University Press, Cambridge, p.151. (Originally published by Longmans, London, in 1926.)

21 Yeo, in JA Jowitt and RKS Taylor (eds) (1980) *Bradford 1890–1914: the cradle of the Independent Labour Party* (Bradford Centre Occasional Papers No.2, Bradford), p.76.

22 Yeo, in P Corrigan (ed.) (1980) *Capitalism, State, Formation and Marxist Theory. Historical investigations* (Quartet Books, London), p.136.

23 'Health Secretary announces new plans to improve health in poorest areas'. Department of Health press release, 20 January 2001; www.doh.gov.uk/healthinequalities; Milburn A (2002) We have to give the voters more than this. *The Times.* 7 **August**: 18.

24 Bloor K, Barton G and Maynard A (2002) *The Future of Hospital Services. Management updates.* The Stationery Office, London. Also see Institute of Health Management, *IHM Management Updates: Health Services and Deprivation* (Institute of Health Management, London, 2000); D Acheson (Chairman) *Independent Inquiry into Inequalities in Health* (The Stationery Office, London, 1996); Office of Health Economics, *Compendium of Health Statistics* (Office of Health Economics, London, 1999); F Drever and J Bunting, 'Patterns and trends in male mortality', in F Drever and M Whitehead (eds) *Health Inequalities. Decennial Supplement,* DS Series, No.15 (The Stationery Office, London, 1997); Department of Health, *Saving Lives: our healthier nation* (Department of Health, London, 1999); R Goodin and J Le Grand, *The Middle Classes and the Welfare State* (Allen & Unwin, London, 1987). See also RG Wilkinson, 'Income distribution and life expectancy' (*BMJ.* **304**: 165–8, 1992); JP Mackenbach, 'Income equality and population health' (*BMJ.* **324**: 1–2, 2002); RF Heller,

P McElduff and R Edwards, 'Impact of upward social mobility on population mortality: analysis with routine data' (*BMJ*. **325**: 134–6, 2002). The OECD data show that countries with social insurance do better overall than we do, and that there is more social solidarity and less class divergence; see OECD publications, op. cit. Also see A Wagstaff and E van Doorslaer, Equity in the delivery of health care: methods and findings, in A Wagstaff, E van Doorslaer and F Rutten (eds) *Equity in the Finance and Delivery of Health Care: an international perspective* (Oxford University Press, Oxford, 1993); D Hobson, *The National Wealth. Who gets what in Britain* (HarperCollins, London, 1999).

25 Leon D (2002) *Wilful Behaviour.* William Heinemann, London, p.139.

26 See four valuable recent pamphlets: S Lawlor, *Second Opinion? Moving the NHS monopoly to a mixed system* (Politea, London, 2001); D Lal, *A Premium on Health. A national health insurance scheme* (Politea, London, 2001); N Blackwell and D Kruger, *Better Healthcare for All. Replacing the NHS monopoly* (Centre for Policy Studies, London, 2002) and Browne, Young op. cit. Also, N Blackwell, 'Milburn's foundation for serious NHS reform' (*The Times*. **23 May**: 2002, p.20); I Birrell, 'Set us free to pay' (*Spectator*. **11 May**: 26–7, 2002). Also, D Marsland, 'Progressing health and healthcare' (*Sociological Papers*. **8**:3). Republished in E Krausz and G Tulea (eds) *Starting the Twenty-first Century* (Transaction, New Brunswick and London, 2001).

27 For example, 'Hospitals in London employ twice as many doctors' (*BMJ*. **325**: 459, 2002).

28 Hoskins WG (1955) *The Making of the English Landscape.* Hodder, London, p.14.

29 Queen Victoria, in her journal, cited by Leapman M (2002) *The World for a Shilling. The story of the Great Exhibition of 1851.* Review, London, p.109.

30 Lees DS (1961) *Health Through Choice. An economic study of the English National Health Service.* Institute of Economic Affairs, London, p.34.

31 Fuller T (1993) The poetics of civil life. In: J Norman (ed.) *The Achievement of Michael Oakeshott.* Duckworth, London, p.68.

32 Oakeshott M (1962) *Rationalism in Politics and Other Essays.* Methuen, London, and Barnes & Noble, New York (new expanded edition edited by T Fuller, published in 1991 by Liberty Press, Indianapolis, IN), p.127

33 O'Sullivan N (1993) In the perspective of Western thought. In: J Norman (ed.) *The Achievement of Michael Oakeshott.* Duckworth, London, p.102. Foucault cautioned us not to be surprised by suspicion of received institutions. He warned that 'We should not be deceived into thinking that this heritage is an acquisition, a possession that grows and solidifies; rather, it is an unstable assemblage of faults, fissures and heterogeneous layers that threaten the fragile inheritor from within or underneath.... The search for descent is not the erecting of foundations: on the contrary, it disturbs what was previously considered immobile; it fragments what was thought unified; it shows the heterogeneity of what was imagined consistent with itself. What convictions and, far more decisively, what knowledge can resist it?' Foucault M (1971) Nietzsche, genealogy, history. In: P Rainbow (ed.) *The Foucault Reader.* Penguin, Harmondsworth, pp.76–100. This will also be true of whatever it is with which we replace the NHS. The concept of 'civil association' is, of course, Oakeshott's; see M Oakeshott, *On Human Conduct* (Oxford University Press, Oxford, 1975).

34 Beveridge WH (1942) *Social Insurance and Allied Services.* Cmnd.6404, HMSO, London.

35 WJ Braithwaite, the civil servant assisting D Lloyd George with the National Insurance Bill, 1911, wanted this approach at the time. See Bunbury H (ed.) (1957) *Lloyd*

George's Ambulance Wagon: being the memoirs of WJ Braithwaite, 1911–12. Methuen, London. See also M Oakeshott, *On Human Conduct*, op. cit., pp.182–3.

36 On the sources and 'rationality' of this apathy see Yeo, in N Parry, M Rustin and C Satyamurti (eds) *Social Work, Welfare and the State* (Edward Arnold, London, 1979, pp.69–71). An alternative view is to see low vote turnout as a disappointment at politics compared with the benefits that working people have seen in markets.

37 Normand C and Busse R (2002) Social health insurance financing. In: E Mossialos, A Dixon, J Fugueras and J Kutzin (eds) *Funding Health Care: options for Europe.* Open University Press, Buckingham. See also E Mossialos, *Citizens and Health Systems. Main results from a Eurobarometer survey* (European Commission Directorate General for Health and Consumer Protection, Brussels, 1998).

38 Yeo, in Jowitt JA and Taylor RKS (eds) (1980) *Bradford 1890–1914: The cradle of the independent Labour Party.* Bradford Centre Occasional Papers, No. 2, Bradford.

39 Webb S and Webb B (1894) *History of Trade Unionism.* Longmans, London, pp.475–6.

40 Quoted by R Harrison in 'Sidney and Beatrice Webb', in Levy (ed.) op. cit., p.55.

41 Yeo, *Mitchell*, ibid., p.49. See also his discussion in N Parry, M Rustin and C Satyamurti (eds) op. cit. of S Reynolds, B Woolley and T Woolley, *Seems So! A working class view of politics* (Macmillan, London, 1911), which includes the following comment: 'the worst tyranny to beware of is that of intellectuals ordering other people's lives. They are so well intentioned, so merely logical, so cruel … [the working man's] democratic leaders flatter him and hold him in contempt at the same time.' See also PHJH Gosden, *The Friendly Societies in England, 1815–75* (Manchester University Press, Manchester, 1961); *Self-Help, Voluntary Associations in Nineteenth-Century Britain* (Batsford, London, 1973); H Pelling, 'The working class and the origins of the welfare state', in *Popular Politics and Society in Late Victorian Britain* (Macmillan, London, 1968); B Supple, 'Legislation and virtue: an essay on working-class self-help and the State in the early nineteenth century', in N McKendrick (ed.) *Historical Perspectives: studies in English thought and society in honour of JH Plumb* (Europa, London, 1974); Yeo, op. cit. In the words of one leading Friendly Society figure (1891), the prospect of state subsidy was to be resisted: 'Care must be taken that the rising generations are not enticed by bribes drawn from the pockets of those who esteem their freedom or forced by legislative compulsion to exchange the stimulating atmosphere of independence and work for an enervating system of mechanical obedience to State management and control – the certain sequence to State subsidy.' Brother Radley, Grand Chief High Ranger, Ancient Order of Foresters, quoted by Yeo, in Parry, Rustin, Satyamuri (eds) op. cit., p.52, from JH Treble, 'The attitudes of the Friendly Societies towards the movement in Great Britain for state pensions, 1878–1958' (*Int Rev Soc History.* **15**: 266–99, 1970).

42 King's Fund (2002) *The Future of the NHS. A framework for debate. Discussion paper.* King's Fund, London. Compare shopping as an empowered buyer with the approach of the following Department of Health documents: *Involving Patients and the Public in Healthcare: a discussion document* (Department of Health, London, September 2001); *Involving Patients and the Public in Healthcare: response to the Listening Exercise* (Department of Health, London, November 2001). And also compare it with the recently established Patient Advice and Liaison Advisory Services (PALS) (Department of Health circular, *Patient Advice and Liaison Services (PALS)*, April 2001). See also, Department of Health, *Shifting the Balance of Power Within the NHS* (Department of

Health, London, July 2001); F Campbell, *Health and the New Political Structures in Local Government* (Democratic Health Network, London, 2001) and the following three Audit Commission publications: *We Hold These Truths to be Self-Evident. Essential principles to guide political restructuring* (Audit Commission, London, 2001); *To Whom Much is Given: new ways of working for councillors following political restructuring* (Audit Commission, London, 2001); *A Healthy Outlook. Local authority overview and scrutiny of health* (Audit Commission, London, 2001).

43 Misselbrook D (2001) *Thinking About Patients.* Petroc Press, Newbury, p.189.

44 Collis JS (1978) *Living With a Stranger. A discourse on the human body.* Macdonald and Jane's Publishers, London.

45 Postrel V (1998) *The Future and its Enemies. The growing conflict over creativity, enterprise and progress.* The Free Press, New York, p.22.

46 See McElvoy A (2002) Why tax and spend is a class issue. *Evening Standard.* **10 July**: 11. See also, G Leech, 'UK is heading in the wrong direction with its fiscal policy' (*The Business.* 30 June 2002); R Douglas, R Richardson, S Robson, *Spending Without Reform.* Commission on the Reform of Public Services. Interim Report (Reform, London, June 2002).

47 See National Association of Primary Care (NAPC) *NHS 2002 Annual Conference and Exhibition for Primary Care. Full Steam Ahead.* 30–31 October 2002. Conference Programme and Registration Form. This offers just such an example. It lists Mr Graham Lister, Chairman of The College of Health, as speaking on 'Ensuring patient empowerment and public participation'. The advance blurb offers: 'Empowerment requires rights, information, choice and support for patients; lessons from other countries; progress in the UK; suggestions for steps to create a more responsive NHS; using the opportunities created by information and communications technology.' All obvious enough. But *money*? This is not even mentioned in the list of necessary conditions for change – in the stress offered by the blurb at least – even by a speaker from a respected source of information about the patient's experience. This itself is very telling on the limits of imagination which the inheritance of the NHS has shadowed in our minds. It is striking, too, that this event concerned with patients and empowerment is not showcased as an important plenary session to which all delegates should be called. It is merely an alternate or parallel session, with delegates offered a choice of sessions of apparent equality of relevance and importance – the new practice contract, creating primary estates, modernising repeat prescribing, and national clinical leads networks. Note, too, that this is not a marginal event in the phalanx of NHS conferences, but one of the most important and influential in the NHS calendar.

48 Fairlie H (1972) *The Kennedy Promise.* Doubleday, New York, p.292. See also A King, 'Disenchantment sets in as New Labour fails to deliver the goods', and G Jones, '2 in 3 voters lose faith in Blair reform. Pace of change too slow, says poll' (*Daily Telegraph.* **30 September** 2002, on YouGov survey; N Hawkes, 'No 10 tells Milburn not to squander NHS cash' (*The Times*, 9 January 2003).

49 Williams R (1976) *Keywords. A vocabulary of culture and society.* Fontana/Collins, London.

50 Manning J (2002) *The Emblem.* Reaktion Books, London, pp.26–7.

51 McGrath A (2002) *In the Beginning. The story of the King James Bible.* Hodder & Stoughton, London, p.285.

52 Young GM (1936) *Victorian England. Portrait of an age.* Oxford University Press, Oxford, p.75.

53 Crichton M (2002) *Prey*. Harper Collins, London, p.212.

54 Burn WL (1964) *The Age of Equipoise. A study of the mid-Victorian generation.* G Allen & Unwin, London, p.47, p.21.

55 Quoted, Yeo S (1995) *Who was JTW Mitchell?* CWS Membership Services, Manchester, p.72.

56 Himmelfarb G (1994) *On Looking Into the Abyss. Untimely thoughts on culture and society.* Alfred A Knopf, New York, passim; L Trilling, *The Liberal Imagination. Essays on literature and society* (Viking Press, New York, 1950).

57 Spiers J (2002) *'Coming, Ready or Not!' Politics and the Future of Health Care. The Potential of Consumer Power to Renovate Health Care.* Edward Everett Root, Brighton.

Chapter 2

Patients, culture and anarchy

Taking a donkey towards his ordinary place of residence is a very different thing, and a feat much more easily to be accomplished, than taking him from it. It requires a great deal of foresight and presence of mind in the one case, to anticipate the numerous flights of his discursive imagination; whereas in the other, all you have to do is to hold on, and place a blind confidence in the animal.

(Charles Dickens)

'Ah, all very well,' you may say. 'But just *look* at the patients. Self-neglect. Obesity. Millions engrossed in watching *Big Brother*. Junk food in both hands. Turning up in A&E drunk and violent. Smoking like chimneys. Mothers with four children, with four different fathers. The men gratifying their senses and taking no responsibility. Many only here going to the GP to get a certificate to say they are too ill to go to work, or can't go to court. Foul-mouthed. Demanding. Ignorant. Unco-operative. Just you try to deal with a surgery full of them on a Monday morning.'

This is the perspective of Matthew Arnold's *Culture and Anarchy*, where he spoke of:

the working-class … raw and half-developed … long lain half-hidden amidst its poverty and squalor, and is now issuing from its hiding-place to assert an Englishman's heaven-born privilege of doing as he likes, and is beginning to perplex us by marching where it likes, meeting where it likes, bawling what it likes, breaking what it likes.[1]

Well, realism about these issues – notably in deprived inner cities – matters. Dealing with such patients *is* a tough job. There *is* lamentable self-neglect, we may think, and foolish incultivation, ignorance and debasement. But the system has encouraged demands without price. There has been no incentive for self-responsibility. And, as Misselbrook shows, the fact is that patients bring with them a culture, values and explanations of their own realities which it is important to respect if any self-responsibility and any better outcomes are to emerge, with greater public awareness and benefits from educated self-understanding. We need to consider how and why some people are as they are – within the system and within themselves. We need to remember, too, that each of us has had a strange journey. And that it is normal for a person faced with disease to think that everything in their sight begins with them, and everything returns to them. Everyone's notion of the best differs. And free will requires the individual to negotiate with destiny. In Dennis Severs' words, 'the choice *between* our two natural leanings: *meant to be* – Divine Providence – and to *take control* – Free Will. It is the inside story of every hour of every day of our lives.'[2] We are, and should be, ultimately responsible for ourselves.

Plato dubbed the medley of messengers in our brains calling for attention 'the rabble of the senses'. Some would use this phrase of patients. But the ultimate choice is whether we rule our lives, or allow our lives to rule us. I submit that the present results that we see in some people's lives are not the consequence of markets, but of their absence. The difficulties they face – some self-imposed – have many roots, in an inherited past of class and of social policies including the 'needs'-led analysis of the NHS, in 'welfarism', and in the lack of incentives for personal responsibility.

The requirement is to find ways to build self-care, self-ownership and self-responsibility, and to continue to invest in effective education at an early age. Anything else is like putting ambulances at the bottom of cliffs. For self-responsibility is a characteristic of a *whole* life. It needs to begin young. Any other approach is disadvantageous to all concerned. I argue instead that we can overcome the worst of perils – in our own lives, and in society – without sacrificing liberty or its values (indeed, by identifying these and enabling them to be the focus of our lives). However, Government offers much market mimicry instead of self-responsibility, patient empowerment and provider competition. Its alternatives, which often ingeniously elude realities, include the following:

- more provider freedoms (for example, 'Foundation Hospitals') but without demand-side change by which individuals secure budgetary power
- devolution, but without leveraged individual financial choice which genuinely captures an expressed local knowledge
- the transfer of NHS assets to 'the local community', but with no individual 'ownership' and no incentives for preventive care
- more accountability through local democracy, but which does not enable an individual to command a specific service when they want it
- more political activism and consultation in planning, but which does not equip the individual to command a specific service
- hypothecated taxation, but no personal mobility of funds
- the money to follow the patient, but without individual control or financially empowered choice – although here, as I have suggested, there is revolutionary change with consumers securing direct cash payments.

Money by itself is not a solution, without direct incentive for self-responsibility, and in the absence of managers or training and cultural change focused on consumers. Meanwhile, there remains a devastating list of unnecessary difficulties. However, I suggest that we can and should still seek to ensure a new approach. Such a renovated system would have specific characteristics, as follows:

1 a system in which every life is valued, and in which everyone is free to live their own life and to make their own decisions – and assess consequences
2 legally guaranteed prompt access to a core package of quality care for all

3 *effective* consumer power enabling the most direct benefits to accrue to the individual – instrumentally, by controlling cash with which to secure these benefits

4 every individual to securely obtain a personal, separable, timely, specific service, instead of merely voting for its promises

5 an 'NHS credit' (from general taxation) for every person, to achieve the equivalence of European-style social insurance to ensure value for money, and social solidarity for all

6 incentives which appeal to individual values, to encourage personal responsibility for the consequences of controllable personal behaviour – which is different from blaming people for misfortunes for which the individual is not responsible

7 incentives for competing providers and competing purchasing organisations to meet the preferences of sovereign consumers – including positive incentives (gratitude, reinforced professional status, honours, fees) which doctors perceive as being for their benefit and excluding perverse incentives (for example, to prescribe ineffective or unnecessary drugs, or – in the topsy-turvy NHS – to fiddle figures) which encourage managers to spend their time jockeying the numbers to please the politicians. For example, as identified by the National Audit Office, and separately by the Audit Commission, recently 'inappropriate adjustment' of waiting lists. Or fiddling of ambulance returns, or the number of operations.[3] These targets encourage managers to focus on current politicised objectives, rather than on preventive care or on what some doctors regard as higher clinical priorities concerning the more sensitive and responsive provision of services. Primary care trusts are bowing under the weight of Government targets.[4] Instead of this hyperactivity from the centre, direct incentives would face individuals with the costs of choices. This means both service users and managers. We need to take incentives seriously. They can release gains in efficiency, productivity, investment, lower costs, higher levels of skills, and improved pay and morale. Incentives alone can prompt the very different tone, attitudes and environment that people encounter when they are sent – as NHS patients, and privately – into the independent sector. Without incentive we shall never release the fullest potentials

8 a system empowering people *as people*, rather than as members of a group or an interest – both on the grounds of liberty and because we know that the ability to increase control of one's own world improves individual health[5]

9 a minimal role for the State, functioning as an umpire and for the enforcement of contracts voluntarily entered into[6]

10 scepticism about the claims of Government when it wishes to limit freedom, on our behalf and in our interest

11 no detailed final master-plan, no inevitable 'progress', no grand visions of perfection, but an adaptive, incremental and evolutionary system which operates through choice.

Here I have made one major, overarching assumption – that liberty is best. And another – that the individual probably best judges their own interests and faces the risks. And another – that the cost of choices cannot be avoided. There is a parade of geniuses who make this case – Kant, Mill, Popper, Jefferson, Tocqueville, Hayek, Berlin, Oakeshott and Nozick among them. They have thought most deeply about its implications. I do not seek to be so foolhardy as to summarise their works, or to seek again here to make the case for liberty as they do with such formidable philosophical power and detail. However, Chapter 8, entitled 'How many doors are open to me?' (*see* pages 85–90), offers a brief statement to support my assumptions.[7]

And, in terms of liberty, this book more modestly offers some ideas about what might be done about healthcare in the UK, within a context of dynamism and liberty. It seeks ideas which can be an initiating, creative, enabling force. As Wellington once said, 'All the business of war, and indeed all the business of life, is to endeavour to find out what you don't know by what you do; that's what I call "guessing what was on the other side of the hill".'[8] Perhaps the ideas that I am exploring can be summarised in one sentence. *Hear the patient speak.* And, in terms of systems, let the Government make the rules and the consumer make the running. And in terms of the individual, trust yourself, but don't forget the costs of every opportunity. It stresses, too, the importance of doctors, particularly of GPs, and of the community as the locale for care. And it makes something of a totem of the importance of the patient judging the experience, reporting on it, and making this a key part of the outcome of any care – including most importantly care at the end of life too.

This book emphasises hearing the fullest experience of the patient, insofar as we can experience anything of the interior life of another. This means hearing more than the words said. Hearing the unsaid, pausing for the spaces between the words, the space between things. Being aware of the silent anxieties, nurturing the expression of tensions, respecting the patient's world, empowering the individual to act upon their insights. It concerns seeking to understand the world of the patient, and admitting to the conversation between doctor and patient those concerns that are conveyed explicitly, and seeking to hear those implications which lie behind the words and gestures used by the patient. This is not psychobabble. It is fundamental to a useful conception of what we each mean by 'health'. The conversation should be conducted by both participants with composure, humour and self-restraint if individual, tacit, usable meanings are to be released. Here I am much influenced by Misselbrook's superb book – recognising, too, that the patient's model of what is happening to them, and of what they can live with – irrational at times, perhaps – is legitimate, meaningful and central to the outcomes of care the patient seeks or prefers. The book will have succeeded in its objectives if it makes some contribution to moving us forward in discussion of how to secure good healthcare for all in these *specific terms* for *individuals*, and not just statistically for 'populations'. And to improving Monday mornings!

Notes

1 Arnold M (1869) *Culture and Anarchy. An essay in political and social criticism.* Smith, Elder, London.

2 Severs D (2001) *18 Folgate Street. The Life of a House in Spitalfields.* Chatto & Windus, London, p.64.

3 National Audit Office (2002) *Inappropriate Adjustments to NHS Waiting Lists.* National Audit Office, London. Also see J Carvel, 'Junior doctors "forced to lie over working hours"' (*Guardian.* **3 July**: 8, 2002). Public Accounts Committee report, *Inappropriate Adjustments to Waiting Lists* (House of Commons. 18 September 2002).

4 King's Fund (2002) *Five-Year Health Check.* King's Fund, London.

5 Evans RG, Barer ML and Marmot R (1994) *Why Are Some People Healthy and Others Not?* Aldine de Gruyter, New York. Also see M Marmot *et al.*, 'Contribution of job control and other risk factors to social variations in coronary heart disease incidence' (*Lancet.* **350**: 235–9, 1997) and D Misselbrook, *Thinking About Patients* (Petroc Press, Newbury, 2001).

6 For example, Government would ensure that the level of the voucher value in tax transfers to the poor is maintained and not eroded over time (as has happened with the NHS voucher in the optics market). Federation of Ophthalmic and Dispensing Opticians (2001) *Optics at a Glance for the Year to 31st March 2001.* Federation of Ophthalmic & Dispensing Opticians, London, p.1.

7 But in case of doubt, the reader should see one or more of the following: JS Mill, *On Liberty* (Longmans Green, London, 1859); K Popper, *The Open Society and Its Enemies* (Routledge & Kegan Paul, London, 1945; revised edition, Princeton University Press, Princeton, NJ, 1950); FA Hayek, *The Constitution of Liberty* (Routledge, London, 1960); I Berlin, *Four Essays on Liberty* (Oxford University Press, London, 1969); M Oakeshott, *Rationalism in Politics and Other Essays* (Methuen, London, and Barnes & Noble, New York, 1962), and others previously listed. Also see R Nozick, *Anarchy, State and Utopia* (Basil Blackwell, Oxford, 1974), and I Kant, *The Critique of Pure Reason* (1781), *The Critique of Practical Reason* (1788) and *The Critique of Judgement* (1790). A Seldon, *Capitalism* (Basil Blackwell, Oxford, 1990) offers a modern statement of the economic ideas. Michel Foucault is very important. For example, see *Discipline and Punish* (Penguin Books, Harmondsworth, 1979), P Rainbow (ed.) *The Foucault Reader* (Penguin, Harmondsworth, 1984) and *The Birth of the Clinic* (Tavistock Press, London, 1973, and Routledge, London, 1989). So, too, is Ivan Illich, especially his *Medical Nemesis: the expropriation of health* (Marion Boyars, London, 1976), revised as *Limits to Medicine* (Marion Boyars, London, 1995). The following two important recent books offer a commentary on philosophical ideas that are directly relevant to our current crises: V Postrel, *The Future and its Enemies: the growing conflict over creativity, enterprise and progress* (The Free Press, New York, 1998); D Misselbrook, *Thinking About Patients* (Petroc Press, Newbury, 2001). Both, I am sure, will disagree with some of my own interpretations.

8 Croker JW (1885) *The Croker Papers: the correspondence and diaries of John Wilson Croker, Secretary to the Admiralty from 1809 to 1830.* John Murray, London, Vol. III, p.28.

Chapter 3

Time, money and capacity

These things happen every hour, and we all know it; and yet we felt as much sorrow when we saw – it makes no difference which – the change that began to take place now, as if we had just conceived the bare possibility of such a thing for the first time.

(Charles Dickens)

All these things cost money. They take time. They require people to be able to give time and care.

This means spending money to make the time available by having the staff in place. It means allowing the patient – and the professional – the social and the political space to express themselves. It means hearing the 'real' meaning of what is being said. It means listening best, not knowing best. It means doctors honing their social skills to see the framework of meaning, and to really hear what the patient seeks to report and explain. This itself means selecting – for attitudes, for behaviours – those capable of bringing these qualities to the doctor role when we consider who to admit to medical school. It means doctors being aware of the personal and social as well as medical information that is relevant, and linking this to the world view of the patient. It means helping people to speak for themselves and to learn to choose. It asks, too, for education about our bodies and about ourselves, from the beginning of formal education as well as within the family. A book like John Stewart Collis's *Living With a Stranger. A discourse on the human body* should be a keystone of the curriculum,[1] as we learn to discriminate on what is beneficial and what is harmful.

What follows addresses how to evolve a dynamist healthcare system which revolves around the specific individual, as well as the traditional philosophical issues about the legitimate bounds of the State and the responsibility of the individual. It urges what Beveridge called voluntary action (or private action), independent of public control. It asks if we can each get much better value from the large sums we each spend on the NHS every year, and if so, how. It focuses on the patient journey, and the patient's ticket for the journey. It goes beyond 'involvement', beyond 'valuing patients as partners', and asks for a new pivot of the system – one in which the user has *the say*, and can walk away to a preferred purchaser and a provider. It asks for a system where any provider will eventually be a good listener and not only a surviving provider because 'there are always more patients where this lot came from' (to quote a senior consultant I heard at Brighton in the mid-1990s). These are real practical as well as genuine theoretical questions, and they call for specific answers. They are actual, not just academic. The late Henry Fairlie, a shrewd analyst of politics, wrote of the issues they raise as 'the problem of collective energy in a democracy',[2] for it is vital – by reference to first principles – to ask how collective responsibilities and individual choice can be successfully linked.

The future of healthcare is the management of chronic illness in the community, and of the very elderly in appropriate and supportive locations – chiefly, when possible, in the home. For this approach to succeed, the informed, empowered, engaged involved patient must be a cardinal objective of public policy. For the objective is management in accord with our own individual values. None of this can be 'delivered' by experts, by management or by politics. It is the result of both individual preference and responsibility, of the commitment of the empowered patient to the shared management of their care, and of the best professional advice and support. That this can all be developed requires a commitment to patient preference, to learning to choose, to self-responsibility *throughout* life. It requires an explicit recognition of the tension between 'internal' views of health and of care (derived from the patient's own perceptions and beliefs) and 'external' views (based on so-called 'objective' evidence, usually from a professionalised perspective). For example, pain – and its management – is quintessentially a matter of self-perception, as is the judgement of preferred outcomes. In addition, 'strength and knowledge come with doing'.[3]

Despite the illusions of Freud, we cannot enter the mind and persona of another and compare the experience of pain, distress or the capacity to cope. Thus we need to support the empowered consumer, who decides what s/he wants, not as a passive recipient of whatever the all-knowing decide s/he *ought* to have. This is not to call for isolated individualism, but for a strengthened sense of solidarity in society. This kind of community cannot be delivered by direction and control from above. It arises from people living voluntarily under the same shared moral obligations.

To achieve this approach to care, I propose two chief instruments of change. Patient-guaranteed care will be a core package of services, legally enforceable by the individual and backed by Government. Second, patient fundholding. The NHS core package would, I suggest, be expected to cover primary care, hospital care, mental healthcare, community care, pharmaceutical spend and emergency care, and deal with serious and long-term illness. Addiction services would be included – for 300 people die each day from smoking-related diseases, and 100 people die each day from the effects of alcoholism, and their impact on hospitals and on Accident and Emergency services is huge. Smoking is the single greatest cause of preventable illness and early death, and there are 13 million people in the UK who have not been deterred by higher prices, likely consequences, educational programmes or smoking cessation 'services'. Of course, to smoke or not is a personal decision, daft as it seems to do it. For the dynamist the issue is that the individual should be free to choose, but not be able to pass the costs on to others – whether in terms of self-imposed difficulties, the costs of care, or passive smoking inflicted on others in pubs and other public places. Government should toughen legislation to protect the non-smoker.[4] Psychiatric care and preventive care – with doctors trained to understand the reasons why people become addicted, trained in ways to cope, and backed up by direct financial incentives for patients – should be a matter of major investment.

We should each of us expect to have to take seriously *personalised* preventive care. It is the best medicine. And when we are ill we need to learn to choose, assess potential outcomes, express preferences, and consider risks, benefits, costs and alternatives. Many of the most painful (and expensive to treat) conditions are largely preventable by lifestyle changes (e.g. cardiovascular disease, lung disease, osteoporosis, diabetes). Smoking is at the root of much of the difficulty. Here we need to tell ourselves many truths about inner and external realities – learning by becoming. There is evidence that people have learned from doctors' advice and from public health messages concerning smoking – but 40 years after the Royal College of Physicians warned that smoking causes lung cancer, society still permits it in public places, and the Treasury condones it (and wider alcohol use, despite a rise in young people's drinking and the number of deaths from drunk driving) in the interest of income.[5]

Then there is the question of broadening the financial base. In a patient fundholding structure there would be incentives for people to contribute additional money if they wish to buy services which the tax base will not afford. The core package will have to specify to which generic and which prescription drugs patients will have access, and this will need to be kept up to date. Each of these is inevitably the subject of downward pressure on costs, exerted by Government. In the USA, elderly Americans fear the dilution of services in this way.[6]

Patient fundholding, or the concept of direct control of cash, argues that the most direct benefits will accrue to the individual if they are given a voucher with which to secure these services.[7] But more cash without self-responsibility will not answer.

Notes

1 Collis JS (1978) *Living With a Stranger. A discourse on the human body.* Macdonald and Jane's Publishers, London.
2 Fairlie H (1972) *The Kennedy Promise. The politics of expectation.* Doubleday, New York.
3 Stewart EP *Letters of a Woman Homesteader,* quoted, Auspitz, op. cit., p.5.
4 Department of Health (2000) *Statistics on Smoking: England, 1978 onwards.* Department of Health, London. See also Department of Health (2002) *Statistical Press Release. Statistics on smoking cessation services in England, April 2000 to March 2001.* Department of Health, London.
5 Royal College of Physicians (1962) *Smoking and Health.* Royal College of Physicians, London. Royal College of Physicians (2002) *Forty Fatal Years.* Royal College of Physicians/ Action on Smoking and Health, London. Alcohol misuse costs an estimated £7 billion annually. See Paton A (2002) Our favourite drug. *BMJ.* **324**: p.1410. Department of Health (2000) *Statistics on Smoking, 1978 Onwards.* Department of Health, London; Department of Health (2002) *Statistics on Smoking Cessation Services in England, April 2000 to March 2001.* Department of Health, London.
6 Charatan F (2002) Healthcare costs hit older Americans. *BMJ.* **324**: p.756.
7 It is striking that when NHS managers (or those whose incomes, self-image and status are inextricably entwined with the NHS) talk of 'the last resort' for achieving NHS reform,

they *still make no mention* of the notion of giving patients money to spend directly. For example, Laurie McMahon, Director of Health and Social Care of the Office of Public Management, 'which helps organisations such as the NHS implement change', says that 'franchising is the last resort in putting things right'. Which, of course, *it isn't*. It is but one management approach, and it does not put patients in charge. See McMahon L (2002) Borrowing from the education sector might help us understand how it could work. *NHS Magazine.* **July/August**: 9.

Chapter 4

To raise all boats

The chief democratic argument [is] that those who wear the shoe know best where it pinches and must be given power to act in their own interest.

(JR Vincent)

Sir Isaiah Berlin told us that we cannot usually have everything.[1] We have to make choices. Both Mill and Hayek, too, told us that learning to choose is what adult life is significantly about.[2] These questions, in the healthcare context, are daunting too because they involve a struggle for influence by many interests, and for the possession of history – past and future – and the tale it tells. We often see the wagons circled, by the BMA, the RCN and Unison – for example, on Foundation Hospitals, and on contracts of service. This concerns control, and who should have it over whom, and why. It concerns individual rights and the State, and who should make specific trade-offs concerning opportunities and costs. It also concerns views of the potential of individuals, and who decides our 'real interests'? Essentially, these questions concern two concepts of social order, which I shall explore in the following chapter. And I offer, too, a stress on liberty, which should be regarded as innocent and normal.

Whence do our difficulties in the UK arise? Many of the endemic difficulties of the NHS are the consequence of the decision to abolish prices in 1948, replacing this by subsidy, rationing and the suffocation of competition. This decision has left patients with virtually no rights enforceable in law. It has proved to be the classic recipe for enforced scarcity. For Government, reform has consistently been about costs, a response to financial crisis, about reacting to scandals – rather than about *guaranteeing* quality or empowering the individual. It is a truism, of course, that healthcare involves price-conscious choices at every level. There is no escape from affordability. Yet patient empowerment is impossible and contradictory without price. Ultimately, there is no escape from affordability and thus from price. The question of where price is placed in the system is an important one – whether it is considered by the individual when negotiating an insurance contract, or at the point of service, or something of both, it cannot be avoided. Price offers an objective, non-political measure of subjective relative value. It shows how much people value a thing. It shows to whom they will voluntarily give the value accumulated in money, and on what grounds. It captures the idea of the actions of people making a bargain, with judgements being freely expressed on both sides of the service line.

The question of where choice is placed in the system is important, too. Choice is about the free expression of ideas concerning the contents of a service, by contrast with such separate political goals as equality of outcome. It is important for each of us to clarify at which point we want to make choices for ourselves, for how you are asked to choose about your care is a health outcome in itself. Choice, too, implies an attitude of welcome to change. There is no way to avoid change. Nor should we want to do so. We should zestfully embrace those creative processes which offer the potential to balance instability and opportunity, and which enhance both dynamism and stability. It is this process which raises standards for all.

What price signals and markets ensure is that individual rights and choices are *co-possible*. This matters when people so often express quite different preferences about similar health conditions and their resolution. When each person expresses a price-conscious decision and acquires a benefit, this does not deduct a benefit from another, given sufficient capacity. By contrast, choices that are made by the political methods of social ordering do not have this characteristic. For models of patterned 'justice' require continuous interference with the actions of individuals and their choices. In the NHS this has consistently included the suppression of information and of choice to discourage unaffordable demand in the rationed system of allocative scarcity.

Three important points bear repetition if democracy is to be persuaded of the case for change.

First, an individual's wishes concerning their necessarily personal, intimate, separable and timely health wants cannot be known in advance or captured in a collective policy. Individual choice is essential, and at the times when it matters.

Secondly, any proposed reforms will significantly and politically be measured by public sentiment in terms of whether they help the poor. There are elemental errors to correct. The campaign for political equalisation since 1948 has not eliminated serious inequalities in care. Indeed, the middle class – throwing cultural power, having contacts, using networks, behaving in the expectation of being taken seriously – has always done better. To that extent the NHS has been an instrument of social exclusion, distancing the poor from services in a way that would not be the case if they were empowered in a market. This has handicapped the poor by further handicapping them in the cultural race we all have to run. In addition, there has been a two-tier system where the rich have been able to secure better clinical care in the private market. In continental Europe this is not the case. There, social insurance has ensured that everyone has better services, and there is no significant private market of the kind represented by Harley Street. But in the UK the more powerful have competed for restricted resources with the less powerful, whereas the poor could have been provided with a voucher, and thus with more equal opportunities.

So a fundamental objective in principle is to ensure that the poorest in society *routinely* receive a high standard of care, and equal access to it. This can be achieved by ensuring that by tax transfers the poor have a personal fund which can only be used for purchasing healthcare insurance. This will secure for them what the middle class would buy when making a cost-conscious choice. Then the grounds of treatment would be on a basis of equity. If the individual wished to consume additional healthcare, this would, too, be a matter of private choice. Meanwhile, redistributive Government programmes which result from democratic elections generally most benefit the middle class, who have the greater capacity to hurry politicians along through public opinion.

Thirdly, there is a pivotal distinction between social solidarity – which is a proper public policy objective – and equality – which isn't. They are not the same thing. *Social solidarity* can be and is achieved in healthcare systems such as those of France, Germany, The Netherlands and Switzerland (where care is especially notably, and successfully, consumer driven). But there is no attempt there to insist upon political *equality*. The issue is equality of *access*. And, indeed, some inequalities are both unavoidable and useful. They are themselves a prompt to emulative improvement. John Rawls has argued, too, that inequalities are justified if they serve to raise the position of the worst-off group in society, if *without the inequalities* the worst-off group would be even worse off. That is, that these serviceable inequalities stem, at least in part, from the need to provide incentives for certain people to perform various roles that not everyone can do equally well. As Rawls says, 'there is no injustice in the greater benefits earned by a few provided that the situation of persons not so fortunate is thereby improved'. And 'The intuitive idea is that since everyone's well-being depends upon a scheme without which no one could have a satisfactory life, the division of advantages should be such as to draw forth the willing co-operation of everyone taking part in it, including those less well situated. Yet this can be expected only if reasonable terms are proposed.'[3]

Rawls argues that the institutional structure is to be so designed that the worst-off group under it is at least as well off as the worst-off group (which is not necessarily the same group) would be under any alternative institutional structure.[4] Nozick states the symmetry: 'The better endowed gain by co-operating with the worse endowed, and the worse endowed gain by co-operating with the better endowed.' But he also fears that the least well endowed will gain more than the better endowed, which may undermine the necessary incentives. And he is suspicious of imposing, in the name of fairness, constraints upon voluntary social co-operation (and the set of holdings that arises from it), so that those already benefiting most from this general co-operation benefit even more.[5]

However, the argument is that inequalities are of much less concern if everyone receives a high standard of care. And provided that the standard of care for the poor is at least as good as the moral minimum which society determines to be the standard to be provided to all. Granted that there are significant theoretical difficulties about entitlements and redistributive justice. But we have to make *some* move if we are to make *any* progress, and this direction seems to offer genuine gains. And, as Steven Henning Sieverts, a senior American healthcare manager now working in the UK, has said, 'Our goal, in fact, should be a system in which some [services/doctors] are much better than others, and in which none are unacceptable.'[6]

Once a structure is in place which raises all boats, and which guarantees the least well off a much better standard of care and assured access to it, then individuals can spend more of their own money on further consumption of healthcare if they wish. At present, the middle class (or the desperate working-class consumer who stretches their resources) are the only ones with any choice, albeit limited by the restricted provision that the independent sector currently offers. In the UK, the independent and voluntary sector merely duplicates rather than supplements the state system. It competes with the public sector, by taking NHS consultants away from public work to part-time private work. But it does not otherwise offer a developed alternative to the NHS in terms of a wide range of good services. In addition, demand for these services from patients is significantly dependent on the denials and deficits of the NHS system itself. NHS waiting lists act as a work-bank for the NHS consultant who also has a private practice. So the independent sector plays a small role. Instead, as in the optics market, we need one system for all, but one which does not lever down standards to the lowest common denominator.

It is a matter of judgement whether the less well off would receive more from a system which is in some respects unequal – but which *guarantees* equality of access – than from a system that is theoretically equal but which is in practice culturally unequal. The NHS meanwhile offers no guarantees of access or quality.

The key question, of course, is what *would* be reasonable terms of the scheme, which would encourage co-operation of the worst off and the better off. What would justice require? And, further, what would be a workable arrangement which could be sold politically, and which would be a necessary condition of benefits for all? Of course, what is reasonable to one is unreasonable to another. But the basis of successful and principled reform would, I believe, be powerfully advanced by the legally enforceable guarantee of a package of care assured for all – my proposed *patient-guaranteed care*. And the best test of a good standard of care is the market test, where a decent standard of care is made available to everybody.

What standard should be expected? I think the only sensible answer is to urge that the poor receive care at the level that the middle classes would buy in a market, using the funds available from a tax-based system – my proposed core guarantee. Everyone, too must have the mandatory funding for the same standard of care – my proposed patient fundholding.

The funding structure

Clearly, by comparison with other advanced systems, healthcare in the UK is underfunded, and the outcomes achieved are generally poor by comparison with other advanced industrial countries. It is necessary to stimulate higher levels of investment. The approach to care which relies on cover by taxation, from a national risk pool, is essential, but the Organisation for Economic Co-operation and Development (OECD) evidence of outcomes and of the optimal funding base suggests that it is not in itself a sufficient answer. Any funding structure which can be politically saleable in the UK must, I suggest, include both a *mandatory* element from public funding and an *optional* element from voluntary additional spending. This need not worsen inequalities in a morally unacceptable way. Indeed, it is the only means by which these can be reduced. The mandatory element is what Government would decide everyone must spend on health – and for which the guaranteed package of care would be accessed through collaborative purchasing. Thus taxation and tax transfers to the poor would remain a major element. Especially so if it is desired to so arrange contingencies that they work for the greater benefit of the less fortunate, as with a weighted voucher providing enhanced financial clout. The voluntary and additional element – which is where we lag so badly behind other advanced countries – would bring us closer to the necessary levels of investment indicated by spending and outcomes elsewhere. In addition, the operation of a more mixed funding structure would itself prompt new funding ideas, offer direct incentives for personal responsibility, and prompt changes in attitudes and behaviours – among both providers and consumers. It is a key challenge to get this relationship between the mandatory spend and the optional spend into better balance.

We should note en passant that culture matters, but that it changes. Nor should we be deterred from reform by being told that market changes in healthcare are 'not English'. For we see around us the revolution in eye care, which I analyse in my chapter 'With eyes to see: one people, one market, one service' (*see* pages 145–61). The contrast in every respect with the tone, feel, environment, morale and professional relations with clients could not be more different in eye care, where the consumer takes part in a continuous process of criticism and correction, and where providers expect services to be compared by the empowered consumer. The revolution in eye care has been a dynamist achievement. And it offers an optimal social and business model for change *throughout* healthcare in the UK, including removing the immoral two-tier system of private care alongside public care – in which doctors drift in and out of the public sector on a daily basis. The continuing but unnecessary difficulties of dentistry in two markets would be addressed by the same approach, and so, too, the position of the disempowered elderly in the social and long-term care sector.

The class system is the one big primary social fact in life in the UK. This has not been entirely without benefits – as, for example, our magnificent architectural heritage suggests. But in healthcare this two-tier system has undermined morality in society by placing us in different pigeon-holes according to class. Here the advances in eye care manifest a different, unified morality. The changes most crucially show that we can be one people, in one market and in one system. And they demonstrate locally in every High Street the truths that come the opportunity, come the investment, comes the service. The eye market demonstrates that, in terms of dynamist evolution, with the effective application of chemistry, materials science, 'high-tech' manufacturing and customised services – and where the individual has a choice and can go down the road to another preferred provider – there is more creativity, not less. Deregulation, financially empowered choice and competition have created the change.

This has occurred within the context of UK 'culture'. We see, too, the development of a global mind, in terms of shared technology and interconnectedness. And generational changes which are shifting ideas about options. These generational shifts represent the closure of an age when voting in a local democracy or in occasional general elections was thought to be sufficient to secure a personal service.

They signal the opening of a new age when democracy will be expressed in a new relationship between protective Government frameworks and user empowerment, through individual financial control. The *patient fundholder* (where each person holds a guaranteed fund entitling them to the core package of care) is central to all of this – as are the direct cash payments which Mr Milburn has begun to introduce. This is the vital incentive both to patients and to management. Money is the essential lever. We all know this, for we know that the everyday democracy of the market has changed all our lives for the better, and in every class, since the end of the Second World War. But no political party has yet proposed to give service users overall direct financial clout in healthcare with an endowed and personal fund in a system of genuine social insurance.

Professors John Dearlove and John Saunders, authors of the leading English introduction to politics, have written:

> *Many critics of the New Right react with horror to the suggestion that ordinary people should be left to judge for themselves the kind of health care they should buy or the kind of schooling which is best for their children. State provision, they say, is necessary in order to ensure that everybody gets the right sort of services. This is because many people are ignorant and do not have the means to gather the information which is required in order to make an informed choice.*[7]

These authors make the point that people are generally capable of making rational choices provided that they are allowed the responsibility to do so, and:

> *When the State decides what we need, we lose the habit of making decisions for ourselves. Of course it is true that many parents know precious little about the schools their children attend, but this ignorance is more a product of a State system of education than a reason for continuing with it. Give parents the means for purchasing education and they will swiftly find out what is on offer. As schools will advertise their wares and parents will seek out the best buy. Under existing arrangements there is no reason for parents to inform themselves, since the Government decides for them what type of education their children should have.*[7]

Dearlove and Saunders make another powerful point:

> *Many socialists claim that 'the working class' is quite capable of running factories and even planning and managing a whole complex economy, yet this same 'working class' is apparently incapable of choosing between different health insurance policies, and cannot be trusted to select an adequate education for its children. People cannot be empowered if you refuse to let them take responsibility for their own lives. New Right libertarians are quite happy to see this happen. For all their talk of transferring power to the working class, socialist intellectuals seem much more hesitant.*[7]

I believe that the right response is that the individual should be in command of a personal fund, and that the availability of this mobility of revenue would itself generate not only appropriate supply but also a different attitude towards self-care, self-responsibility and social relationships. Once it is working, it will allay fears of change. Basic to the potential for change is the vigorous assertion of the importance of a legally enforceable core guaranteed package of care.

Such an analysis makes a further point about people and the results of their free choices. It is that we should value the expression and development of individual abilities, and view talents as a common asset, rather than seek to nullify the natural advantages of some individuals compared with others. As Nozick puts this:

> People's talents and abilities are an asset to a free community; others in the community benefit from their presence and are better off because they are there rather than elsewhere or nowhere. (Otherwise they wouldn't choose to deal with them.) Life, over time, is not a constant-sum game, wherein if greater ability or efforts lead to some getting more, that means that others must lose. In a free society, people's talents do benefit others, and not only themselves. [8]

We, too, need a transformation in management which will not otherwise be attainable. The transformations we need emphasise that it is necessary to have management styles and structures which bring the best from everyone. It is not merely a matter of new organisational systems, revised hierarchical charts, multiple targets and fiddling with figures, with documents issued from the centre, and with committee structures. It means believing in the space for vision and trust in venturesome management which can respond to a new consumer focus and to newly empowered purchasing. It means a new belief in leadership and a new freedom to show it, rather than an insistence on administration alone within a politicised monopoly system. It means teaching new competencies, and retraining or newly hiring people with consumer-focused attitudes, real listening abilities (communications skills), open minds, and the ability to detect and resolve problems. A management style is needed which encourages new expectations (of managers by themselves, and of service users) and the empowerment of participating staff – what they care about, how they work, what they want and what they experience. [9] As the challenge to traditional ways of doing things grows, it means, too, engaging the present NHS employees in carrying forward root-and-branch change. This itself is a vast task. This is not only to evolve a structure that matches the strategy of adaptive local change, but to change the way in which many of the *more than a million NHS employees* see the world and their tasks. For to improve quality, productivity, morale and responsiveness to individuals, with genuine choices, we are seeking changes in attitudes and behaviours among literally *hundreds of thousands of people*. Without direct incentive it is difficult to compel individuals to change, or to put their best efforts into everything that they do. The problem is not only that we are spending too little money – although in European terms we are. It is not only that we spend less than consumers would choose to spend in a free market. It is that we are getting too little for the money, and we are getting the wrong attitudes in the wrong social model, too.

To get change in all this is in itself a gargantuan challenge for the majority of these million individuals. For this concerns both institutional inertia and personal mind sets, as well as accustomed control over other people's bodies and minds. These challenges call for really powerful and direct incentives if a user focus is to become *a quality of the whole* – that is, the primary motif of every employed individual, and not just another add-on to be monitored on aggregate among the 7, or 77, or 777, or 7777 current priority targets. The task is to convert people not merely to action which not only shadows philosophies of free choice, but also to encourage people to capture within themselves and *willingly express new attitudes* in their everyday work. Everyone must 'think user'. This must be the real touch-stone for all involved. It should guide everything – beginning at the beginning. It should guide not only training, but also the very processes of advertising, recruit-ment and selection. Staff should be selected whose attitudes, behaviours and use of time all focus willingly and understandingly on user preferences. And who understand that they must *seek* willing demand if they are to receive revenues.

I do not by any means underestimate these tasks, especially given the anti-competitive mind sets which are so deeply embedded. But there is much know-ledge at the front-line which can be released in a different system. Meanwhile, as they sit at their desks on a Monday morning, and view the incessant and newly gathered piles of central circulars, targets and various kinds of disem-powered autonomies which seek to manage every detail from above, NHS managers must feel as if they are visiting Greenwich Fair with Charles Dickens at Whitsun:

> *Imagine yourself in an extremely dense crowd, which swings you to and fro, and in and out, and every way but the right one; add to this the screams of women, the shouts of boys, the clanging of gongs, the firing of pistols, the ringing of bells, the bellowings of speaking-trumpets, the squeaking of penny dittos, the noise of a dozen bands, with three drums in each, all playing different tunes at the same time, the hallooing of showmen, and an occasional roar from the wild-beast shows; and you are in the very centre and heart of the fair.*[10]

As they open their mail on Monday mornings, as they listen to every new policy diktat, as they ponder every rigorously polished detail, they may, too, think of Proudhon. He gave us this picture of the State's domestic 'inconveniences' (which may be neither rebarbative nor reassuring, as they work):

> *To be GOVERNED is to be watched, inspected, spied upon, directed, law-driven, numbered, regulated, enrolled, indoctrinated, preached at, controlled, checked, estimated, valued, censured, commanded, by creatures who have neither the right nor the wisdom nor the virtue to do so. To be GOVERNED is to be at every operation, at every transaction noted, registered, counted, taxed, stamped, meas-ured, numbered, assessed, licensed, authorised, admonished, prevented, forbidden, reformed, corrected, punished. It is under pretext of public utility, and in the name of the general interest, to be placed under contribution, drilled, fleeced, exploited, monopolised, extorted from, squeezed, hoaxed, robbed; then, at the slightest resistance, the first word of complaint, to be repressed, fined, vilified, harassed, hunted down, abused, clubbed, disarmed, bound, choked, imprisoned, judged, condemned, shot, deported, outraged, dishonoured. That is government; that is its justice; that is its morality.*[11]

So, as we consider healthcare reform, there are thus many complex issues. These concern, among other fundamentals:

- *Political attitudes.* Many people are suspicious of change and will want comprehensive reassurance within a coherent and principled account of guarantees and values. As the US Declaration of Independence says, 'all experience has shewn, that mankind are more disposed to suffer, while evils are sufferable, than to right themselves by abolishing the forms to which they are accustomed'. But despite the requirements of reassurance, we should not seek to offer a master-plan, but instead prefer an evolutionary system.
- *Vision and creativity in an evolutionary system.* This is difficult, even in the free market. It was not so long ago that senior management in industry failed to foresee the digital revolution. Few in the early 1980s, let alone the late 1940s, foresaw either the potential demands created by technology, longer life, informed consumers, international comparison, pharmaceutical and therapeutic innovation, or the genetic revolution. But vision and leadership count.
- *Economic issues.* These concern the fit labour force, the lower tax economy, and the investment choice between welfarism and dynamic economic and service innovation, and the necessary limits on Government expenditure in an innovative economy.
- *Governance issues.* These concern how to promote relevant accountability, higher quality, better standards and essential diversity – prompted by incentive, information, competition and choice – while also achieving professionalism and higher morale. One key to change is the inevitable coalition between professionals and politicians. It is important to provide incentives for doctors and other professionals, who have few under the NHS regime. However, professionals can accept more change if they have more investment, more facilities and greater numbers of professional colleagues. Government and the public must persuade doctors to accept that there will always be external influences on what they do – whether from central Government, or consumers, or both. The commitment, morale and self-image of the people actually delivering care matter. So we need a policy that is both practical and inspiring.
- *Cultural issues.* The context within which politicians address healthcare *is* change – which they wish to survive. This is being deeply influenced by shifts in the cultural context in which information is the most valuable commodity. Cultural shifts of expectations – rising, and difficult to satisfy – and of daily and now routine experiences, notably of a new generation and of new technologies. The exchange of digital and shared information. Large-scale commerce conducted on the Internet. Shared patient experiences of specific and individual practitioners, treatments, drugs and outcomes. This is leading us to online voting, and to shopping for services, including healthcare, on the Internet and over the electronic shop counter.[12]
- *De-medicalisation of our lives.* This means benefiting from medical and pharmaceutical innovation without undermining self-reliance by medicalising every aspect of our lives.

- *Preventive care.* This means learning how to motivate people to consider consequences, without directing their lives through the interventionist 'Nanny State'.
- *Leadership, or the art of politics.* This consists of making what you believe practical.

These are each philosophical as well as practical questions concerning the basis of individual health status, self-care and responsibility, and the nature of society. These problems remain here which are still hardly discussed in the healthcare debate, at least in the popular media. What essential role must price play? What is the nature of knowledge, and who can know what an individual wants? What do we mean when we say that an asset is 'community owned'? What is the right level of spending, and who can know? How? We need to recall again the reminder from Isaiah Berlin, too, that we cannot have everything. There are what he calls 'incommensurables'. The introduction of anaesthetics, for example, allowed more extensive operations, but exposed the patient to the risk of death by sepsis. All possible choices imply losses as well as gains. In addressing these questions and in coming to a resolution of them in a democracy, the most difficult part is changing our thinking – both about how we can each live our own life, and about political structures. But here in the past year we have seen major advances, both in the media and in politics itself (but not yet among public service workers). At least those in power are giving the issues priority. We know Government's answers. But there are others.

Throughout this debate about access and standards we should keep in mind the important comment made by Dr Richard Smith, editor of the *British Medical Journal*, when discussing the necessary de-medicalisation of society:

> *Perhaps some doctors will now become the pioneers of de-medicalisation. They can hand back power to patients, encourage self-care and autonomy, call for better world-wide distribution of simple effective healthcare, resist the categorisation of life's problems as medical, promote the de-professionalisation of primary care, and help decide which complex services should be available. This is no longer a radical agenda.*[13]

The argument which provides a context for this work urges that the way to achieve the necessary changes can be contained in one sentence, namely that there is only one genuine route to ensuring that *everyone* – poor or rich – is guaranteed quality care. And to genuine self-responsibility. That is for Government to make the rules and for consumers to make the running.

Notes

1 Berlin I (1969) *Four Essays on Liberty.* Oxford University Press, London.
2 Mill JS (ed.) (1859) *On Liberty*; G Himmelfarb (1974) Penguin Books, Harmondsworth. Hayek F (1960) *The Constitution of Liberty.* Routledge, London.
3 Rawls J (1971) *A Theory of Justice.* Belknap Press of The Harvard University Press, Cambridge, MA.
4 It remains a problem that this discussion focuses on groups, rather than on individuals. However, this may be the only way to persuade people of the direction of change, and

for satisfaction to be raised considerably above present levels. This is, however, an area of philosophical and practical difficulty.

5 Nozick R (1974) *Anarchy, State and Utopia*. Basil Blackwell, Oxford, p.228.

6 Private communication, July 1995. See also Henning Sieverts S (1996) *No Pain, No Gain: lessons from US healthcare*. Fabian Society, London.

7 Dearlove J and Saunders P (1991) *Introduction to British Politics*. Polity Press, Cambridge, p.331.

8 Nozick, op. cit.

9 For example, how is bad news given to patients? What we know of general medical practice is discouraging. See Eggly S *et al.* (1997) An assessment of residents' competence in the delivery of bad news to patients. *Acad Med.* **72**: 397–9; and Joos S *et al.* (1993) 'Patients' desires and satisfaction in general medical clinics. *Publ Health Rep.* **108**: 751–9.

10 Dickens C (1839) Greenwich Fair. In: D Walder (ed.) (1995 edition) *Sketches By Boz*. Penguin, Harmondsworth, p.140.

11 Proudhon J (1923) *General Idea of the Revolution in the Nineteenth Century* (trans. J Beverley Robinson). Freedom Press, London, pp.293–4, with some alterations from B Tucker's translation in *Instead of a Book* (New York, 1893, reprinted Arno Press, New York, 1972), p.26, cited by Nozick, op. cit., p.11.

12 See *British Medical Journal* 324 (2002) for a sequence of important articles about the Internet, and see Misselbrook D (2001) *Thinking About Patients*. Petroc Press, Newbury, on the values that people bring to consultations.

13 Moynihan R and Smith R (2002) Too much medicine? Almost certainly. *BMJ.* **324**: pp.859–60.

Chapter 5

Dynamism, stasism and two concepts of order

The test of a real society is its ability to differentiate in detail while remaining fundamentally homogeneous.

(Thomas Sharp)

Central to the structure and direction of my argument is the choice between what the cultural commentator Virginia Postrel poses in her book *The Future and Its Enemies*. This is the choice between the search for *stasis* – a regulated, engineered world – or *dynamism* – a world of constant creation, discovery, competition and learning. This is the choice between two concepts of order: stability and control – which means stagnation – or evolution and learning, which reveals many unthought of but emergent potentials. In Postrel's words, the choice is for 'a dynamic future [which] tolerates diversity, evolves through trial and error, and contains a rich ecology of human choices'.[1] The choice is between dynamism and stasism. It is a choice between two different conceptions of human nature. Each differently determines what are 'the facts', their meaning, and our relationship to them.

This dualism is at the root of the issues concerning patients, power, responsibility and reform. Indeed, it is a choice between two incompatible concepts of order. The first is one of control, hierarchy and 'expertise' offered by others who know our interests best. This has been characterised by Foucault as a 'strategy of domination', which he viewed as the prevailing model of modern society. It is this model which the NHS, based in Fabian analysis, represents.[2] This seeks to reduce diverse experience to an unrelenting unitary order, and to limit surprise, innovation, and trial and error, from which new benefits arise.

The second concept of order is one of evolutionary trial and error, deduction and controlled experiment, surprise and dynamism. This is the choice between the design device of ideology and the filter device of experience. It implies quite different principles of latency, or the potential of the individual, and the evolutionary pattern of nature. It suggests alternative ways to consider power relationships, especially those commonly reflected in the different uses of the mirror-words 'needs' and 'wants'. 'Needs'-led analysis (like the camera) is not an innocent eye.

However, the lack of a hierarchical master-plan controlled by central Government does not imply dis-order. As the economist Paul Samuelson said:

[There is] convincing proof that a competitive system of markets and prices ... is not a system of chaos and anarchy. There is in it a certain order and orderliness.

It works. It functions. Without [centralised] intelligence. It solves one of the most complex problems imaginable, involving thousands of unknown variables and relations. Nobody designed it. Like Topsy, it just grew.[3]

This is a choice between two ways of looking at life, about living in the world, and about how human societies grow and evolve. How new patterns are discovered, adaptations enabled, recombinations approved, improvements achieved, surprises valued, moral sentiments expressed, local knowledge empowered, individuals fulfilled, personal good discovered, and complexity evolved – all of which benefits the non-specialist and specialist alike. It is the choice between a concept of life which relies on order achieved by control, and one which sees a different kind of order generated by choices freely made – save that Government should establish a general framework of rules within which choices occur.

The key point to hold on to here in terms of healthcare reform is that a stasist view privileges hierarchy and control, and expects *specific* outcomes which can be predicted and insisted upon in advance. A dynamist view recognises that all progress emerges from *unavoidable uncertainties*, in which adaptations are best discovered and endorsed when they are expressed in the spontaneous order and free exchange that comes from personal choices made in open markets. This is a choice, too, between two views of risk taking. This is a choice endorsing necessary uncertainty and innovation which is seen as fruitful, productive and an inextricable part of life. One in which we all assess risk all the time, and in which we learn from the experience of uncertainty. The alternative is to be controlled, from fear and anxiety.

A dynamist believes in an open-ended future in which spontaneity and choice releases local knowledge, invention and adaptation, and generates unforeseen benefits. And as Postrel says:

Such disagreements have political ramifications that go much deeper than the short-term business of campaigns and legislation. They affect our governing assumptions about how political, economic, social, intellectual and cultural systems work; what those systems should value; and what they mean.' … [And] the distinction between dynamism and stasis is a real and important one that explains much that otherwise appears puzzling in our intellectual and political life.[4]

It is dynamism which lies at the root of human creativity, which enables progress, prosperity, happiness and freedom. It is its absence in UK health systems, based as they are on stasist assumptions about control, which explain their deficits. It is notable that these apparently permanent disappointments – located in the main in public services – exist in a society which is otherwise booming and in which personal choices have grown exponentially. It is one which, through the creative and renewing operations of markets and individual choice, has seen the continuing development of liberal capitalism – in which the standards of life of the great majority, including the poor, have been raised to previously unconsidered and unknown levels. However, the remaining areas of gravest difficulty – in terms of investment, productivity, standards, consumer satisfaction, free choice, safety and security – are in the main still run by Government on monopoly and central-ising lines. Most notably, health and education.

It is stasism which prevents a refocusing on the patient's preferences, despite all of the talk about consultation, patient-centredness, and empowerment through modernisation. We see, too, in terms of NHS outcomes how the results are often dismal when compared with the solutions that are achieved by custom and com-promise, negotiation and trade-offs made by empowered individuals in other areas of life.[5]

Those in charge of the NHS have begun to ask how the existing organisation can engage with the future. This depends, of course, on what you think the future might be, and whether you can and should second-guess it. Meanwhile, there are two competing theories as to why the NHS has not been effective, and how to adjust to 'realities'. Broadly, these are that the NHS needs more public cash and more detailed management – the Gordon Brown view, insisted upon again in the Comprehensive Spending Review of July 2002.[6] Or there is Hayek's notion of the 'extended order', of spontaneous change, of the order which generates itself without control from above. Mr Brown's view is that with massive new funding and better management, the NHS (but without direct incentives and proper markets) can actually deliver both coherent order and individual service. But the mix of more money, more management and more regulation is too short a list of variables to identify the real sources of cultural change. Indeed, in terms of cul-tural change it is a merely cosmetic approach. For the sources of cultural change are to be located elsewhere: in the history of science and in technology, in evolu-tionary biology, in anthropology and in many contemporary contextual shifts – notably in how organisations grow, live and change, as well as in business strategy, in psychology, and in all aspects of social history. And, most crucially, in what people expect of themselves. Here, direct incentives and choice are key.

I suggest that the cultural realities and massive changes which we see around us in the contemporary world of new technologies encourage Hayek's view. They express the 'extended order' in the bottom-up growth of the Web and its com-munications that reach into every home. Fluid international trade is making new connections between people in the development of customised services.[7] It is note-worthy, too, that the Web is one part of the 'lay referral network' of family, friends, media information, personal networks and associations on which people rely when making decisions, including self-treatments and the decision to do without consulting general practice. This is valuable – not least because it avoids symptoms (many of which are self-correcting) becoming 'socially constructed' as 'illness'. And it needs to be set in the balance when medical organisations criticise the information that is available on the Web, and the 'irrational' beliefs of patients.[8]

Here, for us all to benefit from the complex processes by which cultures do change (and especially by which knowledge in all its forms evolves), everyone in the NHS – including patients – needs direct incentives. Without direct incentives we are cut off from the trial-and-error processes of feedback of adaptation, and of personal learning. There is presently no direct incentive for providers to serve the user of services. Indeed, without dynamism and individual choice, what improvement means, and who is to determine value and how, remain elusive. So there *can* be no real changes, if innovation and evolution, choice and competition continue to be stifled. This is a loss of the individual benefits that arise uniquely from the collective wisdom that is only discovered by market processes, and by the neutrality and the co-ordination that arise from price signals. Thus a technocratic approach – by denying direct user feedback and response – makes things worse, and at the expense of both individual self-responsibility, and the security and control which it ostensibly offers. No matter how many billions Mr Brown spends.

Postrel unerringly helps us. She has said that the centralising, 'expert' mentality:

> *overvalues the taste of an articulate elite, compares the real world of trade-offs to fantasies of Utopia, omits important details and connections, and confuses temporary growing pains with permanent catastrophes. It demoralises and devalues the creative minds on whom our future depends. And it encourages the coercive use of political power to wipe out choice, forbid experimentation, short-circuit feedback, and trammel progress.*[9]

By contrast, as Professor Royden Harrison, historian of the Webbs, wrote:

> *Man was an animal who formed committees! The wealth, health and happiness of mankind depended, to a large degree, upon the adequacy or otherwise of the structure of public administration and the scope which was allotted to it.*[10]

The best cure for believing in the present monopoly – to adopt Walter Bagehot's famous remark (on the House of Lords) – is to go and really look at it.

Notes

1 Postrel V (1998) *The Future and Its Enemies. The growing conflict over creativity, enterprise and progress.* The Free Press, New York, p.26.
2 Foucault M (1979) *Discipline and Punish.* Penguin, Harmondsworth. However, Foucault has not been without challengers. See, for example, Wiener MJ (1990) *Reconstructing the Criminal: culture, law and policy in England, 1830–1914.* Cambridge University Press, Cambridge. Professor Royden Harrison, historian of the Webbs, wrote: 'For the Fabians … the dialectic … lay in man as a being whose uniqueness consisted in his being moulded by institutions even while he was the maker of them. What was decisive was the institutional "superstructure" rather than the economic "base".' And Harrison adds: '[Sidney] Webb and his friends saw themselves for what they were: a contingent recruited from *la nouvelle couche sociale*, the rising stratum of modestly placed professional men, civil servants, journalists, teachers, scientists and technicians ... [who] wanted to enlarge the sphere of their own existing usefulness: to change the world so as to give greater scope to the disinterested expert and the professional administrator at the expense of backward politicians and selfish industrialists. They thought of socialism in terms of the gradual eradication of injustice and waste in favour of order and progress: of undiminished inequality and of discreetly regulated freedom.' (R Harrison, in Levy C (ed.) (1987) *Socialism and the Intelligentsia, 1880–1914.* Routledge & Kegan Paul, London, pp.40–2). See also Hobsbawm EJ (1964) The Fabians reconsidered. In: *Labouring Men. Studies in the history of labour.* Weidenfeld

& Nicolson, London. The success of the Webbs is indicated by the fact that all three main political parties at Westminster reflect this image, as does the NHS – which, as Dr Robert Lefever has said, has been in the main a middle-class organisation, run by the middle classes for the benefit of the middle classes (R Lefever, private communication, 18 July 2002).

3 Cited in Kemp A (1964) The mixed US system. In: *Monopoly or Choice in Health Services?* Institute of Economic Affairs, London, p.48. H Spencer made the same case in *The Man Versus the State* (Williams & Norgate, London, 1884).

4 Postrel, op. cit., p.xvi.

5 The NHS language used, the literature produced, the design and the approach in so-called consultation are also often grotesquely unsuitable and hopelessly out of date. They are produced almost as if they are *intended* to be ignored. See (and this is but one of many possible examples) South East Regional Office, Department of Health (2001) *Modernising the NHS: shifting the balance of power in the South East. Consultation on a proposal to establish a new health authority for Surrey and Sussex.* South East Regional Office, Department of Health, Camberley.

6 House of Commons (2002) *Hansard.* **15 July**: cols.21–34; Webster P (2002) Spend, spend, spend. Sell, sell, sell. *Times.* **16 July**: 1; White M and Elliott L (2002) Brown's big gamble. *Guardian.* **16 July**: 1; Pollard S (2002) Brown must stop throwing money at state monopolies. *Guardian.* **16 July**: 20; Kaletsky A (2002) Can Labour give us value for money? *Times.* **16 July**: 7.

7 Hagel J and Singer M (1999) *Net Worth: shaping markets when customers make the rules.* Harvard Business School Press, Boston, MA; Negroponte N (1995) *Being Digital.* Hodder & Stoughton, London.

8 See *British Medical Journal* **324**, 9 March 2002; Misselbrook D (2001) *Thinking About Patients.* Petroc Press, Newbury; Schmidt E and Schmidt K (2002) 'Alternative' cancer cures via the Internet?' *Br J Cancer.* **87**: 479–80; Lister S (2002) Websites for alternative medicine 'dangerous'. *Times.* **21 August**: 4.

9 Postrel, op. cit., pp.xvii–xviii.

10 Harrison, ibid.

Chapter 6

Twelve good ideas and true

We ride the greatest trend of all, the drive to create a bit more than we use, and to leave the world a little bit better than we entered it.

(Julian Simon)

Change will be incremental. We shall, of course, have to build from where we start, but the context is shifting favourably and quickly. Change will nevertheless take time, and it should be such that the older patient is comforted and reassured, not terrified that they will not be covered by the health and social care system. People will need to believe that they will be covered, and that the new system will be better. We need, too, to consider language carefully, and to explain the true value in terms of social justice of concepts such as 'price' and 'markets', which are a turn-off to many. We need, too, to use an essential simplicity of language, and to have a constant sense of the perils of jargon.

At the heart of this book are a dozen linked ideas.

First, that everyone should be free to live their own life and to make their own decisions. The patient and only the patient can know what it feels like to live and experience their own life, and evaluate how appropriate are the choices they face.[1]

Second, that one size fits nobody – care and care relationships are about individualised conversations, negotiations, access and coping mechanisms. The pursuit of uniformity at the average level has discouraged diversity, improvement, investment, creativity, innovation, and the exercise of personal responsibility and choice.

Third, that there is no inevitable and principled conflict between self-ownership and markets. On the contrary, each integrally delivers freedom and autonomy.

Fourth, that it is in liberty – in dynamism rather than in stasism – that we are most innovative, creative and successful in living our own lives and in helping others. Dynamist structures *presuming liberty and self-responsibility* are more fruitful than stasist ones where *experts know best*.

Fifth, that good health relies in part on good relationships with professionals, and if they are to have satisfying and fulfilled lives, they too must be valued in this context and supported.

Sixth, that life is necessarily risky, choices are difficult and they all have a cost.

Seventh, that the biomedical approach which seeks to encompass and offer treatment for every risk and every challenge with which the individual has to cope reduces self-reliance, often hinders 'health', and is damagingly narrow in its conceptual focus.

Eighth, that there will be insufficient improvements in quality, access, cost reduction or sensitivity to patients unless there is genuine choice – which means competition for funding by providers and willing subscription by patients with individual financial leverage. This requires greater capacity, too.

Ninth, that only individuals can successfully limit demand, spending growth and costs, and this requires price controls combined with price-conscious choice presenting clear opportunity costs and testing willingness to pay.

Tenth, that public policy cannot ignore economic objectives and economic instruments – notably direct incentives.

Eleventh, that we have confused an ideal – good-quality health cover for all – with an institution (the NHS) which has represented incorrect ideas about our own nature and about the nature of social realities. We can honour ideals, but the practical results of stasism and its mis-statements about how the social order and the individual function are there for all to see.

Twelfth, that the continued financial structure and the new numbers offered by the Chancellor of the Exchequer continue to undermine the capacity of the individual to provide for themselves, leave the middle class in place as the most successful demanders from the NHS, do nothing to equip the poor to gain better access to care, and are themselves misleading about likely benefits. For even if the economy generates the cash, more money flowing will not by itself bring either the cultural changes – in our relationships to Government, to one another, and to ourselves – nor the specific and individual service improvements that a market-led system gives.

Institutional innovation and cultural change are both vital and inter-related. The NHS represents statist ideas which are in conflict with the basic principles of voluntary exchange, incentive, self-ownership and human nature. And so the present system cannot work, no matter at what level it is funded by the State. This is because the fundamental ideas on which the NHS is based are wrong. These suppose that the State can and should be the compassionate director and controller of individual services (and thus of individual lives), that the State can and should take over responsibility from the individual, that the State should distribute resources according to 'need' (which experts decide), that it can do so with individuals being unaware of costs, and that individuals have rights without responsibilities. These are all fundamental errors, from which much further corrosive distortion follows, including the failure of the State to serve individuals as well as they can serve themselves, both individually and in mutual, voluntary, charitable and co-operative action.

In 1948, Government abolished the individual customer when it founded the NHS. Government crowded out charitable, private and mutual-aid initiatives, and removed the potential development of the provision of health services at lower cost, with the higher quality and greater access that could have been produced. Since its inception, the NHS has claimed to be 'efficient' (i.e. cost-effective – a Treasury perspective). However, from the viewpoint of the individual patient, it is exceptionally inefficient.[2]

There are persistent reminders of disorganisation, of poor management and of a lack of capacity, in a non-market system. The Organisation for Economic Co-operation and Development (OECD) data show that the UK performs poorly in almost every major area of activity. And the media continue to report difficulties. Voters have rarely been content. And governments of all parties have struggled to find ways to empower the consumers, short of giving them the financial say-so. There have, too, been no direct incentives to build self-responsibility, or to take personal responsibility for the consequences.

We should move away from the assumption that the outputs of the NHS are more valuable because *its institutional and political structure* is more valuable. And towards the new reality that a reformed health system is more valuable because its *results* are more valuable.[3] Choice is *both* an instrument *and* a moral result.

Notes

1 At its strongest – for example, as in R Nozick's classic *Anarchy State and Utopia* (Basil Blackwell, Oxford, 1974), this is known as the libertarian principle of self-ownership, where individuals enjoy over themselves and their powers full and exclusive rights of control and use, and owe no service unless they have contracted to provide this.

2 See, for example, Birrell I (2002) Set us free to pay. *Spectator.* **11 May**: 26–7.

3 Redwood H (2000) *Why Ration Health Care? An international study of the United Kingdom, France, Germany and public sector health care in the USA.* Civitas, London, p.122. Also see *OECD Health Data 1998: a comparative analysis of 29 countries* and *OECD Health Data 2001: a comparative analysis of 30 countries* (10e), both published by OECD Electronic Publications, Paris; Jabubowski E (1998) *Health Care Systems in the EU: a comparative study. European Parliament Working Paper.* SACO 101/revised; European Parliament, Brussels; World Health Organisation (2000) *World Health Report 2000.* World Health Organisation, Geneva; Freeman R (2000) *The Politics of Health in Europe.* European Policy Research Unit Series, Manchester University Press, Manchester; Smith D (2001) So how do you want to pay for it? *Sunday Times.* **2 December**; Green DG and Irvine B (2001) *Health Care in France and Germany: lessons for the UK.* Civitas, London. But see also the letter from H Bramley, an NHS-trained nurse who has worked in the French health service ('NHS care row', *The Independent*, 25 January 2002).

Chapter 7

First principles and their context

We must, for the most part, choose how to act as individuals on the basis of moral beliefs which are merely fairly grounded, but when we make these choices we are exercising *our freedom, whereas when governments choose, they are diminishing our freedom.*

(John Marenbon)

We began with the fundamental principle, which is the rule of law – and its associated principles of the freedom of the individual and the personal rights of property. By this we can achieve a free society in which good healthcare is guaranteed to all.

I suggest that the principles of a free society in which individual fulfilment is possible include social solidarity, the protection of the poor, the defence of property, individual responsibility, and safeguards for choice and competition, with respect for adaptive change and surprises. In terms of healthcare, these principles can increase individual freedom, control costs, improve productivity, focus the culture on responsive service, raise standards, ensure universal access to quality care, and expose poor performance to scrutiny and direct incentive for improvement.

Individual responsibility matters. But it cannot be commanded. It should be viewed as the right of the individual to determine which of a range of possible options concerning some preferred goods or services will be realised in their own lives. The protection of property rights is pivotal. As Richard Pipes has written:

> *Historical evidence indicates that the liberties of individuals can only be protected when property rights are firmly guaranteed, because these rights constitute the most effective barrier to State encroachments. The recognition by the State of the right of its subjects and citizens to their belongings – with respect shown to this right – is tantamount to acknowledging limits to State power.*[1]

Thus we should diminish State interference in the lives of people, subject to securing the basic patient-guaranteed care that we must ensure is provided to all. However, that provision itself need not necessarily and inevitably be by a central or local bureaucracy, as we seek to balance freedom of choice with the requirement that money raised by taxation is well spent. How we define 'well spent' also remains open to debate, and is directly linked to consumer wishes.

Here there is an important moral point about the nature of our humanity and the nature of knowledge. John Marenbon summarises this as follows:

> *Many would agree that, besides their ability to understand and reason, what is best about human beings is their capacity for moral decisions and actions – a capacity which can be exercised only when people have freedom to choose how to act (in particular, whether to act well or badly).*[2]

To protect this value means seeking practical ways to ensure that choice works so that individuals can secure uniquely personal, intimate, separable and essentially timely individual care benefits. This requires mechanisms which guarantee choice to the *specific individual*, rather than offering a generalised 'choice' in elections or in planning and various 'consultations'.

The liberation of supply is part of the picture. Marenbon has said that:

> *Education and healthcare are Basic Social Goods and no one should be deprived of them, but they need not be provided through public healthcare and education free to all at the point of delivery, nor even through public services at all; indeed, they are better provided in other ways ... without the extra resources which a non-public system will bring, and the flexibility to adapt, to meet people's wishes, to innovate where necessary and to preserve what deserves to be preserved, doctors and hospitals, teachers and schools will continue ever more to disappoint the public.*[3]

So the first principles and governing axioms should be as follows:

- the rule of law
- social order which arises from evolution rather than from central direction
- respect for private property and private decision making
- the central value of voluntary exchange, in which individuals co-operate with others to satisfy wants
- respect for the individual and reliance on personal responsibility, individual action and mutual-aid, while valuing the differences between people
- the ultimate protection of consumers through choice and competition
- social solidarity (as in social insurance)
- compassion and concern for others, and the protection of the poor.

These commitments require the following:

- the maximum degree of freedom for the individual consistent with one person's freedom not interfering with another's
- the maximum dispersal of power compatible with a democracy
- resistance to the idea assigned to Government of those functions which can be performed more effectively in competitive markets
- the State as umpire – in a Government of laws, not men – for the enforcement of contracts voluntarily entered into, supervising a framework of rules limited to supporting first principles
- otherwise, scepticism about the claims of Government when it wishes to limit freedom on our behalf and in our interest

- the avoidance of coercion being substituted for voluntary action where possible
- respect for the individual and reliance on individual action
- healthcare for all as a pillar of a society of liberty, and a healthcare system which reinforces these foundations
- openness and accountability
- an evolutionary, incremental system responding to consumers' wishes, with incentives, and with freedom and individual choice valued as such
- the avoidance of coercion where possible
- no detailed final master-plan.

These principles will express, endorse and encourage the following essentials:

- the maximum degree of freedom for the individual to live their own life in dignity, consistent with one person's freedom not interfering with another's
- the ultimate protection of consumers, through choice
- a core package of good care for all, including the poor, the disadvantaged and the unlucky – difficult and controversial with regard to precise content, although the proposed new contract for GPs in the UK makes a start in terms of defining a core of essential services
- a framework of rules that are set (and watched over) by the State, which limits rules to supporting first principles – otherwise the State is to keep out, save for the role of umpire and the enforcement of contracts that are voluntarily entered into
- an evolutionary system that responds to consumers' wishes, with incentives, and with freedom and individual choice valued as such
- quality care, dignity, efficiency and social responsibility
- the maximisation of economic and social mobility
- a major shift away from the exclusivity of the biomedical model.

In order to *achieve* these principles in practice, I believe that we require the following:

- legally guaranteed prompt access to a core package of quality care for all
- *effective* consumer power from devices for individual financial leverage
- social insurance (and thus social solidarity) for all
- incentives for personal responsibility and understanding of the consequences of behaviour
- incentives for competing providers and competing purchasing organisations
- a minimal role for the State in purchasing and provision, based on belief in an open market, but functioning as an umpire and for the enforcement of contracts that are voluntarily entered into
- Government to ensure that the level of the 'NHS credit' or voucher value in tax transfers to the poor is maintained and not eroded over time (as has happened with the NHS voucher in the optics market)[4]
- a much reduced emphasis on the biomedicalisation of every aspect of our lives, in place of greater self-reliance.

The tie-beam of change should be a legally guaranteed entitlement to a core package of good-quality care, and legally guaranteed prompt access to it. The conditions of success include the following:

- direct incentives
- *effective* consumer power
- the introduction of price and market mechanisms.

It is fundamental to identify these moral and operational first principles in order to make sense of the current NHS debate – and to structure and explain possible new policies. This is especially pertinent if voters are to be persuaded to accept the merits of voluntary exchange substituted for state monopoly. There is, too, the debate between two concepts of order, namely hierarchy or choice. I argue that a system of liberty which privileges the autonomous citizen can be at least as inspiring as the comfort that so many have apparently derived from the notion of the over-reaching interventionist state.

The point is that freedom is not merely a means, but also an end in itself. This principle depends on Berlin's concept of 'negative liberty' – of being left alone to live your own life. This, by contrast with 'positive liberty' – or being controlled by those who know your interests better than you do. To be left alone to live our own lives we require *effective* consumer power. This must not be merely 'consultation', or some politically determined 'partnership', 'involvement' or some other political or linguistic substitute for enabling individuals to control money in order to secure a preferred and costed service. It means money – in individual hands.

The first of first principles are thus twins – liberty and equality are companions. This is to value freedom and individual choice *as such*, as an end and not merely a means. *And* it is to legally guarantee that all, including the poor, shall have prompt access to high-quality care. These are the first principles of justice by which we should regulate activity, test proposals, and subject institutions to criticism and reform.

In addition, it is important to be sceptical about the claims of Government to limit freedom, and to do things on our behalf. Especially those things which we can do for ourselves, or which can be supplied by a variety of institutions other than Government, and for which payment can be tendered – as we see done effectively and efficiently in many OECD member countries, with better results than we achieve. We see this situation now in the UK itself with regard to eye care. Thus, in Mill's words, it is a first principle to widen and not to narrow the areas of life in which we allow people the greatest liberty to choose how to live their own lives which is consistent with not doing harm to others.[5]

These questions involve us in thinking about the structure of healthcare. We require a theory in order to see what it is we have before us. We need to re-examine the merits and problems of a structure of medical care in which decision making is concentrated in the centre, and by which Government monopolises medical services and supplies them to the public 'free of charge', with the funding coming almost wholly from direct taxation. We need to do this urgently, as the Chancellor of the Exchequer continues to insist on enlarging this funding by taxation and restricting more diverse and balanced funding approaches.[6] Government remains dominant with regard to funding, purchasing and provision. The self-responsible individual remains highly marginal. This contradiction, as I have said, is becoming increasingly obvious and difficult for Government to manage.

Nozick reminds us that we take a risk even by asking for first principles by which we should be guided. He warns us of:

> the great ingenuity with which people dream up principles to rationalise their emotions ... [and] ... One persistent strand in Utopian thinking ... is the feeling that there is some set of principles obvious enough to be accepted by all men of good will, precise enough to give unambiguous guidance in particular situations, clear enough so all will realise its dictates, and complete enough to cover all problems which actually arise.[7]

Debate is made difficult because opposing sides usually offer *one* moral universe in which only *their* moral concepts apply. And, as Commissario Brunetti noted in Donna Leon's novel *Wilful Behaviour*, 'I'm afraid it costs people too much to abandon what they believe.... If you give your loyalty and, I suppose, your love to ideas like that then it's all but impossible to admit what madness they are.'[8] Evelyn Waugh wrote in *Remote People* that 'criticism only becomes useful when it can show people where their own principles are in conflict'. But one of the greatest difficulties of reform is that it requires shifting people from one particular moral judgement – 'the State knows best' – to another which has seemed alien – 'trust the consumer'. This especially asks managers and professionals to consider another judgement which they have in recent times refused (or at least not been much encouraged) to make. That is, that voluntary action and self-organisation are as optimal as we can get. The alternative is described by G Bernard Shaw: 'Later on, liberty will not be ... enough: men will die for human perfection, to which they will sacrifice all liberty gladly.'[9]

Notes

1 Pipes R (2001) *Communism: a brief history.* Weidenfeld & Nicolson, London, p.153.

2 Marenbon J (1997) *The Dominance of Centrism and the Politics of Certainty.* Politeia, London, p.45.

3 Letwin O (1999) *Civilised Conservatism* passim., and Marenbon J *Little Platoons or a Free Society.* Politeia, London, pp.37–8.

4 Federation of Ophthalmic and Dispensing Opticians (2001) *Optics at a Glance for the Year to 31st March 2001.* Federation of Ophthalmic and Dispensing Opticians, London, p.1.

5 Mill JS (1991) In: J Gray (ed.) *On Liberty and Other Essays.* Oxford University Press, Oxford. I am also indebted to the discussion offered by J Marenbon, in Letwin and Marenbon, op. cit.

6 Health Trends Team (2002) *Wanless Report. Securing Our Future Health: taking a long-term view. Review of the trends affecting the health service in the UK.* Health Trends Team, HM Treasury, London. On the Budget, see the following: Hall C (2002) Spending

must double for the NHS to recover. *Daily Telegraph*. **18 April**; Crooks E and Groom B (2002) Brown raises taxes by £8.3bn to fund health. *Financial Times*. **18 April**. For a variety of perspectives, see Pollard S (2002) If we really do have the best possible system, why isn't everyone else trying to copy us? *Independent*. **18 April**; Theory and practice. Milburn's challenge is to implement flexibility and choice. *The Times*. **19 April**; Miles A and Baldwin T (2002) NHS not bound to cost £184bn, says cautious Wanless. *The Times*. **19 April**; Insurance at a premium. *Daily Telegraph*. **19 April**; Mr Milburn is saying the right things about patient power. But can he deliver? *Independent*. **19 April**; Orr D (2002) Now let the health service get on with its work. *Independent*. **19 April**; Hey, big spender. *Sunday Times*. **21 April**; Smith D, Cracknell D and Rogers L (2002) So much for prudence. *Sunday Times*. **21 April**; Pollard S (2002) The great health gamble could backfire fatally. *Sunday Telegraph*. **21 April**; Worse than income tax. *Sunday Telegraph*. **21 April**. Two recent commentaries on social insurance alternatives are L Craven, *A Radical Alternative to Wanless* (Bow Group, London, 2002) and A Browne and M Taylor, *NHS Reform: towards consensus* (Adam Smith Institute, London, 2002). See also Lord Desai, You're wrong, Gordon, this isn't the way to heal the NHS (*Sunday Times*. **28 April**).

7 Nozick R (1974) *Anarchy, State and Utopia*. Basil Blackwell, Oxford, p.240.
8 Leon D (2002) *Wilful Behaviour*. William Heinemann, London, p.211.
9 Shaw GB, cited in L Trilling (1936) *Matthew Arnold*. Unwin University Books edition, London (1963) p.252.

Chapter 8

How many doors are open to me?

Nature delights in diversity.

(Latin tag)

Berlin (in his 'Two Concepts of Liberty', reprinted in *Four Essays on Liberty*) sets out the basic scaffolding of principle. And he maps the territory within which we should consider how to ensure access to good care for all. As we read him we can see, too, what kind of approach to liberty the NHS itself represents.

Berlin says:

> There are two separate questions. One is 'How many doors are open to me?'; the other is 'Who is in control?' These questions are interwoven, but they are not the same, and they require different answers.
>
> How many doors are open to me? The question about the extent of negative liberty is to do with what obstacles lie before me. What am I prevented from doing by other people – deliberately or indirectly, unintentionally or institutionally? The other question is 'Who governs me?' Do others govern me, or do I govern myself? If others, by what right, what authority? If I have a right to self-rule, autonomy, can I lose this right? Can I give it away? Waive it? Recover it? In what way? Who makes the laws? Or implements them? Am I consulted? Does the majority govern? Why? Does God? The priests? The Party? The pressure of public opinion? Or tradition? By what authority? Both questions, and their subquestions, are central and legitimate. Both have to be answered.... Both are genuine questions. Both are inescapable. And the answers to them determine the nature of a given society.[1]

We can see that we must privilege and protect what he calls 'negative liberty', or the freedom to be ourselves, and resist the idea of 'positive liberty', or of being forced to be some such self as others above us seek to realise on our behalf. Crucially, if choice is to be real for the individual it needs to connect to the imaginative perception – the direct inner vision – of the person concerned. This is the distinction that the historian John Lukacs offers between understanding and knowing. This concerns that tacit knowledge on which we all call in crisis. As Pascal said, 'We understand more than we know.' Understanding is *not* only the result of knowledge, although it can follow knowledge. Yet, as Lukacs says, 'there are myriad instances and examples when understanding precedes knowledge, indeed, when it *leads* to knowledge'.[2] People can *understand* a thing which they do not yet *know*. Indeed, they can understand and think about something about which they do not wish to know! Yet these perceptions inform our choices. This is not to countenance unbridled licence, not to suggest that we can insist on our own preferences without bearing the cross.

We need to be alert to these admittedly difficult and perplexing points as we consider whether or not an 'expert', a planner, an official or a manager can truly make these decisions about personal, timely, intimate healthcare questions on our behalf. We should keep a steady 'eyes-front' in addressing the idea that choices should ultimately come from within ourselves. From the mental pictures we each conjure, from intuitive consciousness within our own being. From how people feel experiences *from the inside*. From their own 'values' in a diverse society, rather than from values which others assume on their behalf as being common to us all. Indeed, the best of all possible worlds for you will not necessarily be that for me. And in Nozick's summary, 'What else can matter to us, other than how our lives feel from the inside?'[3] This recognises the *reality* of how the individual relates to their *own* consciousness, for we relate to our own world, not to the *whole* world. We relate not to naked reality, but to those aspects of reality to which our own temperament and values enable us to link. Those from which we can make sense of what is happening to us. Those on which we found our 'lived only once' lives. We need to consider carefully the implications of this approach for the principles of institutional design, if we are to try to open up the potential for each of us to achieve the most favourable eventualities for ourselves, within a moral structure of mutual respect.

Thus choices concerning healthcare are not merely technical matters concerning the professional 'expertise' of 'decision makers'. Ultimately the choices that individuals have to make are shaped from within. They not a priori truths like those of mathematical science. Instead, we should recognise the transforming power of the imagination and the creative process, too. It is also an iterative process – of linking the inside and the outside world. And we need to find the shapes and structures which enable the individual to do this. It is not a matter of getting it right once, either, but of adaptation and evolution. The East End novelist Israel Zangwill, author of *Children of the Ghetto* (1892), puts the point succinctly in *Without Prejudice* (1896):

> *human documents are made up of facts. But in human life there are no facts. This is not a paradox but 'a fact'. Life is in the eye of the beholder. The humour or pity of it belongs entirely to the spectator, and depends upon the gift of vision he brings.*

As Isaiah Berlin's biographer, Michael Ignatieff, noted, Berlin believed that 'Fighting injustice was essential, but men "do not live only by fighting evils". They live by choosing their own goals – a vast variety of them, seldom predictable, at times incompatible.' It was individual freedom, to choose well or ill, which had to be defended, not some ultimate vision of the human good. Since no disposition was faultless, no disposition was final. His motto in politics, he concluded, was '*surtout pas trop de zele*'.[4]

Thus what begins for many with an apparently simple question, such as 'Why can't I get my hip done quickly by the NHS?', leads to deep (and often frightening) questions concerning faith in human reason itself, the potential of each of us, and our relationships with our inner selves. Such questions concern a high or low view of human potential. They engage our relationships with our inner selves, with one another and with Government. They concern the nature of values, their relativity and their source – notably, who should decide moral questions, and how. They concern the legitimate or illegitimate, moral or immoral significance of differences between people, and the moral value of autonomy. That is, should individuals be perceived as sentient and self-conscious, rational and capable of learning to choose, possessing free will, and guiding their own behaviour by moral principles as a moral agent? Are they capable of engaging in the mutual limitation of personal conduct? And of doing so with regard to some picture of what counts as an appropriate life for themselves and for others?

If we answer 'yes' to all of this, then it is essential that the individual should be permitted to make autonomous choices among options – even if we would not make these particular choices for ourselves. As Mill said, the freedom to fail is the guarantee that the successful experiment will be made. If we deny all this, in order to privilege an 'expert' system of management of healthcare in a hierarchical structure from above, we must make some startling (although surprisingly common) claims. As different value systems guide individuals, and as people make decisions for themselves (amid the complexities of life, their own personalities, and diverse cultural strands), they make decisions which we might not make for ourselves but which are legal and valid for them. This is the old chestnut that a free person could sell him- or herself into slavery. Of course, it is good choices which make for good outcomes, and bad choices have a price. Indeed, as Berlin says, *all* choices have a price. However, this is a risk which is part of the price of freedom. It is one unavoidable aspect of its opportunities. And we each constantly make our own assessments of a price worth paying in making *any* choices.

This is difficult ethical and conceptual territory because it concerns the meaning of life – which Nozick calls 'that elusive and difficult notion'. However, I think we can agree with his formulation that 'a person's shaping his life in accordance with some overall plan is his way of giving meaning to his life; only a being with the capacity so to shape his life can have or strive for meaningful life'.[5]

This discussion shows the inadequacy and hazardousness of the project for politicised equality, which is different from the project for equality of access. And it concerns the value of the differences between people being allowed to show and live. My thesis is that if we are to enable individuals to choose how they shall live, we need to find ways to *make differences between people count and be legitimate*. And that healthcare systems must privilege this approach if they are to deliver access to high-quality care for all. We need to help people to articulate their differences legitimately in ways that they understand and which can directly influence in order to secure a satisfactory personal service. And to do so while also (but incidentally, in a market) influencing for the better services that can be secured by others. Individuals need to expect to be capable of drawing distinctions, making personal assessments, and differentially and legitimately acting upon them. None of us does so without advice, and there is every prospect of this being available to us.

However, the NHS demonstrates that it is very difficult to enable people to live and support self-chosen lives without markets. Its 'needs-led' prescriptiveness contradicts this possibility. And it is, too, becoming increasingly clear in a diverse Britain that there is no one right way to live. However, from the beginning the NHS itself represented an aspect of Utopian temptation – of 'knowing best'. It offers a realm based on centralising beliefs, as a remedy to the choices that are implicit in healthcare. Yet it is self-referring, and makes no use of other explanations for why things are as they are. It is chilling to recall that Sidney Webb, the Fabian draughtsman of the original Labour Party Constitution and subsequently a Cabinet Minister, said 'We have no right to live our own lives.'[6]

We should therefore be sceptical about the call for master-plans and for highly detailed policies or new 'systems' that are prescriptive in their details to resolve all of our difficulties. We should be suspicious of great systems and their moral architecture. Incredulous about the very bricks and mortar. Wary of the plans that precede their marriage. Indeed, the twentieth century should have taught us the consequences of being required to merge ourselves into some 'higher reality' offered by the vanguard, by 'experts', by 'the Party' or by the Plan. In addition, consider the perspective offered by Nozick:

> *I believe there is also a place and a function in our ongoing intellectual life for a less complete work, containing unfinished presentations, conjectures, open questions and problems, leads, side connections, as well as a main line of argument. There is room for words on subjects other than last words.*[7]

This is not to say that we cannot at least establish the outline and the shape of an approach which will enable the structure to evolve in response to consumers' wishes, when they make price-conscious decisions. For this is the present objective. One, too, which will correct the injustices embodied in the inadequate outcomes and poor access of the State monopoly system. Here, free and self-responsible choice is fundamental to liberty *in principle*, and to constructive change *in practice* – so that there can be better healthcare for all. What this better healthcare means in actuality is, to some considerable extent, a matter for individuals to decide upon for themselves. Resistance to the medicalisation of our lives, persistence in self-reliance, and preference for personality above prescription – all these make the case.

None of this is impossible. Of course, changes on a large scale of the kind required usually look easier in retrospect than they do at the time of asking. I do not underestimate the challenges. The changes on the ground will necessarily be complex, slow-moving and dauntingly voluminous – for example, in the administrative tasks of freeing us from bureaucracies. Not least in constructing new contractual arrangements. Changes will take more than one generation, even if we begin the evolutionary processes now. The power of staff and vested interests is considerable. Public service union opposition is entrenched. Bad ideas are deeply embedded. Lost historical opportunities are only now being uncovered again. Vested interests, too, benefit from specific injustices and defects in the NHS structure. For example, the waiting list caused by inadequate funding and capacity serves as a bank which benefits particular vested interests from which the demand for much private work derives. The detailed work of sorting out new systems and setting them workably in place will take a very long time. However, this is an argument for starting sooner, rather than realising later.

No master-plan. But it is still necessary to set out a framework for an approach to policy, rooted in understandings about how things work and how they might change. In doing so we should keep in mind and cherish what Peter Lilley called 'the inconvenient diversity of the real world'.[8] Reliance on a master-plan is the perspective of the centraliser, not the dynamist. There has to be an *outline* of policy which is credible, and persuasive – which satisfies the mind and the heart, and which relies on reassuring people that services will be there and evolve in response to the wishes of consumers. This commitment must be based on the world-view expressed by Oakeshott. It should be rooted in first principles which ensure that we do not get lost in the maze of incident, individual cases and shocking events as we consider change. And so the real issue is not how we will *definitively* solve the problems, but how we *pose them*; the terms of the dialogue that we establish, and whose point of view is emphasised. That, of course, must be the service user's. And here it is impossible for there to be just *one* story – either one 'system' or one conception of the wishes of others – derived from the push of the past and the pull of the future.

So, the folly of dogmatism might be evaded. The memory of all those final truths now abandoned – the ideas which governed men's minds, once so inevitable, so encompassing, and now so unfamiliar – is itself chastening. But, of course, there have to be sufficient details about a new system to indicate how devices for change would function. This is essential for persuasion in a democracy, but there must be space, too, for readings which we have *not* conceived, which are prompted by the 'reader', which are introduced by users, which are imagined by new providers who offer new ideas for testing. The structure must allow others to challenge it, test it, amend it within the general framework of rules regulated by Government. This, a framework which grants the floor to the users of services. The approach must enable different readings, variants and revisions to come about. Here we should value *innocence* as well as *process*, and spontaneity as much as prediction. We should, too, value surprise, and learn from the biologist and angler Julian Pepperell, who wrote: 'No matter how much we might think we know about the marine life in our waters, there's always something that pops up now and again which shakes us up and gives us a surprise.'[9]

Instead of a master-plan – if we want user-led services – we should rely on the power of evolution, of adaptive trial and error, of spontaneity and innovation. For the approach – not 'the system' – is being established for millions of users still to come. It is not being organised as a penance for past error, but for its future potential. We should not conceive of posterity only according to the model of what we know. An open system should create opportunities that its authors cannot yet imagine. This is the very opposite of the concept of 'positive liberty', where we are forced to become someone that others have imagined on our behalf.

As the cultural critic Jane Jacobs has shown, economies also make themselves up as they go along. Instead of a master-plan we should facilitate this, while setting out an approach and standards. We should outline the results that we would like to achieve. This is the part that takes the hard thinking: what is to be the framework of the underlying rules? And the devices (notably in purchasing care) which will express these successfully? We need to consider these issues from first principles, and to see how these can be carried into practice with effective devices and incentives. How can we make them actually operational, as the means to achieve the vision in our earth-bound actual life? For we need to bring abstractions down to earth, if we are to argue a case. And as Jacobs says (and Postrel illustrates), 'Economic history is stuffed with expensive duds undertaken by people who thought they could predict the future by shaping it.'[10]

Notes

1 Berlin I (1969) *Four Essays on Liberty.* Oxford University Press, Oxford.
2 Lukacs J (2001) *Five Days in London. May 1940.* Yale University Press, New Haven, CT.
3 Nozick R (1974) *Anarchy, State and Utopia.* Basil Blackwell, Oxford, p.xii.
4 Ignatieff M (1998) *Isaiah Berlin: a life.* Chatto & Windus, London.
5 Nozick, ibid., p.xii.
6 Beckson K (1992) *London in the 1890s: a cultural history.* WW Norton, New York.
7 Nozick, ibid., p.43.
8 Lilley P (2001) Speech, 23 June 1993, quoted by N Timmins in *The Five Giants: a biography of the Welfare State.* HarperCollins, London, p.524.
9 Pepperell J (2001) *Fish Tales. The mystery of the Snapper Bump and other stories from Australian waters.* Random House Australia, Milsons Point, New South Wales, p.8.
10 Jacobs J (2000) *The Nature of Economies.* Modern Library, New York, p.139; Postrel V (1998) *The Future and Its Enemies, The Growing Conflict over Creativity, Enterprise and Progress.* The Free Press, New York.

Chapter 9

The meaning of 'equality'

Before it is just to say that a man ought to be an independent labourer, the country ought to be in such a state that a labourer by honest industry can become independent.

(Lord Beveridge)

There is also the question of equality. What can this mean in healthcare? It's clear what it *cannot* mean. It cannot mean equality of outcome, since we are all different. As Professor Macneile Dixon wrote

> 'Both health and illness are in part a matter of inheritance.... In a word we inherit our genes, upon whose combination and distribution everything depends. In our genes lies our destiny.... We are partakers in a gigantic lottery' – even to have entered upon life at all – for 'in each family a few, a very few, out of legions of possible human beings come into existence. They are, shall we say, among the favoured few. Why were they, like ourselves, so singled out? And at what moment did this self of yours, so precious to this "I", this individual person, attach itself to the chromosomes from which our bodies have sprung? And are there somewhere souls awaiting their opportunity to be born?'
>
> 'I stand terrified and amazed,' wrote Pascal, 'to see myself here rather than elsewhere, for there is not the slightest reason for the here rather than for the elsewhere, or for the now rather than for some other time.' And we may add, 'or any time at all', no reason why your 'I' or mine should ever have entered into the world or life.[1]

So prisoners of our genes – and of our times – as we are, the most startling inequalities are beyond our influence, and even our ken. It's clear, however, that there are others which we can *enable*. Here lies the *useful* meaning of that Gladstone bag of a word – 'equality' – for it should mean equality of opportunity, which the State should guarantee in law and make effective in practice. However, it should do so without driving standards down by artificially suppressing funding. Everyone should have access to a 'moral minimum' of patient-guaranteed good care, as a patient fundholder – and otherwise be able to spend their own income on whatever extras for which they wish to pay.

Here the issue of personal self-esteem is important. For the political attempt to eliminate differences between individuals – by insisting on equality – actually harms individual health status. And thus disempowerment of the poor is not the *result* of markets, but it is due to their *absence*. This means the suppression of market signals and, due to failure to use tax transfers, a lack of income with which to secure good healthcare. It has been a tragedy of Wagnerian immensity. And the NHS requires the poor to compete with the middle classes for scarce and rationed NHS services. It represents deprivation reinforced by social engineering on a large scale. This has recently been analysed by Dr Ellie Lee of Southampton University, as the State interfering in our lives to such an extent that many lose the ability to cope on their own, instead of (as Hayek argued was so essential) learning to choose in order genuinely to be an adult.[2]

Self-esteem is one of the vital foundations which the State undermines by 'knowing best'. The State reduces people's confidence in their own abilities. Yet health economist Robert Evans has shown that much disease is an expression of other, non-medical factors. Self-esteem and the feeling of individual worth as a unique person are vital factors in good health, in feeling in control of one's own life, of being an effective actor in choices. Nozick says that 'self-esteem is based on *differentiating characteristics*; that's why it's *self-esteem*'.[3]

So opportunity is essential to self-esteem. It is a genuine pivot of good health. The political attempt to eliminate differences between individuals limits opportunity, reduces diversity, and thus hinders the basis of self-esteem where it arises *from comparisons with others*. Nozick argues that different people need to be able to see themselves as doing well on varied axes. If someone is less good at something, they are at least good at something else. Empowerment can renovate self-esteem, by fortifying demand with money in individual hands. And it can show people that they can do well with respect to their preferences, as they as consumers predominate over providers. Here individuals will explore their own tacit knowledge, and as they learn they will discover that they can secure their choices. And the power of self-esteem should be given significant weight, alongside the inflated claims made for medicine itself.[4]

Of course, the strong have an obligation to aid the weak. Here we come across old-fashioned but directly relevant words like 'duty' and moral obligation. And, as Francis Maude recently stressed, 'Obligations freely undertaken and cheerfully discharged are the bonds that bind society and the community together.'[5] It is a fundamental principle that social justice matters when we consider healthcare. This surely means that no one should be denied care. However, this does not imply imposing politicised equality, nor – once a guaranteed 'moral minimum' of quality care is legally ensured for all – does it imply that people should be forbidden to spend their own money on additional consumption of care if they want to do so and if professionals can legally provide that care.

Much of the discussion about healthcare is focused on successful relationships between patients and doctors. This is an important question, but it will be seen that at the heart of ensuring these fundamentals – and thus of discovering real answers to outstanding questions – is the more fundamental issue of the relationship between economic freedom and political freedom, of our relations with ourselves, with one another, and with Government. Here there are strongly held views about controverted ideas of how the world works, what it is that motivates people, about 'values', and about how the world should work. This is why there is so much basic disagreement and so little unanimity. For these are ideological debates, not technical ones. As Dr Irwin M Stelzer says, these disagreements are 'merely a subset of a broader debate concerning the extent to which Government should be asked or allowed to interfere in the lives of its citizens'.[6]

These differences are as much about morality as about 'services', and the potential for disharmony, for accusations of bad faith and for angry flouncing is huge. For different assumptions situate people in different corners with regard to such choices as intrusive central Government or voluntary exchange, paternalism or individual responsibility and freedom of choice and action, risk taking (or its avoidance at all costs), equality of opportunity or of outcome, decisions taken by 'expertise' – the prescient few controlling the irresponsible many – or from the individual's learned capacity for choice, the protection of 'the public interest', and of individual and public welfare (and morality). Arguments of this kind, too, are about 'fairness' and equality, particularly concerning how wealth is distributed, the potential of officialdom or of individual decision making, the desirability of economic growth (and thus of rising incomes, higher material standards of life, and the generation and diffusion of wealth) to pay for services, the importance of direct incentives or of central guidance related to output and results. Often what is evidence to one persuasion is invisible, irrelevant or miscast (in terms of values) to another persuasion. And this is why it is so difficult to persuade. This is the origin of disdain, of accusations of bad faith, of the allegation of the abandonment of the poor.

The search for politicised equality is often seemingly underpinned by the re-distributive idea that *any* economic differences and the existing distribution of property are illegitimate. Yet there is a genuine sense in which the NHS has itself caused poverty, by rationing available funds which have been limited in the main to taxation, and by reducing healthcare chances while at the same time suppressing choice and competition. The NHS has, too, had to respond from an unnecessarily weak base to the consequences of other causal factors in society. The insistence on politicised equality has made a bad case worse.

Notes

1 Macneile Dixon W (1938) *The Human Situation. The Gifford Lectures delivered in the University of Glasgow 1935–1937.* Longmans Green, New York, pp.136–47.
2 Lee E, quoted by Frean A (2002) Can't cope, won't cope? Blame the nanny state. *The Times.* **20 July**.
3 Nozick R (1974) *Anarchy, State and Utopia.* Basil Blackwell, Oxford, p.43.
4 Nozick, ibid.
5 Maude F (2002) A phoenix, not a dodo. *Spectator.* **23 March**.
6 Stelzer IM (2001) *Lectures on Regulatory and Competition Policy.* Institute of Economic Affairs, London, p.16.

Chapter 10

The meaning of 'choice'

Isn't there such a thing as a natural monopoly? The only one I can think of is the sun.

(Jane Jacobs)

We should be clear what we mean by *choice*. It is a word often used to cloak smuggled goods – notably its substitution by 'consultation'.

The word is used very loosely in politics. It is often a label to conceal rather than an instrument to reveal. Essential to genuine choice is the precise idea expressed in economics – that is, that by expressing *costed* preferences, *financially empowered* individuals can test out specific adaptations against *competition*. We need this possibility if we require choice. But this is exactly what is suppressed in State monopoly provision. Yet change and adaptation, together with choice, are fundamental to our nature.

So, too, the art of beachcombing – or the observation upon which choice depends. And which is supported and prompted by dynamism and keen-eyed competition. We are each the result of dynamism and of its cumulative processes. Or, as Oscar Wilde's Lord Illingworth says in *A Woman of No Importance*, 'Discontent is the beginning of the success of a nation.'

We need to consider too the effect of choices, and those instruments which achieve the précis of the economist and the sensibility of the patient. It is by the expression of preferences that successful and timely adaptations spread because their possessors spread, or are emulated in timely fashion. Later is too late for the provider who does not adapt. Choice is thus both moral and operational. This is to argue that choice is one of those properties by virtue of which a being has the full rights that human beings have. It is not merely an operational or technical issue, but a philosophical fundamental. Even so, operationally – in the words of cultural critic Jane Jacobs – 'opportunity, not necessity, is the mother of invention. The necessity is seen by hindsight.'[1] Choice, too, implies an attitude of welcome to change. There is no way to avoid change. And so we should zestfully embrace those creative processes which offer the potential to balance instability and opportunity, and which enhance both dynamism and stability. It is this process which raises standards for all.

Such an analysis makes a further point about people and the results of their free choices. We should value the expression and development of individual abilities, and view talents as a common asset, rather than seek to nullify the natural advantages of some individuals compared with others. As Nozick puts this:

People's talents and abilities are an asset to a free community; others in the community benefit from their presence and are better off because they are there rather than elsewhere or nowhere. (Otherwise they wouldn't choose to deal with them.) Life, over time, is not a constant-sum game, wherein if greater ability or efforts leads to some getting more, that means that others must lose. In a free society, people's talents do benefit others, and not only themselves.[2]

Therefore there is a powerful moral and a practical case for health policies based on the principle of liberty and free choice which is fully empowered financially. And we should create a system where there is *effective* consumer demand, by contrast to the present position within the NHS, in which service users have virtually no choices that matter. Indeed, if the language of 'stake-holding' is to have any meaning, it must recognise that no one has a greater stake in their own life than the individual. We should each have the opportunity to exercise personal choices which are at present undertaken on our behalf by Government and its agencies – doctors, professionals, civil servants, health authorities, agencies of various kinds, Ministers of the Crown, the National Institute for Clinical Excellence (a disguised governmental rationing body), and so on. This is both a moral and a practical question – for it concerns the nature of our personal reality, as well as the pragmatic reality of services which are either delivered or denied, compromised or commanded by the user of the service.

Notes

1 Jacobs J (2000) *The Nature of Economies.* Modern Library, New York, p.90.
2 Nozick R (1974) *Anarchy, State and Utopia.* Basil Blackwell, Oxford, passim.

Chapter 11

The prerequisites and framework of change

Propose to an Englishman any principle, any instrument, however admirable, and you will observe that the whole effort of the English mind is directed to find a difficulty, a defect, or an impossibility in it. If you speak to him of a machine for peeling a potato, he will pronounce it impossible; if you peel a potato with it before his eyes, he will declare it useless, because it will not slice a pineapple.

(Charles Babbage)

Babbage might be proved wrong. But for there to be a successful approach to change, there are a number of political and economic essentials which must be in place.

Political essentials

- Public consensus that things have reached the point where politicians must act to change things fundamentally.
- Anxiety among politicians that if they don't act, they will suffer. As William Blake said, 'The tigers of wrath are wiser than the horses of instruction'.
- Decisions about what can and cannot be left to the market.
- A guaranteed core package of care to build support for change, and to create confidence in a secure service, rather than allow opinion to be driven by anxiety about change and fear of being abandoned.
- Understanding in society that if a commitment to change is made, then we must expect the inevitable opposition of powerful interests.
- Political and media support, explanation and leadership.
- A regulatory framework which protects competition and encourages new entrants.
- Deliberate and thorough implementation of policies, despite political temptations to stray.
- Dynamist contextual shifts – in new technologies, generational changes in expectations, and so on.
- A society-wide commitment to voluntary exchange and to adaptive development, taking the view that whatever arises from a just situation as a result of free voluntary transactions on the part of all participants is itself just.
- A persuasive case for change made by reference to first principles.

Economic essentials

- Incentives to ensure that resources flow to the organisations that do the best job, in terms of quality, access, cost and consumer satisfaction.
- Genuine market forces which empower significant consumer choice and motivate insurers, purchasers and providers:
  - each of these must earn their incomes by satisfying consumers
  - purchasers must be of sufficient size to achieve gains from their buying power
  - there must be freedom for purchasers to buy selectively, rather than in bulk and from NHS sources only
  - there must be free access to capital markets for providers and purchasers
  - direct incentives are needed for individuals to participate thoughtfully and to join economical health plans
  - facilitation of choice by good information, on quality and cost.

We can be encouraged that much of this is now incrementally falling into place. It is a major opportunity for political leadership to secure incentives, choice and genuine change. In the next chapter I suggest that Mr Milburn has taken some much under-estimated steps. He has carried forward the battle, but without declaring war. He seems, too, to be a 'lucky General'. The consequences have their *own* momentum.

Chapter 12

Cash on the nail

I am not so much seeking to regulate the industry as intervening at a particular moment of time in order to promote conditions in which the 'invisible hand' of market forces, driven by competition, will ensure that an industry performs efficiently and in the interests of consumers.... But regulation is a last resort. Wherever possible, the instruments of competition policy aim to remove restrictions on the effective working of competition.

(Sir Gordon Borrie)

We can already see and analyse the specific devices which will make each of these dreams come true. These can make individual choice real and attainable, in a co-operative, conscious and socially concerned structure. Mr Milburn's initiatives on direct payment and on choice show us both the direction and the destination. These can lead to more extensively experienced individual empowerment, which can be the framework for our coming together in co-operative purchasing, serving both the general and the particular interest. It can resolve many issues of production, distribution, education, understanding and government. This is the beginning of *patient fundholding*.

Direct control of cash, or the voucher, is not a new principle for the NHS. We can see some good working examples of what we can regard as pilots for the patient fundholder. The most important and informative UK evidence comes from the approach seen in the optics market. And there are two recent Government schemes which are now opening the door wider to patient fundholding. These employ direct incentives. And one of them gives patients direct control of cash. This will change provision and purchasing, and it will open new doors. For it offers recognition that it is very difficult, without the deployment of direct incentives, to persuade people to do what they perceive to be against their short-term interests. But when direct incentives have been used – even with the limited approach that relatively small cash payments out of pocket represent – research has demonstrated that significant changes in behaviour occur, as the well-known Rand Corporation Study showed as long ago as the 1980s. And this without harming the health of the individuals concerned.[1]

These are the genuine, incremental beginnings of a new axis of care. They can be broadened to include such important and specific areas as all elderly care, mental healthcare, dentistry, aids to the hard of hearing, and other specialist services – as an extension of a principle, and as educative steps in themselves towards the wider and continuous reform of our health and social care.

First, there is the new scheme designed to give some 400 000 older people direct cash payments of up to £200 a week to buy help in the home in order to keep pensioners out of hospitals and care homes. This scheme, announced on 24 July 2002, follows on from the success of the scheme of giving direct cash payment to some 4000 disabled people, who have proved how well they can exercise this power, supported by advice and assistance in the voluntary sector. This new and wider scheme in Social Services is to replace having to have care supplied through a Social Services department with no user choice. There are more than 11 million older people in the UK – and extending direct payments to this group represents a hugely significant shift in purchasing and in provision of services, in self-responsible action, and in what will prove to be a cultural revolution.[2]

It will be compulsory for local authorities to give older people a choice between provision of services and a cash grant that can be used to pay a relative or alternative home help. This will increase Social Services budgets for older people by £1 billion by 2006, over and above the amount that is needed to keep pace with inflation and the gradual rise in the number of pensioners being given support. The chief innovation is that for the first time local authorities will be obliged to offer direct payments on a large scale. Mr Milburn said that 'Every older person assessed as being in need of care – whether for rehabilitation after a hip operation or for a bit of help with household chores – will be given the choice of receiving a service or receiving a cash payment to purchase care for themselves that better suits their individual needs.' This adds to the current arrangements where a few younger disabled people receive cash grants of up to £600 a week.

This requirement to go to the local authority, to be assessed and then to be given money is not the same, of course, as each individual as of right having a lifelong and accumulated patient fundholding fund and the assurance of patient-guaranteed care. And the Government is not openly considering social insurance. Indeed, Mr Brown derided it during the debate on the Wanless Report, and is instead seeking to spend his way to security. However, this introduction of more cash payments will necessarily exert some pressure on providers, as did GP fundholding. This took financial reality down to the front-line, if not quite to the patient. Direct payment is the revolution itself.

Second, there is the pilot scheme – not yet offering patients direct control over funds – which enables some heart patients who have waited for more than 6 months for surgery to go to any hospital, even if it is abroad, to be seen quickly, under an initiative announced by Mr Milburn on 1 July 2002. This is modelled on the Danish Government's health voucher. Cardiac patients who had been on the NHS waiting lists for at least 6 months were able to opt for treatment at another Trust or outside the NHS from 1 July 2002. This initiative is restricted to a relatively small number of 1000 patients – although it is expected to be extended soon to cover other conditions, including cataracts, hip replacements, ear, nose and throat operations, and general surgery. There is now, too, a pilot in London on cataracts. In January 2003, Mr Blair extended the scheme to cover hip, knee and hernia surgery as well as cataracts – throughout the NHS by summer 2004, and to almost all elective surgery in London by summer 2003. All this is not yet linked to patient control of funds by direct cash payment. But it easily could be – it is, effectively, 'the voucher'. Indeed, I expect this incremental development. It could, too, encourage publication on the Internet of detailed information about the performance of individual doctors.[3]

In terms of patients actually being able to exercise the promised choices, and effective empowerment, frustration at the lack of capacity and thus of choice will, I believe, lead to the specific demand for individuals controlling the funds necessary to make choices and to buy the service in cardiac and other care. I expect Mr Milburn will point to the blockages in the system and introduce direct cash payment to shift it. 'The more complex congenital cases' have already been excluded since the promise of choice was made. In addition, the population that is receiving heart surgery is getting older and is likely to have other medical problems. This will necessarily limit patients making the decision to travel, and this in turn will restrict choices. We shall see whether an administrative plea of being unable to balance choice and capacity is also entered. As Martin Roberts, Director of the London Patient Choice Project, has said, 'We shall be looking at the balance between the demand to move somewhere else and capacity, what choices people exercise and the information they need to exercise them.'[4] Is this management deliberately introducing ambiguity and evasion? If so, it will, I suggest, result in demand for direct cash payments as patients are frustrated by the denial of choice.

Direct control of cash is different to control of the patient by the system. A decision to bundle the patient up like a parcel and post them to a provider with Government money attached is not the same as the patient deciding how much care they wish to have, what kind of care, what it costs, what the costed alternatives are and when the care will be supplied. This is the distinction which we need to keep in mind when we consider the proposals that elderly people should be given direct cash payments, and that heart patients should be given the option of receiving immediate treatment elsewhere when they have been waiting at least 6 months for treatment. This could indeed be a start to patient fundholding – with demand being met in public, private or overseas hospitals.

As Mr Milburn said in the House of Commons on 23 July 2002, when introducing direct cash payments for social services:

> I want to empower older people. People should not just be passive recipients of services. They should have the choice and the ability to shape services for themselves. I cannot think of a better way in social care services than direct payments. There will be direct payments on offer for all. Of course, it is for the elderly person, their carers and families to decide whether to take advantage of that.... [And] In time, we want to get to a position where patients have control not just over the time of their appointment and location of the hospital, but they will also have information on individual clinical teams and how well they are performing.[5]

For this to be a real choice, patients must control their fund. This would seem to be a perfect opportunity to go for patient fundholding – if on a pilot basis. And as the programme of making choice real for cardiac patients unrolls, the logic will become obvious, especially if restraints of capacity require supply which the NHS cannot deliver. For then patients will start to be treated for these serious conditions by European providers – which will carry us beyond the relatively straightforward (but at the time courageous) initiative of hips-and-cataracts provision so far undertaken for NHS patients, for example, in Lille.[6] These initiatives offer the basis for a much wider strategy for change. They could, for example, be rapidly extended to the mentally ill, where significant changes are wanted by patients themselves with regard to the approach to their treatment – reducing stigma, reconciling the care of vulnerable individuals with the protection of society, and emphasising choice and advocacy in the least restrictive settings.[7]

First, they enable us to avoid resorting to a 'big bang' solution. Instead, Government can test out systems that work. This itself is persuasive to the electorate. Incremental change is persuasive and unthreatening. It enables Government to demonstrate an evolving and adaptive system which visibly improves outcomes and user satisfaction. It, too, shows empowerment in action, and exemplifies a dynamist approach.

Such initiatives exemplify first principles. They give people direct cash control. I urge this as the basis for a broad-based plan of guaranteed care, individual empowerment and choice with a core package purchased through social insurance by each of us.

It is important that Mr Milburn is making changes using direct cash payment and placing them *within* the rhetoric and traditions of working-class co-operation and self-organisation, even though that enriching inheritance of mutual-aid, self-responsibility and personal choice has long been submerged by the centralising drive of the first post-war Labour Government and its 'welfarist' successors of all parties. However, these new initiatives can open the door to much wider direct cash payment, with the power being given to the individual, as in patient fundholding.

To the NHS, the concept of the quality controller being the user of services is revolutionary, as I stated earlier. However, the battle of ideas can be won. In the words of one leading disability activist, Philip Mason (who became disabled in 1972 as a result of an accident, and then led a local authority and housing authority to make direct payments to enable disabled people to buy their own support in the community), 'At the moment we have politicians saying that they care for us and then they decide how and where, when and to what extent. But we've got to say, "That's wrong. If you care for us, then we should define and decide".'[8] The disabled and the elderly can now buy social services direct, instead of just taking what they are given by Social Services departments. It is the campaign by the disabled movement, long fought, and bed blocking in acute hospitals with the political embarrassment that this brings, which have forced the door. Government looked to the British Council for Disabled People (BCDP) to work it out on their behalf. This has led to the foundation of the National Centre for Independent Living (NCIL), which is playing an important role alongside other forums, groups and consultants associated with independent living, helping both the disabled and those without disability.

Direct payments, which had been illegal since the National Assistance Act of 1948, were introduced in 1997. This change 'is solely attributable to the disability movement', and after a long campaign.[9] People who used or could use

Social Services support were given the option of receiving cash to organise their own support, instead of using 'traditional' Social Services. Direct payments are made to individuals by a local authority Social Services department, either as an alternative or in conjunction with direct provision of services by that department. The sum is based on an individual assessment of 'need' [sic]. There is no nationally agreed amount – each local authority makes its own decisions with regard to calculating the money that they will give to a particular individual. Thus the social worker is the rationer of Government money, but once the money is obtained it can be used to organise support for services of one's own choice, at a time and in a way that one prefers. The money is paid into a separate account, opened specifically for that purpose, and is untaxed and does not affect the assessment of income for social security benefits. However, it cannot be used for NHS services or for local authority housing services.

The money is intended to support independent living. The individual decides what they prefer. They have much more freedom and control. They can recruit people of their choice to work with them, and make their own arrangements with them. Any staff that the individual employs report directly to them. If, in a crisis, they need more or different help they do not have to rely on inflexible social provision, or necessarily have to go into hospital. If they do go into hospital, their discharge does not depend on waiting for Social Services to act on their behalf. As the NCIL says, 'Another advantage is that they support independent living and can enable people to lead fuller lives in the community than they might do otherwise.' It also improves relationships, including those with carers. Support, advice and advocacy are available from a number of Centres for Independent Living to help those who may initially find the responsibilities problematic. These centres include the NCIL and the Centre for Mental Health Service Development (CMHSD).[10]

The Secretary of State is now making wider use of the provisions of the Health and Social Care Act 2002, enabling him to require local Councils to make direct payments to people who meet specified criteria. Effectively, this means that Councils will have a duty to provide a direct payment to any eligible person who requests one. This is hedged about with all types of conditions, but the *principle* has been established. We shall now see pushing at the door.

This important innovation arises from the dichotomy resulting from the separation of responsibilities and funding between the social welfare system, which provided services, and the social security system, which provided cash. First, direct payments were made to the disabled, and now they are being made to older people, too. Older people have been able to claim some direct payments since 2000, but figures from the Department of Health show that between April 2000 and March 2001, of the 5000 people who received these payments, 88% were aged between 18 and 64 years, with only 500 individuals over 65 years of age receiving them.[11] Now, however, it seems likely that direct control over cash and thus over personal care will be more widely taken up. Thus someone who wants services can opt to receive their value in cash from a local authority, together with the Independent Living Fund for larger packages of service. The individual can organise their own care along lines that they want personally. Direct payments can be used for 'anything which meets the objectives of the care plan'. This itself is a personal challenge, a learning challenge, and a developmental challenge both for the individual and for voluntary and patient support groups. These have willingly taken up that challenge.

The patient fundholder concept is introduced, and a consumer co-operative undertakes this direct purchasing on behalf of its subscribers. Indeed, the expertise which is already accumulating in support of the disabled and the elderly in making decisions for themselves will itself be invaluable in this context. The Government's aim to increase home care, too, could be helped by patient fundholding which, if it included some portion of domiciliary care cost, would shift the responsibility away from unwilling local authorities, many of whom limit how much care they will provide and pay for at home (this costs an average of £10 an hour, compared with around £280 paid for residential care). Direct payment also makes it clear who is the client – and it may have an impact on the mentalities of care home providers, too, where the incentives now are to please the local authority in order to keep the contract.

The initiative of direct payment will also be a test of the old idea that people are not competent to make judgements about their own lives when it comes to medical and social care. And as a report in the care journal *Registered Homes and Services* stated in July 2002, reporting on a visit to the NCIL:

> *Autonomy, non-disabled workers need constantly to be reminded, becomes most important when it is threatened. Direct payments and the access that they give to control over one's own affairs have truly transformed lives.... [And] The second reason for the popularity of direct payments with service users is that many Social Services departments are hopelessly inefficient or desperately insensitive, or both, when it comes to tailoring packages of care to individuals. Decisions have to be referred up through a hierarchy of care managers and budget holders, systems are rarely geared to people with multiple impairment, there are long lines of communication through commissioning and providing agencies, detailed contracts of service are difficult to revise as quickly as needs [sic] change, ensuring continuity of helpers is impossible with high staff turnover, and health and safety regulations are horribly restrictive.*[12]

A series of projects have since sprung up – in an adaptive market – to help people who elect for direct payments, and to shift the axis of what were bureaucratic tasks. These include Personal Assistance Support Schemes, Centres of Independent Living, and so on – dynamism in action. They provide information, and offer advocacy, peer support, advice and training in getting the best from the new system. People are generating solutions for themselves, in mutual-aid. Frances Hasler, Director of the National Centre for Independent Living, commented that 'It's about choice, it's about control, it's about autonomy.'[13] She also suggests that the system might seem to favour articulate individuals, but that people have become more articulate by achieving independent living precisely because they had had to become effective self-advocates – Hayek's 'learning to choose'. People with learning difficulties, especially those with additional impairments, have been major beneficiaries. The scheme for the disabled offers individually selected services in place of the previous options, which were often limited to 'a family or a residential home or nothing'. For disabled people, one of the criteria for receiving a payment has been being able to manage it, either alone or with assistance. Thus a support structure has evolved, involving advocacy, family, friends and a Centre for Independent Living.

The advent of direct payment – now extended to older people, carers, disabled people aged 16 and 17 years, and the parents of disabled children – has had a significant impact on domiciliary care. As Francis Hasler says, 'We've never said that direct payments are the only way of producing a flexible and responsive service, but direct payments are a jolly good way because the quality controller is the service user.' In one area, thanks to the new competition, the home care workers suddenly discovered that – yes – they could work later than 8.00pm.[14]

This example shows the difference between the broad concept of 'the money following the patient', and the patient controlling the money. As mentioned earlier, a decision to bundle the patient up like a parcel and post them to a provider with Government money attached is not the same as the patient deciding how much care they wish to have, what kind of care, what it costs, what the costed alternatives are and when the care will be supplied. The money following the patient leaves the decisions with the person or institution buying care for them and on their behalf. The two approaches are diametrically different.

In addition, the specific cash plans which have developed in the private market enable people to see that they can come into a relationship of mutual respect in the market, and for specific services which they can afford and by which they can be empowered. Here the importance of such plans as an aspect of trade union membership should not be underestimated. And this is a constituency and a tradition to which innovative politicians can make more appeal.

Mr Milburn has underlined the need to recognise the merits of a coalition of charities, churches, public and private sectors – and the extra capacity that they could supply if revenues were provided. He will also continue to encourage investment and development in the independent sector, which has shown that it is capable of managing investment well. The long-term care story dramatically highlights this, as does the hospice movement, itself entirely the result of charitable endeavour. The interest in mutual-aid organisations represents more than just an opportunity to increase capacity. It also offers the revival of old co-operative and working-class traditions and the legitimacy of individual choice. In this sense the innovation of mutual-aid is a survival which itself carries cultural messages – including a structure which challenges both State control by independent co-operative action and Mr Brown's analysis of the way forward for the NHS.[15]

The move towards genuine patient empowerment has been incremental, gradual and cumulative, but no less genuine for that, and no less a programme for being apparently un-programmatic. It remains an adaptive, trial-and-error project, and this is one of its strengths. For we want incremental, adaptive, dynamist change. It remains a political initiative in that it responds to events and draws its meaning from them. It remains innovative in that it shapes the next step that events imply. It remains a surprise because politicians do not always know how to benefit from surprises. It offers genuine movement towards a public domain which is not political. *Experience* of empowerment will empower others.

Notes

1 Newhouse JP and the Insurance Experiment Group (1993) *Free For All? Lessons from the RAND Health Insurance Experiment*. Harvard University Press, Cambridge, MA.

2 US consumers have this information in many states. See Twisselmann B (2002) Disciplined doctors. *BMJ*. **325**: 226. See also Philpot T (2002) The right to choose wrongly. *Community Care*. 21–27 November.

3 Smith J (2002) The quality controller is the service user. *Registered Homes and Services*. See also Carvel J (2002) Elderly to get option to buy home care. *Guardian*. **24 July**: 9; Milburn A, House of Commons (2002) *Hansard*. **23 July**: cols.869–72; Meikle J (2002) Cash fine to clear elderly from hospital beds. *Guardian*. **30 July**; Maglazlic RA, Bryan M, Brandon D and Given D (1998) Direct payments in mental health – a research report. *Breakthrough*. **2**; Heslop P (2001) Direct payments for people with mental health support needs. *Advocate*. **May**: 6–9; Glasby J (2002) Independence at a price. *Community Care*. **4 September**: 30–1. Liberal Democrat MP Paul Burstow, spokesman on older people, is one of the few politicians who has openly argued this case: 'I'd want to look at the whole issue of direct payments – they're very underused, undervalued, and poorly advertised. Some of the research I've seen suggests it's a very cost-effective way of providing services. I think the reason it hasn't taken off in older people's services is because Social Services have difficulties with the idea of giving someone control over their own pot of money. There are some professional and employment reasons within local authorities, some staff are not very enthusiastic about it or feel a bit threatened by it. And there are still some places with a very paternalistic attitude to services' (quoted by R Winchester (2002) Age old story. *Community Care*. **20 June**). Mr Burstow urged Mr Milburn to extend direct payments to those currently in nursing and care homes (House of Commons (2002) *Hansard*. **23 July**: col.876). The Audit Commission hinted at direct payments for Social Services in 1997, and in 1998 the Independent Healthcare Association asked for this. See Audit Commission (1997) *The Coming of Age. Improving care services for older people*. Audit Commission, London; Independent Health Care Association (1998) *Caring Into the Future*. IHA, London, p.25. On extension of action – scheme for those waiting more than six months, see H Studd (2003) Blair promises health spending will deliver. *The Times*. **24 January**.

4 Charter D (2002) Heart patients to pick their own hospital. *The Times*. **1 July**; Wilkinson P (2002) Patients' right to choose. *NHS Magazine*. **July/August**: 18–19; Department of Health (2002) *Extending Choice for Patients. Heart surgery. Your guide to your choices*. Department of Health, London; www.doh.gov.uk/extendingchoice.

5 Quoted in Wilkinson P (2002) Patients' right to choose. *NHS Magazine*. **July/August**: 18–19.

6 'Older people's services', statement by Secretary of State for Health, House of Commons (2002) *Hansard*. **23 July**: col.882.

7 Charter D (2002) Heart patients to pick their hospitals. *The Times*. **1 July**; Rogers L (2002) Patients to get treatment funded by NHS in Europe. *Sunday Times*. **11 August**: 22; York Economics Consortium (2002) *Treating Patients Overseas*. York Economics Consortium, York.

8 See Department of Health (2002) *Mental Health Bill. Consultation document*. Stationery Office, London; *The Independent on Sunday* Mental Health Campaign, 2002; Muitjen M (2002) The priority with a new mental health bill is not to hurry, but to get it right. *NHS Magazine*. **September**: 19; press release from Consumers' Association/Office of Fair Trading, *Consumers' Association Makes First Supercomplaint to OFT and OFT Launches Major Investigation into Private Dentistry; super-complaint on private dentistry: preliminary findings on the issues raised by the Consumers' Association*, Office of Fair Trading, London, 23 January 2002. See also Department of Health (2002) *NHS Dentistry: options for change*. Department of Health, London, which is concerned with payment systems.

9 Campbell J and Oliver M (eds) (1996) *Disability Politics. Understanding our past, changing our future*. Routledge, London, p.164.

10 Campbell and Oliver, ibid. See also Department of Health (1996) *Community Care (Direct Payments) Act 1996 – policy and practice guidance*. Department of Health, London; Department of Health (1998) *Guide to Receiving Direct Payments*. Department of Health, London (with Wales/N Ireland versions). Also see Values into Action (undated) *Funding Freedom. Direct payments for people with learning difficulties*. Values into Action, London.

11 National Centre for Independent Living (NICIL), ncil@ncil.org.uk; Values into Action, VIA@BTInternet.com; UK Advocacy Network, ukan@can-online.org.uk; British Council of Organisations of Disabled People, bcodp.org.uk; Centre for Mental Health Service Development, website under construction (September 2002): IAHSP, Deborah.Davidson@IAHSP.kcl.ac.uk; doh:doh.gov.uk.

12 House of Commons (2002) *Hansard*. **5 July**: col.883–8; Leason K (2002) Can the Government deliver on its ambitions for older people's services? *Community Care*. **August**.

13 Smith J, ibid.

14 Smith J, ibid.

15 Smith J, ibid.

Chapter 13

Lord Beveridge and what is really at stake

Social security must be achieved by co-operation between the State and the individual. The State should offer security for service and contribution. The State in organising security should not stifle incentive, opportunity, responsibility; in establishing a national minimum, it should leave room and encouragement for voluntary action by each individual to provide more than that minimum for himself and his family.

(Lord Beveridge)

There is much at stake besides better health and social care. The argument is not just about a *system* as such – the NHS – but also about our fundamental selves. It is not about selfish*ness*, but about the nature of our being, and, too, about the wonder of being. Here I urge that we should not be frightened to say so. Nor should we be frightened of our own shadows – for example, in making difficult decisions. We should be grateful for the opportunity to make them, for this is what makes us human. Risk is integral to life.

So we are exploring ideas of how to reform the relationship between individuals and professionals, how to consider the relationships between Government and the individual, how to reflect upon our relationships with our own selves, and a new structure for reforming health and social care services. Crucially, this offers the choice of a dynamist, market-focused approach rather than a statist or Government-directed approach to living life and to discovering personal identity and the meaning of a life, and of one's own life. In making sense of one's own life it is for the individual to consider and transform the multiplicity of personal experiences into some ordered unity of thought and action. This is the consciousness of an animal coming to knowledge of itself, which is both a wonder of the universe and our own responsibility. Above all else, we should respect this and value it both in ourselves and in others.

In a debate of exactly this kind and tone, the words at the head of this chapter were quoted by Beveridge himself – they were his *own* words – on the first page of his 1948 book, *Voluntary Action*. They are from his report entitled *Social Insurance and Allied Services* ('the Beveridge Report'), published in 1942.[1] They identify the following inescapably intransigent issue. When is it appropriate to make a choice on a communal basis and when is it appropriate to make one on an individual basis? It underlines the questions that Mr Milburn has explored and acted upon. It is easy to talk of giving people choices, and of refocusing the

NHS on the patient, but how is the thing to be done? Direct cash payments (the patient fundholder) represent a more certain route than those which the NHS has tried so far.

We should try to sort out once again what has to be done through and by the machinery of the State, and what the individual (and perhaps *only* the individual) can do. As Beveridge said:

> The community, through the machinery of the State, has the duty of doing those things which can only be done by the State, of so organising itself that there is fair opportunity for all men at all times.... [But which things are which? And] This does not absolve the individual from the duty and responsibility of thinking and planning for himself.

With regard to the State making the rules, it was for the State to 'ensure to individuals the maximum of freedom and responsibility'. This did not mean that there would not be co-operation between public and voluntary agencies. On the contrary, this was a special feature of British public life. For social advance involved action by the State and action by the individual – in Personal Thrift and Mutual Aid (his capitals). Beveridge followed this – and many will find this a surprising echo of Adam Smith – by writing:

> The other (motive) is the Business motive; the pursuit of livelihood or of gain for oneself in meeting the needs of one's fellow citizens; from the interplay of this motive with that of Mutual Aid or Personal Thrift have sprung organisations which are in some cases of portentous scale.[2]

Beveridge did not expect there to be any doubt about the value of these motives, or of the organisations which embodied them. Indeed, he wrote:

> It is needless to emphasise the importance of the subject whose study is attempted here. In a totalitarian society all action outside the citizen's home, and it may be much that goes on there, is directed or controlled by the State. By contrast, vigour and abundance of Voluntary Action outside one's home, individually and in association with other citizens, for bettering one's life and that of one's fellows, are the distinguishing marks of a free society. They have been outstanding features of English life.[3]

This approach indeed saw the dynamic individual, family and group actively shaping their own histories, and not merely being the passive victims of poverty, or dependent on welfare. Well into the twentieth century there was widespread mutual-aid and self-provision by large numbers, shared networks of conviviality and reciprocal support (as well as access to voluntary hospitals). Between 40% and 60% of adult males were probably members of a Friendly Society in the last quarter of the nineteenth century and into the early twentieth century, thus making private provision for their own and their family's wlfare. In addition, there was membership of co-operative societies, trade unions and savings banks, and provision via commercial insurance.

There are two chief mental barriers to returning to this approach to an open-ended future. The negative stasist approach which requires someone always to be in control. And the anxiety that change means disaster. Here – despite the many evident deficits and denials of the NHS and the pain that this causes to millions – the cultural memories of insecurity, and of truly being of no consequence like the Victorian pauper, run deep. Some still fear the modernity of commercial costings in healthcare – the traditional (if falsely based) horror story from the USA. And they recall the history of what the historian Alan Kidd has called the patchwork 'economy of makeshifts' and the world of 'less eligibility' – an anxiety expressed by the poet Thomas Noel: 'Rattle his bones over the stones, he's only a pauper whom nobody knows.'[4]

Beveridge himself called for political invention to find new forms of fruitful co-operation between public authorities and voluntary agencies. These included – and should now include again – those organisations of mutual-aid that were formed in order to secure voluntary exchange in the competitive marketplace, on behalf of their subscribing members. And of course 'of Mutual Aid, of Personal Thrift, and of Philanthropy' – the themes of Beveridge's report on voluntary action. If Lord Beveridge were here today, I would hope that he would be invited to become President of any network linking competing patient-guaranteed care associations (PGCAs), which I propose as a vital part of reforms. These will be in an ideal position to offer to purchase contracts for individual patients for primary, community and other health and social services. The combination of an ageing population and new opportunities for treatment increases the number of patients who are facing complex diseases that require co-ordinated help from various professionals. The emphasis will then be on fully integrated care, on preventive care, and on medical and nursing services in the community, where most people prefer to be treated. And the PGCA would insist upon basics such as booking hospital appointments actually working, instead of still being merely an ambition more than 50 years after the foundation of the NHS.

However, we should be frank about the fact that people do fear change, and we should consider why this is so. The next chapter will explore this question.

Notes

1 Beveridge WH, *Voluntary Action*, ibid, p.8; Beveridge WH (1942) *Social Insurance and Allied Services*. HMSO, London.

2 Beveridge WH, *Voluntary Action*, op. cit., pp.7–8. Also see Beveridge WH and Wells AF (eds) (1949) *The Evidence for Voluntary Action*. G Allen & Unwin, London. There is a significant and valuable historical literature, especially the following: Yeo CS, several works cited; Gosden PHJH (1961) *The Friendly Societies in England, 1815–75*. Manchester University Press, Manchester, and *Self-Help: voluntary associations in nineteenth-century Britain* (Batsford, London, 1973). See also Pelling H (1968) The working class and the origins of the welfare state. In: *Popular Politics and Society in Late Victorian Britain*. Macmillan, London; Supple B (1974) Legislation and Virtue: an essay on working-class self-help and the State in the early nineteenth century. In: N McKendrick (ed.) *Historical Perspectives: studies in English thought and society in honour of JH Plumb*. Europa, London; Crossick G (1978) *An Artisan Elite in Victorian Society: Kentish*

London, 1840–1880. Croom Helm, London; Gladstone D (ed.) (1999) *Before Beveridge. Welfare before the Welfare State.* IEA Health and Welfare Unit, London; Jewkes J and Jewkes S (1961) *The Genesis of the British National Health Service.* Blackwell, Oxford; Seldon A (ed.) (1974) *The Long Debate on Poverty: essays on industrialisation and the 'condition of England'.* IEA, London; Green D (1984) *Working-Class Patients and the Medical Establishment.* Temple Smith/Gower, London; Prokashka F (1988) *The Voluntary Impulse: philanthropy in modern Britain.* Faber & Faber, London; Hanson C (1996) Self-help: the instinct to advance. In: Seldon A (ed.) *Re-Privatising Welfare: after the lost century.* IEA, London. On self-help and education, see West EG (1994) *Education and the State.* Liberty Fund, Indianapolis, IN.

3 Beveridge, ibid., p.10.

4 Noel T (1841) The Pauper drive. In: *Rhymes and Roundelays* (1841), cited by Kidd A (1999) *State, Society and the Poor in Nineteenth-Century England.* Macmillan, Basingstoke, p.119.

Chapter 14

Why people hesitate about change

Men are quite without the sort of prescience which can determine which amount of human happiness a specific action may ultimately achieve, and before the burning house – to rescue a person, or a masterpiece by Rembrandt? – conscience will be a surer guide than any attempts at utilitarian calculation.

(Michael Innes)

If reform proposals are to persuade, they must honestly address anxieties. People have genuine concerns. These include:

- What happens if I get a catastrophic disease? Will the 'core' fund pay the costs?
- If the NHS changes to patient-guaranteed care, how stable will this changed system be?
- Will it change again, disadvantageously (for example, by excluding specific conditions, or the poor)?
- Will I end up paying more? If so, how much more, and for what?
- How can I be reassured that we will all be in one market, as you say?
- What about the problem of people making 'unwise choices' – those who often buy suboptimal services or goods because they do not know about better alternatives, or because alternatives have not been brought to market?
- The market works in optics, I can quite see that. But how different is the optics sector from the rest of healthcare, and to what extent are its lessons applicable or non-applicable?
- Will insurance be like common experience when premiums are paid but insurers are reluctant to pay out?

These concerns are real in people's minds. They make some people hesitate about change. Here we should be honest and admit that all change has a cost – nothing is for free. And better healthcare will cost more. If we want more than we presently get, we will have to afford it. And if we want the poor to benefit in the same way, the better off will have to pay more in order to finance that gain, too. On balance, however, the changes will bring many advantages. Of course, one simple (and often absolutist) principle – which the NHS represents – is often more persuasive and more easily grasped than a more complex and nuanced set of ideas. Even so, we should resist the temptation to offer a set of simple solutions.

Regulation – however structured (for example, providers being enabled to choose between regulatory bodies) – is part of it. We need to make sure that the regulatory process functions so as to reassure people that Government will make appropriate rules, and that these will be independently maintained. Enfolded in this question is the anxiety about how we can ensure that there will be one market in which all are empowered, and that a change will not be the 'thin end of the wedge' for the poor.

One of the important sources of anxiety is that a system which connects individual behaviour with payment might worsen the position of the poor – even if we use tax transfers to significantly 'beef up' individual buying power and guarantee a core package of good services for all. It is essential not only that the structure prevents the wealthy driving the system over time to exclude the poor as an expensive bad risk. And also to persuade people of this, as it is vital to be so robust about this problem that people are convinced that it cannot and will not be allowed to happen. This belief is essential if the psychological shift towards a different system is to occur and to be deliverable politically. And the sums transferred must buy care in a guaranteed package that is at least as good as – and in many respects much better than – that which the NHS offers at present. A free market solution can be fully beneficial to the poor, the unlucky and the disadvantaged. They can come in, out of the margin. It is a moral, a practical, and a philosophical and political question.

Some argue that the poor are marginalised as an expensive bad risk in other areas of insurance. Government must act convincingly to prevent this situation from occurring in healthcare. It must protect the poor more successfully than it has done with the NHS, where they do significantly less well – especially if they are poor and old, poor and female, poor and black, poor and disabled, poor and Scottish, or poor, old, female, black, disabled, gay *and* Scottish.

There should be an independent Patient-Guaranteed Care Commission to ensure that the market is protected, and that it works for all. It must be independent, and not an arm of the executive or of the Department of Health. It must be fully at arm's length from Government. This Commission would be more specific than the Council for Quality of Healthcare that was proposed in the Government's response to the report of the Kennedy Inquiry into heart surgery on children at the Bristol Royal Infirmary, or the subsequent proposals concerning new regulatory bodies.[1]

A Government guarantee may even by itself in some extreme circumstances still be insufficient. If the answer is that Government is the rule maker to guarantee care and access, we need to consider further how *Government itself* can be motivated to sustain the right rules. Here I think we need to ask how can the regulatory process function to reassure people that Government will make appropriate rules and that these will be independently maintained? The only wholly reliable way to ensure that the rules are maintained is for society as a whole to appreciate and articulate dynamist attitudes. Key is the rule of law.

The idea of everyone being in one market – with no two-tier model – was strongly expressed by Canon Samuel Barnett, founder of the East End Settlement Movement, as long ago as the 1880s. For Barnett the answer to poverty and demoralisation was 'the abolition of the space which divides the rich and poor.... Not until the habits of the rich are changed, and they are again content to breathe the same air and walk the same streets as the poor, will East London be saved.'[2]

The chief psychological difficulty causing resistance to change is, I think, concerned with risk aversion. This is a widespread cultural constraint – one of the largest changes in our country since the Victorian era, and one of the massive losses of 'welfarism'. For the Welfare Society has encouraged the idea either that risks are avoidable or that the consequences and costs can be passed to others. We have lost the idea that successful living is about risk, its management and its necessities – that we should expect to make our own decisions.

However, the poor may still believe that a change will be for the worse. And even if this anxiety is not rational, on what basis is it so real to many? If wealth and power coincide, the problem is what will stop the wealthy moving to exclude the poor, in whole or in part, from particular parts of services. In a system which sets up purchasing co-operatives based on individual tax-based funds, price and payment will come more directly into focus. Some people fear this as a consequence.

People do fear change, and for many reasons. Getting older is one of them, and the scariness of the unknown is another. The herd instinct – as a defence against predation – is another. The greater changes in lives that technology (despite all of its benefits) can bring, the uncomfortable shift in cosy routines, and a possible return to old patterns of deprivation. We saw examples of this fear of change with regard to the awful, degrading, inhumane institutions that were occupied by the handicapped and the mentally ill up to the late 1980s and early 1990s. Parents often opposed their closure, in part reasoning that they wished to hold on to what they had, with all of its faults, since a known service might be better than a new one that promised higher quality, but which was to be provided by a local authority which might cut it or close it. The parents' fears were often correct. The individual did not control the personal funds, and thus had no comeback. There is, of course, a natural predisposition to prefer the known to the unknown, especially when knowledge of alternatives has been restricted by a State monopoly for more than 50 years. Lees pointed out the parallel with post-war food rationing. Its abolition was initially unpopular. Food prices rose, and consumers had to make their own choices for the first time in more than a decade. However, the advantages of free choice soon manifested themselves, and today any attempt to reintroduce food rationing would cause riots.[3]

As one earthwork against the fear of change, we ought to be able to rely on social solidarity. But it is a problem that social solidarity is much less well developed in English socio-political culture than it is, for example, in Scandinavia, other western European countries, or further afield – in Canada. We are talking here, of course, about class at the root of the problems. Oddly, the half century of the NHS has undermined social solidarity (which has otherwise been sustained in Europe by social insurance), rather than strengthening it, by encouraging twin markets, twin employers for consultants, and a class-based two-tier system in which consultants have two employers simultaneously, and depend upon unnecessary scarcity as one recruiting sergeant, with clients displaced from the NHS lists by anxiety as well as opportunity. This breaches the moral code.

However, if you want to have some wires and levers, too, in the interim, in order to try to ensure the independence of the Commission, it will have to be funded separately from Government, probably by fees charged to the bodies that it regulates, and not controlled by the Department of Health or another Department of State. It will need to have enforcement powers, by Act of Parliament. Its exercise of its powers will be tested in the courts. Its board will have to be appointed by a separate body, and not within the ambit of the Department of Health itself or the patronage powers of the Prime Minister or the Secretary of State. I envisage an independent Commission, chaired not by 'Lord Mansion House' but by a noted and radical consumer champion, someone like the late Glynn Vernon, with a board of predominantly lay voices – not 'representatives' of vested interests. There will be clinical and other advice on tap. This Commission would have the task of ensuring that Government is unable to change the rules to permit the exclusion of the poor, and that insurers, purchasers and providers must stay up to the mark. It would also be the policeman of the content on the patient-guaranteed care package that I shall discuss below. The sanction of the Commission on Guaranteed Care (one hesitates to add to the regulatory machinery!) would be to de-register – and thus outlaw, and send out of business – any organisation found to be in breach. However, if the Government itself seeks to change the rules by stifling or closing down the Commission, we then face the ultimate of all political problems.

David Lloyd George has said that 'you cannot build navies against nightmares'. The American 'Founding Fathers' considered the problem of so forming a constitution by which to attract wise and discerning rulers, and to keep them virtuous. Virtue in the governing depends on virtues in the people.[4] We have to assume good will and some sense in the situation, backed up by the sanctions of electoral landslides and by the rule of laws, not men, by legislating for the conduct of public life and policy, and by thus seeking to prevent policy from becoming subject to the day-to-day whims of political authorities. The Commission would be a permanent body with the status and independence of the judiciary, and backed up by its presence as a court of appeal to test cases and to redress grievances. Ultimately, however, any Government can change any rules by closing such a body. Fortunately, in an electoral democracy there is always a price to pay for Government doing such things. But we cannot guarantee that a Government which abolishes elections will never appear, although the renovation of mutual-aid, the strengthening of self-responsibility, a dynamist system, the informed consumer, the rule of law and the autonomous independence of the judiciary are the only known (non-military) defence.

This Commission would ensure that access to service by the poor is maintained, once it is in place, and that the poor would enjoy access to improvements as an evolving system made them available. The challenge is to persuade people that this would be so, in order to convince them to support change.

With regard to the question of how different the optics sector is from the rest of healthcare, and to what extent its lessons are applicable or non-applicable, we should notice that for most of us good eye care is a containable cost. But acute and long-term residential and nursing care often is not. For example, consider the cost of spectacles. In the year ended 31 March 2001, spending was as follows: on the least expensive spectacles, £53.24; average spend with the NHS, £41.04; average private spend, £133.16; average spend overall, £119.25.[5] No one person is going to have to spend thousands of pounds a year on drugs, as they might if they had cancer. If people experience serious eye problems, they are referred on to the NHS. For example, if glaucoma is discovered. But if someone develops diabetes, cancer or AIDS, the funding and service challenges look different to most people. These differences must be allowed for, while benefiting from the cultural changes that we see in evidence in the optics market. The answer lies in ensuring that the core package of guaranteed care covers these serious diseases, that it does so with funding provision from the tax base sufficient to offer high-grade services, that there are incentives for private supplementary insurance, and that there is also catastrophe cover for special cases. This is of great political and psychological importance, as random chance has been identified by patients as a frightening concept.[6]

Emergency care would be covered by the patient-guaranteed care package. In addition, the option should remain of adding further personal money – by supplementary insurance or cash in pocket – for lifestyle extras which make life more comfortable but which clinically may not be absolutely 'necessary'. An example might be a state-of-the-art but more costly hip joint, compared with the decent standard offered by a general service. All of this is in fact achieved by the social insurance systems in continental Europe, and we can learn from these about what works, how it works best, and what you should do about the detail. This reassurance is important personally, psychologically and politically. And people must be absolutely convinced that if a new system is brought in they will have this security, and that it will be *maintained* in the future. Without this, the proposals for change will not persuade.

There remains the problem of what is known as 'unwise choice'. The reader who has come with me this far will have formed a view about paternalism, and about 'experts' making our decisions on our behalf. In addition, what may seem irrational choices to some can in fact be quite rational to those who are making them. The problem of the cumulative effects of bad lifestyle choices is a tough one. For example, is the behaviour of what the Victorians called 'the undeserving poor' – those who apparently impose new difficulties on themselves – simply wilful or ignorant? Or do they view this as rational? If we want to encourage what we may prefer as 'rational' behaviour – by incentives and education – we need to consider the extent to which people who smoke, drink and use drugs (or who buy branded trainers for their children but do not feed them properly) are making rational decisions, albeit in difficult circumstances – or believe that they are making rational decisions when or if they reflect on their decisions. This is only in part the old argument that whisky is the quickest way out of (Victorian) Manchester. There may also be differences in class attitudes which feel right to those within the group, but not to those outside it. We need a structure which gives people every opportunity to escape both deprivation and punishment of various kinds, and if they are to do so the acts must make sense in their terms. We may think that the poor suffer from several types of punishment – those that they impose on themselves by certain lifestyle choices, those that a class-biased health system imposes on the disempowered, and the punishment of poverty itself (which has many sources).

Equally, people should have more than one chance of getting it right, and not be condemned to perdition because they get it wrong once. An insurance system of biannual review, with incentives for a programme of improvement (including provision of smoking cessation services, banning smoking in the workplace and in public places – thereby outlawing environmental tobacco smoke) may be one key to incremental and developmental personal change. But I admit that a programme of improvement now seems to be very much a middle-class concept, although such an idea was at the heart of nineteenth-century self-improvement, autodidactism and mutual-aid. This older working-class structure itself must be recovered. And the purchasing co-operatives I urge financially empowered subscribers (poor and rich) to join will themselves be an educative and social force.

There is also the question of the cumulative nature of choices. Here again 'experts' warn us that we should not be allowed to take decisions of whose consequences we do not have a full picture. But then who does? I shall discuss the alleged problems of 'consumer ignorance', consent, capacity and autonomy shortly. Choosing wisely is itself a value judgement. Consumers may indeed have a poor understanding of risk – spending money on mineral water but smoking cigarettes, for example. However, education, preventive care, incentives to self-responsibility, and especially price, can signal risk. Ultimately, self-responsibility means living your own life, but assessing the costs, risks and benefits as you do so.

Notes

1 Bristol Royal Infirmary Inquiry (2001) *Learning from Bristol: the Report of the Public Inquiry into Children's Heart Surgery at the Bristol Royal Infirmary, 1984–1995*. The Stationery Office, London. This made *198* recommendations! See Hobson D (1999) *The National Wealth. Who gets what in Britain?* HarperCollins, London, pp.647–8; and also House of Commons (2002) *Hansard*. **17 January**: col.96; Department of Health (2002) *Learning from Bristol. The Department of Health's response to the Report of the Public Inquiry into Children's Heart Surgery at the Bristol Royal Infirmary, 1984–1995*. Department of Health, London; www.doh.gov.uk/bristolinquiryresponse; Senate of Surgery of Great Britain and Ireland (1998) *Response to the General Medical Council Determination on the Bristol Case*. Senate of Surgery of Great Britain and Ireland, London; Klein R (1998) Regulating the medical profession: doctors and the public interest. In: A Harrison (ed.) *Health Care UK 1997/98*. King's Fund, London (but see my comments on this insufficient analysis in Spiers J (1999) *The Realities of Rationing: 'priority' setting in the NHS*. Institute of Economic Affairs, London, pp.43–5).
2 Cited in Kidd A (1999) *State, Society and the Poor in Nineteenth Century England*. Macmillan, Basingstoke, p.102. See also Briggs A and Macartney A (1984) *Toynbee Hall: the first hundred years*. Routledge, London, p.6.
3 Lees DS (1961) *Health Through Choice. An Economic Study of the English National Health Service*. Institute of Economic Affairs, London, p.34.
4 Cooke JE (1972) *The Federalist*. Middletown, CT, p.384.
5 Federation of Ophthalmic and Dispensing Opticians (FODO) *Optics at a Glance for the Year to 31 March 2001*, op. cit., p.1.
6 Blaxter M (1983) The causes of disease: women talking. *Soc Sci Med.* **17**: 59–69.

Chapter 15

The importance of relationships

The Space Between is the invisible, shared element that lies between any two sides. It contains all we have in common with anyone else. Good or bad, it is the place where sharing being alive happens. Without its recognition, there can only be one-sidedness, selfish ignorance and war. Like the varnish over a painting, a healthy space brings together, bonds and protects the whole picture.

(Dennis Severs)

This structure is not intended to generate a merely instrumental change – that of patients holding money, and unreasonably demanding services with no concern for relationships, others, price or benefit. Nor does it rely on economic theory alone, although it offers this to try to give 'bite' and explanatory meaning to observable experience. It is concerned as much as anything with tone of voice, and with 'the space between' in relationships. I do not wish to emphasise the mechanical at the expense of the spiritual. It is their symbiosis – their concord – which is constructive. For we are concerned both with cultural changes and with what John Stewart Collis called 'the force of life' – the energy and the uniqueness of human consciousness – and its working out in conversation and in relationships with professionals. This concerns each acting with the other in mind, as we consider who does what, how and why, and who takes responsibility for what, why and how.

At the heart of what I hope we can build are good *relationships*. Of course, in relationships with medical professionals, patients should be participants and partners. But ultimately they must be the decision makers in medical and social consultations about their lives. The key point about partnership is not only to recognise that the patient–doctor partnership is pivotal, but that no partnership is real unless the individual has the power to secede from it to another. Both individuals and institutions need to have adequate autonomy. Institutions and their management must have an unrelenting and inevitable responsiveness to consumers' wishes, and the capacity to utilise appropriate freedoms. As the biologist and angler Julian Pepperell says, 'May the fish that get away lure you back again.'[1]

To privilege the patient is not to denigrate the professional, whose intuitions as well as technical expertise will be valued by the patient in considering what course of action to take. Both doctor and patient will wish to blend technical information and humane judgement. Both types of expertise must be valued and developed – the doctor, technically, and with accumulated experience, and the patient, as the expert on their own life within their own skin. As Bryan Lask, Professor of Child and Adolescent Psychiatry at St George's Medical School, London, has said:

> *The time has come for us all to participate in 'concordance' – an agreement reached after discussion between a patient and healthcare professionals that respects the beliefs and wishes of the patient in determining whether, when and how medicines [and other treatments] are to be taken. It is obvious if we want to achieve optimal treatment.*[2]

Good doctors are seeking to build partnerships with patients by means of strategies for care that are consistent with the knowledge, attitude and values of the patient. One of the best examples concerns Parkinson's disease, which also presents many challenges – notably to supporting people, to prevent them losing self-confidence and self-respect, and to the consequent losses of relationships and their way of life. As Mary G Baker, President of the European Parkinson's Disease Association, said in a recent *British Medical Journal* special issue on neurodegenerative disease:

> *Parkinson's disease is an excellent example of the challenges of caring posed by people with neurodegenerative disorders. It is insidious in onset, inexorably progressive, of unknown cause, incurable, yet amenable to management with pharmacological and other interventions. With the ageing of the population, the prevalence of Parkinson's disease is projected to increase in the years ahead.*[3]

What patients want is often not what doctors focus on. Medical professionals do not all understand the expectations of patients and their families, or introduce their perspectives to the framework of scientific practice and evidence-based care. How people are treated (protocols) derives in the main from medical research and not from understanding of the daily burdens in the lives of sufferers. This barrier hinders better outcomes – in terms of coping strategies – and probably hinders the effectiveness of clinical care guidelines. Research concerning these other 'domains of care' (such as levels of optimism and the quality of communication) suggests that most variations in perception of health-related quality of life by patients concerned this issue, and not the severity of the disease or the effectiveness of drug treatment.[4] In other areas, too, outcome measures used by doctors correlate poorly with the patient's perceived benefit from treatments.[5]

As Mary Baker has said:

> *Apart from effecting a cure, maintenance and improvement of the health-related quality of life are the objectives of any treatment programme for neurodegenerative disorders. The message for clinicians from this and other studies is that, contrary to prevailing opinion, a single-minded focus on severity of disease and the effectiveness of drugs will not adequately address the changes in the health-related quality of life expected from encounters between patients and doctors. Undergraduate and postgraduate medical education must provide a broader framework that includes the complexities of factors that are interwoven in their efforts to improve quality of life.*[6]

There is much similar commentary in medical journals concerning patient choice, patient expectations and patients' insights about preferred outcomes (and about informed consent, and resistance to this by doctors). Yet without a major change in healthcare funding and considerable increases in capacity, this is going to be difficult to achieve swiftly. To do it properly will take time, and it cannot be done properly in very brief 10-minute encounters. Patient centredness, patient partnership and patient empowerment are not cheap, quick options. They require time, staffing, money and education,[7] and insufficient funding and incentive contribute to an already conservative attitude of resistance and delay.

The Patient-Guaranteed Care Association (PGCA) which I propose as the purchasing co-operative (developed in the main from primary care trusts) would intrude more urgency, more money and more insistence to improve services, change attitudes, enhance counselling and also require by contract that appropriate staff structures were in place. For example, with regard to treatment of Parkinson's disease, the effectiveness of specialist nurses in general practice has been shown to contribute significantly to preserving patients' sense of well-being, even though health outcomes remain unchanged. Their major role in communication, counselling and education of patients and carers should be the subject of investment and support, in addition to shifting boundaries more so that they can undertake much of the work done by GPs. The PGCA could indeed require this on behalf of its subscribers by specifying this in contracts. It could also encourage patients to visit pharmacists, who are widely trusted and whose skills could be beneficially deployed in addition to their present work. No doubt all of these points are often made in 'consultations' with relevant organisations. But the change needs to be made – with the insistence of a Tony Adams and the accuracy of a Robert Pires. The PGCA would be able to attain these objectives. Greater efficiency would increase resources. It could also lower taxes.

Notes

1 Pepperell J (2001) *Fish Tales. The mystery of the Snapper Bump and other stories from Australian Waters.* Random House, Milson's Point, NSW, p.8.
2 Lask B (2002) Concordance respects beliefs and wishes of patients. *BMJ.* **324**: 4125. See also Downie R and MacNaughton J (2000) *Clinical Judgement. Evidence in practice.* Oxford University Press, Oxford; Ikomi A and Kunde D (2002) Patient values are crucial for good medical decision making. *BMJ.* **324**: 50. See also Marinker M (ed.) (1997) *From Compliance to Concordance: achieving optimal shared goals in medicine taking.* Royal Pharmaceutical Society, London, and Merck, Sharp, Dohme, London; Moscrop A (2001) Expert patients will help manage chronic disease. *BMJ.* **323**: 653.
3 Baker MG (2002) Treating neurodegenerative diseases. *BMJ.* **324**: 1466–7.
4 Baker MG, ibid.
5 For example, Edwards SGM, Playford ED, Hobart JC and Thompson AJ (2002) Comparison of physician outcome measures and patients' perception of benefits of inpatient neuro-rehabilitation. *BMJ.* **324**: 1493.

6 Baker MG, ibid. See also Jarman B, Hurwitz B, Cook A, Bajekal M and Lee A (2002) Effects of community-based nurses specialising in Parkinson's disease on health outcome and costs: a randomised controlled trial. *BMJ.* **324**: 1072–5.

7 Dunn N (2002) Commentary. Patient-centred care: timely, but is it practical? *BMJ.* **324**: 651.

Chapter 16

Money talks, preference walks

Rattle his bones over the stones, he's only a pauper whom nobody knows.

(Thomas Noel)

That the poor, like Thomas Noel's victim, have done least well from the NHS is predictable rather than bizarre. This is the reality concealed by the participatory slogans of 'consultation' with patients. The corrective resides in four words. Money talks, preference walks. Cash compels. Conversation with consumers in a real market concerns what they want. Cash provides security and opportunity.

Cash gives the individual help in the most directly useful way. It empowers the specific individual. It is directed specifically at securing services, individual responsibility, information and choice. It emphasises *personal* responsibility – which is not a bad lesson for managers either. It brings us all into one market for one service. And it can be combined with incentives to help people to help themselves, by topping up if they want to spend further personal income on healthcare. Cash makes explicit the cost borne by the taxpayer. With cost-consciousness and prices, it operates the market. It requires providers to seek revenues. It puts *the* premium on satisfaction. It changes attitudes, behaviours and environments. It makes every detail count. It affects how people are heard, whose voice matters, how people are listened to, and how what they try to say matters as well as the words that they actually use. *It empowers the silent* as well as the vocal. And the elderly, the poor, the ethnic, women, the disabled, the unlucky, the mentally ill and the poor – or those often identified as the victims of discrimination within the NHS. It is directed specifically at securing freedom, individual responsibility and choice.

It is, in short, a much more compelling factor than the general promises of a well-meaning system. As the former King's Fund official Angela Coulter recently noted:

> *Improving responsiveness to patients has been a goal of health policy in the UK for several decades. Until now, most initiatives in this area have failed to change noticeably the everyday experience of most patients in the NHS. The harsh [*but self-induced. JS] *realities of budgetary pressures, staff shortages and other managerial imperatives tend to displace good intentions about informing and involving patients, responding quickly and effectively to patients' needs [*sic] *and wishes [*tick. JS.]*, and ensuring that patients are treated in a dignified and supportive manner.*[1]

The money – it is a notional computer entry, derived from general taxation as an 'NHS credit' – can only be spent on healthcare, not on lottery tickets. However, the individual can secure the required personal, separable, intimate and timely service, instead of merely voting for a political promise. This, too, will help to correct what we know from the social and economic lesson of public intervention – in medicine, in housing, too, and in other subsidised activities – where Government has made things worse which might have been better, and where these interventions have had many unexpected consequences. This change to patient fundholding can accomplish what the limited 'internal market' of the 1990s, and the continued purchaser/provider split, did not achieve, which is to give the individual choices. Political markets empower pressure groups; open markets empower individuals.

The imperative of individually empowered choices will ensure that all of the other 'tools to empower patients' come together, enabling both the individual to be encouraged in self-care and self-responsibility and the services to do much more to meet the wishes of service users. These tools should include the following:

- recognising (and not merely 'recognising', but empowering) patients' expertise, values and preferences
- offering informed choice, not passive consent
- making available research to assist decisions by patients[2]
- investing in public and doctor education with regard to interpreting clinical evidence
- enhancing counselling, support and advocacy
- legally entitling patient ownership of electronic health records
- funding research on patients' experiences, and publishing the results of this
- encouraging openness and accountability with regard to error, but properly identifying it by an independent Medical Inspectorate, which will research medical practice and identify the harm caused by interventions, as well as the benefits in general, and by *specific* practitioners
- ensuring public access to comparative data on quality, outcomes and the individual performance of doctors and clinical teams[3]
- financial empowerment as the first principle of truly voluntary exchange. David Smith (of *The Sunday Times*) reminds us that: 'In his excellent book *The Armchair Economist*, Steven Landsburg writes: "Most of economics can be summarised in four words: People respond to incentives. The rest is commentary".'[4]

Financial empowerment is the first principle of truly voluntary exchange. But for this to be possible there are at least four pre-conditions:

1 Duty respected and undertaken, both by the State and the individual.
2 Voluntary exchange through choice and competition.
3 Dispersal of power.
4 Individual control over a specific personal fund.

First, duty. Let me cite Beveridge just once more here, and then leave him. He said:

> *All three texts [they are quotations which he himself cited] have one thing in common. They are all assertions of duty, either of the community [for Beveridge, its leaders], or of the individual. Emphasis on duty rather than an assertion of rights presents itself as the condition on which alone humanity can resume the progress in civilisation which has been interrupted by two world wars and which remains halted by its consequences.*[5]

Secondly, voluntary exchange. This is only possible when nearly equivalent alternative providers exist. In our contemporary context of NHS reform this means that the capacity must be available to permit contracts to move, so that the individual has the liberty and power to effect this, and so that Government protects the rules of choice and competition to secure it. It will, of course, take time to grow this new capacity. There is also the question of what remains of appropriate institutions in the localities to which power could be devolved, when so many of the initiatives and institutions of 'civil society' have been centralised or dismantled, discouraged and debased. Here a revived structure of the institutions of voluntary, charitable and mutual-aid for co-operation is wanted. The hospice movement is the outstanding example. And such a development can only be prompted by devolved choice in markets. However, there are some encouraging signs of voluntary effort already being made in healthcare, notably by trade unions. These themselves are market responses.

Thirdly, and perhaps this is the most salient point, the sine qua non is the necessity of the dispersal of power – not only into *localities*, but also into individual hands. For democratic choice to be genuine, it must be individual as well as collective. It must be real and individual in every life. And for choices to be respected, they must be genuinely available, To be available, they must be attainable when the individual wishes.

Fourthly, for this to be so, as I have suggested, money is needed – not from the yearnings of avarice, but because it releases the individual from pain and suffering by enabling him or her to secure specific, timely, intimate and personal service. And, as I shall argue in detail shortly, occasional voting does not do the job. There must be economic power in individual hands. Only this can make a reality of the discussion of local action and local power which is apparently offered by 'decentralisation' or 'the new localism'. But what is this practice to be? The issue is not that money without real reform will not work, but that reform is only possible if money changes hands. I do not believe that patients will command specific, personal services by participatory politics alone, and there is no evidence that they can and that they do so. The choice is between money in the hand and the rhetoric of modernisation, as has been well expressed by Labour pollster and strategy adviser Philip Gould:

> *We need to build a participatory democracy in which self-confident citizens are fully engaged in the political process, and in which politicians respect this engagement and use it to fuel change; a democracy that understands the first principle of modern politics – the more empowered the citizen, the more powerful the leader.*[6]

Notes

1 Coulter A (2002) At Bristol: putting patients in the centre. *BMJ.* **324**: 648.
2 Haynes, Devereaux and Guyatt propose the term 'research-enhanced healthcare' instead of 'evidence-based care', for it more easily accepts patient input and decision making. Haynes RB, Devereaux PJ and Guyatt GH (2002) Physicians' and patients' choices in evidence-based practice. *BMJ.* **324**: 1350.
3 Compare with the list in Coulter, op. cit., which (apparently unconsciously) includes the statist idea of the *training* and socialising of patients in shared decision making.
4 Smith D (2003) *Free Lunch. Easily Digestible Economics, Served on a Plate.* Profile Books, London, p.26.
5 Beveridge WH (1948) *Voluntary Action, A Report on methods of Social Advance.* G Allen & Unwin, London, p.14.
6 Gould P (2002) Power to the people. *Spectator.* **18 May**: 23–4.

Chapter 17

'Needs' and 'wants'

*When, therefore, I identify myself with my office or title, I behave as though
I myself were the whole complex of social actors of which that office consists ...
I have made an extraordinary extension of myself and have usurped qualities
which are not in me but outside me. 'L'etat c'est moi' is the motto for such people.*

(CG Jung)

All power is based upon 'need'. This is among its attractions to planners, who
tend to see the unfolding of 'history' as an orderly process, controlled from
above. But there is a fundamental distinction between 'needs' and 'wants'. The
frequent failure to notice this – and, often, in surprising quarters – is at the heart
of much misunderstanding.

First, we meet the experts. Experts, planners and healthcare officials do not
exist in a world entirely of their own. They are (complainingly) subject to politicised
or governmental pressure. This they resist, appealing defensively from their
'independence', their technical character and their accumulated 'expertise'. They
struggle to be seen as the consumer's champion (recognising 'needs', especially
'unmet needs'), rather than as just another part of Government bureaucracy,
overly dominated by the Department of Health. However, they are a professional
class with its own interests, as Friedman, Yeo, and the Virginia School of Economists
(studying 'the economics of politics') have each shown. It is a realisation, too,
that was reached at the end of the nineteenth century by working-class critics of
Fabianism. For example, Belfort Bax, a collaborator of William Morris, wrote in
1901 – criticising Beatrice Webb – that 'Fabianism is the special movement of
the government official, just as militarism is the special movement of the soldier
and clericalism of the priest'.[1]

A more strongly put contemporary statement, in Marxist 'class' terms and
from the harder left, comes from Mike Hales, in his *Living Thinkwork* (1980):
'For the working class the Professional Managerial Class holds a threat; the
systematic undermining of conditions of autonomous working-class practice;
sabotage of working-class cultures, even identity.'[2]

Here, Hales is challenging *both* the state (as the 'agency' of the working class)
and the replacement by a professional class of administrators of working-class
self-organisation and mutual-aid, a substitution led by 'the Party' (in this case, the
Labour Party). And we should notice that as Alan Milburn seeks to appeal to
older traditions of co-operation, he too will find that he is confronted both by
the State machinery and by the professional managers as an elite in their own
right.

Mr Gordon Brown, by contrast to Mr Milburn, is a centraliser in the tradition of the socialist elitism of Sidney Webb, which relies on 'needs analysis', or expertise from above, rather than a consumer focus, or expertise from within the life of the user of services. Webb represented what the Marxist Bakunin referred to as 'the direct command of state engineers who will constitute a new privileged scientific–political class'.[3] We seek instead reform in an older, working-class tradition of mutual-aid and co-operative solidarity – of collective action without collectiv*ism*. One which trusts individual decision-making.

There has long been tension within working-class movements between working-class self-activity (in co-operative action and mutual-aid) and reform from above, even when that is itself led by an organisation like the Labour Party, which Yeo, Hales and others have seen as disabling the imperatives of working-class self-organisation. Here lies a fundamental fissure along which we have to decide upon the true source of discovering individual preference, and the location of satisfactions. Are we to place our trust in our own instincts about our own lives, or in the judgement of others made on our behalf? It will be seen that this concerns not only results, but also the nature, the character and the presence of choice and of self-ownership. It is an example of the 'problem of agency', and of the large space to be occupied either by the individual or by his or her 'representative'.

The planner has several different problems concerning relationships, position and social prestige – first in relating to the service user, and in seeking to deter the alternative organisation of consumers' interests (for example, in co-operation and/or in private purchasing), and secondly, in relation to Government and its interests. It seeks to ensure that these all coincide, but the nature of knowledge makes this an impossibility. The planner must tussle with the irreconcilable and conceptual contrast between 'internal' views of health and of care (derived from the patient's own perceptions and beliefs) and 'external' views (based on the so-called 'objective' evidence), from both a professionalised and a planning perspective.

The job is made more complex by the political requirements of governments that are seeking re-election. And as the economist Dr Irwin M Stelzer says, '[We may have] governments of laws, not men, but the way the laws are administered (and, indeed, drafted) by men will determine the balance drawn between regulation and competition as protectors of consumer interests.'[4] And 'There are a great many able and honourable men and women who sincerely believe that they can protect consumers better than can an unregulated marketplace. They see market imperfections under every bed, and do not believe that imperfectly but nevertheless effectively competitive markets can do a good job of balancing the interests of consumers, producers and investors.'[5] By contrast, both voluntary co-operation and markets ensure a choice both of price – the message which tells providers whether the public wants more or less of a service – and quality, above a moral minimum.

Meanwhile, the health system, managed by professionals and statist experts, still generally confiscates power from the individual. It often undermines them psychologically. And it still does not know very much about what it achieves in terms of outcomes, save on the aggregate where the message itself is discouraging. This, despite the significant new investment in measurement, regulation and assessment.

Secondly, we meet the service users. Here the patient has begun (reluctantly) to be considered as a customer, or continues as the fortunate recipient of services provided by those who know. But there is still no power of sanction or direct incentive controlled by the individual. The private professional world also remains self-regulated and is still unaccountable to ordinary people. This may be unavoidable to some extent in political and social reality. However, this is all the more reason for passing power which people *can* understand – cash and personal choice, supported by information, by other patients, by advocacy services and by the voluntary sector – back into their control. This is especially so with regard to the ethical vision of the NHS which, despite its deficits in practice, people still hold in their minds and imagination as one definition of what it is to be British in a world of constant change. And that the actions of all managers and professionals should be given definition in terms of the patient's wants and values is less exceptionable than it was in the early 1990s. Yet, it is an imperative that is still not fully backed by cash (the patient fundholder, or voucher) on the nail. And for the patient there is still no visible link between care and costs, between investment and outcome, and between personal behaviour and consequences. The fundamentals of price signals, opportunity cost, risk and benefit, cost and outcome remain submerged.

Fundamental to the evolution of a structure which puts the patient's view and preference at the centre is an awareness of the necessary devices which genuinely give people sanctions. As, too, is cognisance of the alternatives to the often harmful medicalisation of our lives. For this leads away from self-reliance to a pathological society, to expansionist 'needs analysis', to enlarged power by the few over the many, and to the leadership of 'experts' who plan on our behalf and then 'consult' with us in the margins. This 'consultation' project, to make the NHS patient-centred, is regrettably still the man on horseback. It is directed by 'needs-led' stasist planners and medical authorities ('experts' who know our interests best). These seek to intrude their own concepts of 'normality' and 'health' – what Illich called 'medical imperialism' and what Skrabanek calls 'lifestylism' – upon our entire 'physical, mental and social well-being'.[6]

The truest trust is in our own instincts about our own lives. And this asks us to think about 'wants', which we decide, balance and consider in terms of cost–benefit, risk and outcome. Here we decide between what we understand that we must do and what we feel we want to do. We make the trade-offs. This, as opposed to 'needs', which other 'experts' decide on our behalf and 'in our interest'. 'Needs' are driven by the expansionist biomedical model. This is a permanent outreach project, into every corner of our lives. 'Wants' are the patient's own account of the 'real' problem, and their consideration necessarily implies cost-consciousness. Without this, indeed, we are lost. 'Wants' is a multifactorial construct of psychological and social determinants, which are often of more consequence – both to the diagnosis and to the solution – than any biomedical factors. They should still be considered by the individual in a framework of opportunity cost. The patient's decision is also as likely to be right, in responding to what they know of themselves.[7] Remember, too, the words of one clinical commentator, LD Willard, who wrote 'of the "results of prejudice, preference, professional blindness, failure of moral nerve, and conditioning which parade as the grand and obvious discoveries of objective scientific method." In making many judgements, patients are as likely to be right as professionals'.[8]

The health system still generally confiscates power from the individual, often undermines them psychologically, and does not know very much about what it achieves in terms of outcomes. This is despite the significant new investment in measurement, regulation and assessment. And it is despite the movement towards 'concordance' between professionals and patients, to seek balance, harmony, even a compound intelligence, to push two defined sides together to stand as one. This state of regulated harmony – just right – is an ideal, but there still remains the ultimate question, in Leigh Richardson's phrase: 'Who decides who decides?'[9] And how does it *stay decided*? Here Dennis Severs helps us again: 'And – oh – what a touchy subject is taste! *What is "just right"? Where does it begin? Where does it end?* And that question that anyone who is unsure of themselves has to ask: *"Who says so?"'*[10]

This distinction between 'needs' and 'wants' helps us to appreciate the importance of autonomy, choice, and competition. And its impact on securing modern, integrated services. The language of 'needs' contradicts and obstructs these fundamentals. 'Needs' have been falsely contrasted with 'ability to pay'. But if services continue to be tax-funded it is time to empower self-responsible 'wants'.

As we consider the shape of services, the requirement expressed by many patients is to shift care into community settings, to increase local influences on local services and to empower the user, with the individual being seen as the most local of all locales. 'Wants' has many dimensions in seeking for the individual to receive the highest quality of *individual* care, in harmony with their values and preferences. This challenge engages each of us with self-management of care, with support from services in the local community setting, notably in one's own home, with the awareness of what the individual can do to prevent disease, and with mutual-aid, co-operation and learning to choose, using the mind, *to think*.

Here, I believe, there is no conflict between the first principles I have identified and the ten core commitments spelled out in *The NHS Plan*, save that the plan speaks of 'needs' rather than 'wants'. These commitments are a universal service based on 'need', a comprehensive range of services shaped around patients' 'needs', responsiveness to the 'needs' of different populations, continuous improvement of services, support for staff, public funds devoted to NHS patients, co-operation with others, work to reduce health inequalities, and open access to information about services and treatments.[11] These commitments and principles are the foundations of successful voluntary exchange, competitive provision and individual choice. 'Wants' are, too, I suggest, more likely to be achieved through competition than through control from above. And the most important contemporary responsibility in politics is to ensure that everyone, rich or poor, comes into one market, with all the powers of choice in networks enjoyed by the middle class. It is to this conversation that this argument is addressed. The argument is that by giving consumers a wide range of choices *and* by empowering them to select from among those choices, competition leads *both* to the desirable goal of greater efficiency in satisfying customers' wishes *and* to social solidarity. And that giving choices to consumers is itself an important *social* goal of competition, for this and other reasons. It directly corrects the defects of the centralised system. But its justification is not in the main instrumental, for this is a by-product of the greater good of a free society. It is a moral problem, focused on 'wants'.

The general argument is that competition combines many benefits. It tends towards greater material equality, and it promotes freedom. It is more efficient than monopoly (public or private) and more socially desirable than central control or private domination. The burden of proof lies on the shoulders of those who wish to argue that monopoly is more beneficial. This case, as we have seen, is usually pressed on ethical and political grounds (fairness, equality, etc.), and I suggest that in UK healthcare it is contradicted by its practical results. Here the middle class – who are capable of providing more for themselves – compete for a restricted pool of services with the poor, who are unable to provide for themselves and who compete less successfully. In summary, if we prefer 'wants' to 'needs' the ultimate protection for consumers lies in choice. Here I believe that competition and the benefits of mutual-aid and co-operation in working-class self-organisation can be combined, in the Patient Guaranteed Care Association. If Government gets the right rules in place to produce effective market competition revolving around individual choice, it is then quite unnecessary to evolve simultaneously a complex and costly bureaucratic regulatory structure concerned with prices, resource allocation and 'fairness'. For to do so encourages the idea that consumers should continue to *look to Government* for protection, rather than to their own knowledge, skills and co-operative and mutual-aid endeavours, and to the preservation of competitive markets. It is hard cash which does most to protect choices, and it is competition which secures these, with quality services at fair prices. It, too, offers the economic incentives to competing providers, to entrepreneurs and risk-takers who must secure revenues from willing consumers and offer services in the most efficient way – minimising costs, maximising access, dealing with over-manning, raising productivity, maximising the rate of innovation, and doing without what the economist JR Hicks noticed as the greatest profit from monopoly, namely 'a quiet life'.[12]

Earlier I cited the words which Lord Beveridge quoted on the first page of his *Voluntary Action*: 'Before it is just to say that a man ought to be an independent labourer, the country ought to be in such a state that a labourer by honest industry can become independent.' They were the words of his own grandfather, William Akroyd of Stourbridge, a descendant of another of the same name, from Marston in Yorkshire, and himself the founder in 1518 of the provision of university scholarships 'to the end of the world'.[13]

The touchstone test – of individual self-responsibility and the power to be self-responsible – is revealed (without any need for further refinement) in Akroyd's words. It concerns the separation of ownership and control, or of self-ownership and self-responsibility. It is by Akroyd's words that any proposal for decentralisation or 'consultation' or any other substitutes for consumer choice should be tested. My argument is that all other substitutes are political kites. They will remain insufficient because they are evasions. So, too, are such substitutes for individual responsibility (although offered as half-way houses) as private–public partnerships and limited contracting out of services to the private sector. For none of these, nor decentralisation, will reduce the range of issues *that will still be decided by political means*, or minimise the extent to which Government (national or regional) retains the power of choice for itself. Substitutes will not correct over-government and the imperfections of 'Government failure'. And while economic power remains joined to political power in healthcare, then the actual decentralisation of control and the necessary prompts to spontaneous order are beyond our reach.

Normative control over patients – 'needs'-led analysis, 'expert' dominion and limited reform from above – takes us in the wrong direction. Surveillance of populations and the purchasing for populations in bulk does so, too. The medicalisation of our lives has the same roots, and with the same negative effects. The attempt to discover every 'unmet need', to intrude upon everything which experts regard as abnormal and worthy of medicalisation, is at odds with autonomous choice and with self-responsible living. The boundaries of 'unmet need' inevitably move incessantly, for this is an imperial project, if underpinned by a detailed critique of 'late capitalism'.[14] The emphasis on 'needs' offers, too, compelling incentives for organised groups to compete in order to establish their own 'needs'. This, rather than offering incentives to encourage people to take responsibility for themselves and on their own account. Worse still, this is a 'beggar-my-neighbour' structure in an NHS that is organised to ration care, for it asks one group to pursue limited funds at the expense of another. Further, it offers no incentive to the individual to consider opportunity cost, nor is there any measure of capacity to benefit. And as Dr Robert Lefever has said:

> Perceived needs become relative rather than absolute. Meeting a need does not satisfy: it merely shifts attention to another need. Instead of the individual patient not being able to afford treatment, the State runs out of money so that either the individual cannot get treatment at all or, alternatively, the treatment that he or she can get is not worth having.[15]

More activist politics, more 'consultation' and 'user involvement' – as if patients were not already involved – is no solution. And it has not worked (which is unsurprising, since it can only appeal to activists), as a recent report, *Every Voice Counts*, by the King's Fund (which very much wants it to work) has shown.[16] The publication's title and intrinsic message in fact contradict its own conclusions. Even when some information was gathered, from user groups and active interests, most NHS organisations did not know how to feed this information back into the corporate process. This itself, too, is unsurprising, for there have never been any incentives to do so, unlike with businesses, which go bust if they don't do it pronto. The real issue is not to rely on politicians but on ourselves. And to evolve healthcare organisations which expect us to do so, and who seek our business. We must encourage politicians to stand aside, save to represent the interests of consumers by protecting choice, competition and a core package of what I call *pretty good care* (or *patient-guaranteed care*) – which ophthalmology clearly now delivers in a new environment. A good society must be able to translate its ideals into practice. Further, people must be able to believe that the gap between ideal and reality can be narrowed if cynicism is not to prevail.

'Experts' (most extremely, in the World Health Organization definition of the scope of 'health' as being 'not merely the absence of disease or infirmity, but a state of complete physical, mental and social well-being') have undertaken widespread surveillance of the population. They have identified 'needs' (many of them 'unmet', in the utopian biomedical gaze), remapped illness and its definition, problemised normality and 'redrawn the relationship between symptom, sign and illness, and the localisation of illness outside the corporal space of the body'. The effects of medicalisation of non-medical problems include undermining the ability of the individual to resolve these problems for themselves, by managing their own resources, their time and the boundaries in their lives. This 'expert' stasist mentality has spread out beyond places like the King's Fund, where it is institutionalised, into an attempted suzerainty over many non-medical aspects of our lives.[17]

The proclaimed concern with patient 'needs' is formulated around a model of the 'expert knowing best' – there is no genuine stretching out to understand *individual preferences* and to empower them. The NHS still buys in bulk, and for 'populations'. However, there is a conjunction between moral imperatives, an actual social agency and specific devices for individual empowerment. It is this unity which by its very nature can carry us forward to a new social order. If we want to rely on choice as the instrument of change, to move away both from the biomedical model and from the triple monopoly of the State as funder, purchaser and provider, we should sharply distinguish between 'needs' and 'wants'. This is not linguistic Lollardry. It is focal to the issues.

Notes

1 Cited by Yeo, Levy (ed.) (1987) *Socialism and the Intelligensia 1880–1914*. Routledge & Kegan Paul, London, p.225, from an article by B Bax in *Justice*, 9 March 1901.

2 Hales M (1980) *Living Thinkwork. Where do labour processes come from?* CSE Books, London, p.110. I owe the reference to Yeo, in Levy (ed.), op. cit., p.226.

3 Cited by Yeo, in Levy (ed.), op. cit., p.220.

4 Stelzer IM (2001) *Lectures on Regulatory and Competition Policy*. Institute of Economic Affairs, London, p.16.

5 Stelzer, IM, ibid., pp.17–18. Also see Stelzer IM and Shenefield J (1998) *The Antitrust Laws. A primer*. AEI Press, Washington, DC.

6 Illich I (1976) *Medical Nemesis: the expropriation of health*. Marion Boyars, London, revised as *Limits to Medicine*. Marion Boyars, London. Skrabanek P (1994) *The Death of Humane Medicine*. Social Affairs Unit, London.

7 See, for example, Birrell I (2002) Set us free to pay. *Spectator*. **11 May**: 26–7, which contains an account of discussion of treatment for his daughter, who suffers complex epilepsy that has left her blind and unable to walk or talk.

8 Willard LD (1982) Needs and medicine. *J Med Philos*. 7: 259–73. Andre J (1991) Learning to see: moral growth during medical training. *J Med Ethics*. **18**: 148–52.

Also Lettwin SR (1992) *The Anatomy of Thatcherism*. Fontana, London, p.204. And see the following commentaries by Dr W Pickering: Medical omniscience. *BMJ*. 1998; **317**: 19–26; Does medical treatment mean patient benefit? *Lancet*. 1996; **347**: 379–80; A nation of people called patients. *J Med Ethics*. 1991; **17**: 91–2; Patient satisfaction: an imperfect measurement of quality medicine? *J Med Ethics*. 1993; **19**: 121–2. Alas, 'needs' is found used instead of 'wants' (and apparently as an equivalent) in the most surprising places. See, for example, Independent Healthcare Association, *Caring into the Future*, op. cit., passim. Even Misselbrook, op. cit., falls into this trap. See, for example, op. cit., p.vii. Yeo, although a people's advocate, also makes the same error. See Yeo, in Corrigan (ed.) op. cit., p.112.

9 Richardson L (1997) *Promoting Patient Participation in Portsmouth*. MBA Consultancy Project, Ashridge Management College, Ashridge.

10 Severs D (2001) *18 Folgate Street, The Tale of a House in Spitalfields*. Chatto & Windus, London, p.140.

11 Secretary of State for Health (2000) *The NHS Plan: a plan for reform*. Stationery Office, London. Audit Commission (2002) *Data Remember. Improving the Quality of Patient-Based Information in the NHS*. Audit Commission, London.

12 Hicks JR (1939) *Value and Capital*. Clarendon Press, Oxford.

13 Akroyd W, at a dinner of Poor Law Guardians of Stourbridge, April 1841, quoted by Beveridge WH (1948) in *Voluntary Action, A Report on Methods of Social Advance*. G Allen & Unwin, London, p.7.

14 For this approach see, for example, Barnes C (1996) Foreword. In: J Campbell and M Oliver (eds) *Disability Politics. Understanding our past, changing our future*. Routledge, London. The new Patient Forums are expected to pursue the search for 'unmet need', too. See Eames L (2002) In on the Act. *NHS Magazine*. **September issue**: 128–9, and comment by R Lefever, op. cit.

15 Lefever R (2002) The philosophy of the National Health Service is wrong. Unpublished paper.

16 Anderson W, Florin D, Gillan S, Mountford LA (2002) *Every Voice Counts: primary care organisations and public involvement*. King's Fund, London. The report's conclusions directly contradict its own title.

17 King's Fund (2002) *The Future of the NHS. A framework for debate. Discussion paper*. King's Fund, London. See also my discussion in *Coming, Ready or Not!* (2002) Edward Everett Root, Brighton.

Chapter 18

Incentives to change: in whose interest?

The problem is doctors – paid enormously for private work and a pittance by the NHS for the same work. No other professional group has such a huge incentive to maintain the status quo. And it will be tricky to persuade the voter, too. They are fine about all this until someone asks them to actually pay for healthcare. There is then stony silence. True choice means that you can choose to spend your money on other things, like cellphones, drinking, white goods, and holidays in Ibiza. That's what people will do if you give them choice. Look how tricky it is to get people to put money aside for pensions – it's boring, and we all know we are being ripped off by intermediaries.

(A senior NHS surgeon)

These are the words of a very senior doctor, internationally known in his field. He wrote them to me in a private letter in June 2002. No government will improve health services unless those working there are persuaded that changes are in their best interests. However, we can expect orchestrated opposition to change from doctor organisations, in their own interests. The history of such opposition is well known. The issue of incentives – for doctors and for consumers – remains a serious difficulty. So, too, does political leadership.

First, reward. Doctors are poorly paid within the NHS. And Professor Julian Le Grand has pointed out that the system of rewarding NHS consultants is perverse, arising from the respective payment systems for private and public practice. In the private sector, consultants are paid by fee for service, according to the work that they do. In the public sector they get a salary:

Hence, when faced with patients needing operations who have the means to go private, the incentive is always to encourage him or her to do so; for the consultant will then get paid for the extra work. It is no coincidence that the longest NHS waiting lists are in those specialities where consultants have the highest private earnings. Nor is it surprising that in recent years consultant productivity in the NHS has been falling.[1]

The usual solutions are to ban private work, or to pay consultants on a fee-for-service basis, or (Professor Le Grand does not mention this on this particular occasion, although he has previously favoured the idea of the weighted voucher) to introduce patient fundholding for all, with us all in one market. For then the inducement to go private would vanish.[2] It is striking that there is no private market (and no waiting list) in Europe in social insurance systems, for no one thinks there is any need for this. No one is ever asked the question commonly put to patients by many UK consultants, 'Do you have insurance?', because in Europe the bewildered reply would be 'Of course. Social insurance, with the State. Doesn't everybody?'

Second, quality (and morale). A northern GP wrote to me in June 2002:

> *I look at medicine from the bottom up rather than from the top down. Did it work? I am of the view that a break has to be put on demand. It is currently unreasonable. Patients must pay, one way or another, to force them to think. The top-down approach has given us patchy service, with staff who largely hate their lot. The top-down has also given us a medical modus operandi which dissuades initiative. It dissuades efficacy, too: if the herd do it, it is right, and, besides, I still get paid. This is all typical of bureaucracies, of course.*[3]

I have proposed a market-led structure in which we will see responsible personal choice among competing providers who can only secure incomes by seeking subscriptions from consumers with a free choice, and who can only retain their loyalty by satisfying them. This is not in itself original. Professor Alain C Enthoven, for example, has led the way in developing and arguing for these understandings in our approach to healthcare reform, and in seeking practical steps towards change.[4]

Direct incentives – together with national support for Government to insist on change – are essential. If we seek to reward the efficient, encourage the patient centred, improve quality, curtail cost, introduce price sensitivity and move away from the wholesale medicalisation of our lives – which we must if we want the healthcare system to survive – we need to set in place the motivating forces which enable the right kind of purchaser to succeed. Many initiatives for change have run aground on the rocks of the medical establishment, which has been able to set new ideas aside and refuse to co-operate with change. As an article in *The Times* reported recently:

> *Some hospital managers accuse consultants of operating 'cartels' enabling them to control the prices they charge and ensure a plentiful supply of patients prepared to pay to go private, an arrangement that would be destroyed by the introduction of rival colleagues from abroad [under the International Fellowship Scheme led by Sir Magdi Yacoub].... [And] this was a scheme in which Mr Blair had invested a great deal of political capital and Whitehall officials are understood to regard the collapse [of the scheme] as the latest example of consultants protecting their interests at the expense of patients.*
>
> *The Office of Fair Trading made a series of dawn raids in recent weeks on consultant anaesthetists in Oxford, Reading and Wales after complaints that some were acting as a cartel to force up prices for private practice by limiting their NHS work. Ministers are understood to be studying academic evidence that the more consultants there are, the less work they do. This research, by Professor John Yates of Birmingham University, suggests that there has been a significant decrease in surgeon productivity, and Professor Alan Maynard of York University has said 'There probably are cartels operating in some areas ... the medical profession has a great deal of power'.*[5]

Vested interests (and policies of naked power) have been enthroned within the NHS since its creation. To get the NHS up and running, Aneurin Bevan found that he had to allay opposition from doctors by placing control of the service in the hands of consultants, who were also allowed two employers at the same time – the State and the private sector.[6]

Two things will encourage professionals to consider that change is in their interests, namely greater trust in their professionalism, and direct economic incentives. Together these can improve quality (including access and the experience of care), achieve fundamental restructuring in the delivery of care and achieve value for money. Crucially, every individual must have effective financial leverage, and the opportunity to make responsible choices. And at the same time be sensitive to costs. This requires incentives to encourage individuals to take care of themselves, and to consider the consequences of their behaviour. The problems of managing doctors are, in an important sense, an aspect of the less-discussed issues of 'Government failure' – which we have to set in the balance with the well-discussed issues of 'market failure'.

Enthoven, reflecting on several decades of seeking this in two continents, recently said:

> *Markets for health insurance and health care services are beset by the well-known causes of market failure – uncertainty, moral hazard, adverse selection, asymmetry of information, plus the implications of a moral judgement that nobody should go without needed medical care for lack of ability to pay. This makes creation of a market in health care that drives improvement a particularly complex undertaking. The details are important and must be got right. Not any thing that sounds like 'competition' or 'markets' or 'private sector' will necessarily improve economic performance.*[7]

This must be right, although market failure must be set alongside Government failure – exemplified by the NHS – and this is much more difficult to correct. There is of course such a thing as market failure, although it is more easily and swiftly corrected by markets themselves than is Government failure (and the unintended consequences of Government action), which is embedded in a context of vested interest and inertia. In markets we rapidly learn by our mistakes.[8]

One of the difficulties is the 'un-obviousness' of the obvious. And as TS Eliot said, 'Humankind cannot bear very much reality'. But we will not get good answers unless we ask the right questions. One of the most important is the issue of how doctors can and will change. We must resolve this issue, if we are to get to the basic problem of introducing markets. For the fundamental question concerning resources is how to co-ordinate the activities of large numbers of people, to allocate and make best use of scarce capital and resources, to give consumers what they want at acceptable prices, and to maximise welfare by ensuring that all can benefit from opportunities in healthcare. This is not only an economic question about how to deliver efficiencies most effectively. It is also a question about relationships, as well as a moral and a social question. It is about how to attain social and political ideals – such as voluntary exchange, uncoerced co-operation, the diffusion of both public and private power, social solidarity and protection of the poor and unlucky, and the maximum opportunity for self-responsibility and self-expression for living our own lives without breaking into unbridled selfishness. This, too, is about promoting a *social* system which is fair and equitable, which is perceived to be so, which can coincide with *economic* efficiencies, and in which patients *and* doctors respond to incentives.

Incentives are vital if we are to persuade people to do things which they do not believe are in their interests, at least in the short term. I remain of the view (which I have argued from 1991, and which is explored in my books *The Invisible Hospital and The Secret Garden* and *Who Owns Our Bodies?*) that everything should start with the patient and focus on what happens to patients. That we should assume that we can all act in our own best interests. And that it is the individual (often confused, often maddening, and often apparently perverse) who can best define and give weight to these, as we balance other choices, risks, costs and benefits.

When I challenged medical practice, outcomes and the Kafkaesque institutions of the NHS in the early 1990s, it was easier for people to say that we should leave all of these questions 'to the professionals – *they* know'. This was before Bristol (where 29 babies died between 1988 and 1995), before Alder Hey and the body parts scandal, before the case of gynaecologist Roderick Ledward, before the loss of confidence in the General Medical Council, and before the dreadful revelations about the GP Dr Harold Shipman, who killed a large number of elderly people (where the system for issuing death certificates and other fail-safe controls failed to reveal the truth or to provide effective safeguards against a determined killer within the medical profession). The Shipman Enquiry heard in December 2002 that the structure 'in place at the time did not permit criticism to be made without a backlash'. Some still insist that these were isolated examples, and that they could not happen again. One hopes so. But no one really knows.[9] And no one is looking in the necessary ways to identify error, as Dr William Pickering has pointed out in his persistent call for an independent Medical Inspectorate. This is certainly needed, as is an improvement in the morale of doctors. The two objectives are not contradictory but complementary. And, indeed, as Terence says, 'Nothing is so difficult as to be beyond the reach of investigation (*Nil tam difficile est quin quarendo investigari possit*).' Few things now unknown to us remain a mystery for ever.

There is, too, the question of the quality of *clinical* practice, in the services regulated by the National Care Standards Commission, and in the wider NHS context itself where, I fear, this remains uninvestigated in our society – despite the cases of Bristol, Alder Hey, Dr Roderick Ledwood and the scandals of gynaecology, and the long-overlooked (and hardly overseen) career of Dr Harold Shipman. There are up to 850 000 adverse events in hospitals every year.[10] No one knows how many there are in primary and community care, including long-term elderly care and other areas regulated by the NCSC. However, Labour MP Laura Moffatt, a State Registered Nurse prior to her election in 1997, told the House of Commons during its care homes debate in July 2002 that there were too many admissions to the acute sector 'from older people who have not had their medicines reviewed for a long time'.[11] We know little of the general quality of medical care or of nutrition in care homes. The necessities of incentives for practitioners to change are obvious.

'Governance' is no answer in itself, for it generalises the challenge and side-steps the necessity to scrutinise *individual* practice. Clinical accountability should be about someone else looking at your practice routinely, and remarking upon it, especially with regard to errors. However, communication by itself is not a panacea. Dr Shipman and the Bristol surgeons were good communicators. As the medical negligence expert Dr William Pickering has written in the *British Medical Journal*:

> The multiplicity of recommendations of the non-medical reporting of the performance failures of the heart surgeons at Bristol Royal Infirmary prompts [some to] repeat the slogan 'put patients at the centre'. The primary issue – that of poor clinical practice going unchecked – has again been obfuscated. The failure of clinical self-regulation caused the serial disasters at Bristol; smothering this uncomfortable truth risks its remedy.[12]

Dr Pickering has consistently urged the foundation of an *independent* Medical Inspectorate. Re-accreditation and revalidation are themselves necessary but not sufficient. An Inspectorate of the kind Dr Pickering has urged is, I believe, an initiative that doctors should support, endorse and campaign to see made real. It is directly relevant to the remit concerning standards. Currently there is no means available to prevent medical errors from being repeated, and from remaining undiscovered until it is too late. For all serial disasters begin with one occasion, and the one occasion in itself is a disaster for the individual concerned. An emphasis on openness, or on patients at the centre, does not address this deficit. Nor does an emphasis on improved communications itself do the job. As Dr Pickering says:

> Many cases of bad clinical practice have shown that the offender was actually a skilful (or wily) communicator. Patients will tolerate a doctor's social inadequacy or even poor outcome if they believe that reasonable professional competence prevails and clinical rudiments are not neglected. Their only assurance would be a strong system of clinical accountability for all doctors.[13]

Dr Pickering recommends that copies of all complaints and their written medical responses should be seen by an independent medical inspector who, when necessary, would examine the medical records. The resulting increased attention by doctors would make them clinically accountable. It would also 'simultaneously solve the unfashionable issue of patient accountability. Poor medicine, the expense of litigation and the cost of patients' unrealistic expectations would all decline.'[14] This in itself is an incentive for doctors.

As I urged in the Introduction to this book, we need to catch people doing things right, as well as catch people doing things wrong. Good doctors must be properly rewarded, whereas they are poorly rewarded in the NHS. Good doctors must be enabled to do medicine, and not be social cogs in everyone else's Ferris wheel. Good doctors create something in their own right, which is good care and faith in care itself. Yet if this goes unrecognised, good people will remain poorly motivated and patients will feel stranded. Yet it is necessary to ensure that those with such power over others – a prime motive, in my experience at Brighton, for some individuals becoming hospital consultants – are appropriately inspected and accountable, as Dr Pickering has proposed.[15]

This realisation is not in conflict with the fact that patients, too, are not rational desiccating calculators. There is a deep need for mystery, romance, spirituality and faith. Reason alone cannot allow for this, or see or empower it. Further, as a new study in the *New England Journal of Medicine* recently suggested, it works.[14] Equally, however, as Macneile Dixon says, 'Of what value is any attempt to explain the world till you have faced the facts of the world?'[16] Progress in good part relies on incentives for the professions to change.[17]

Notes

1 Le Grand J (2002) New contracts for NHS consultants. *The Times.* **17 June**: 19.
2 Le Grand J (1989) Markets, welfare and equality. In: J Le Grand and S Estrin (eds) *Market Socialism.* Oxford University Press, Oxford.
3 Personal communication, 7 June 2002.
4 Enthoven AC (1978) Consumer choice health plan. *NEJM.* **298**: 650–58, 709–20. Enthoven AC (1991) History and principles of managed competition. *Health Affairs.* **12 Supplement**, 24–8. Enthoven AC (1988) *Theory and Practice of Managed Competition in Health Care Finance.* North Holland, Amsterdam. Enthoven AC and Singer SJ (1994) The Clinton Health Plan. A single-payer system in Jackson Hole clothing. *Health Affairs.* **Spring issue**: 81–95. Enthoven AC (1994) Why not the Clinton health plan? *Inquiry.* **32**: 129–35. Enthoven AC (1993) Why managed care has failed to contain health costs. *Health Affairs.* **12**: 27–43. Enthoven AC (1985) *Reflections on the Management of the National Health Service: an American looks at incentives to efficiency in health service management in the UK.* Nuffield Provincial Hospitals Trust, London. Enthoven AC (1999) *In Pursuit of an Improving National Health Service.* The Nuffield Trust, London. Enthoven AC (2000) In pursuit of an improving NHS. *Health Affairs.* **19**: 102–9. Enthoven AC (2002) Commentary: competition made them do it. *BMJ.* **324**: 143. Enthoven AC, Schauffler HH and McMenamin S (2001) Consumer choice and the managed care backlash. *Am J Law Med.* **27**: 1–15. Enthoven AC (2002) *Health Plan.* Beard Books, Washington, DC. On Health management organisations, see also McLachlan G and Maynard A (1993) *The Public/Private Mix for Health.* Nuffield Provincial Hospitals Trust, London.
5 Baldwin T and Miles A (2002) Blair initiative runs aground on rock of medical establishment. *The Times.* **13 June**: 13. Also see Yates J (1995) *Private Eye, Heart and Hip. Surgical consultants, the National Health Service and private medicine.* Churchill Livingstone, London.
6 Timmins N (2001) *The Five Giants. A Biography of the Welfare State.* Harper Collins, London. Revised edition.
7 Enthoven A (2002) Introducing market forces into healthcare: a tale of two countries. Paper delivered to 4th European Conference on health economics, Paris, 10 July.
8 See Seldon A (1998) *The Dilemma of Democracy, The Political Economics of Over-Government.* Institute of Economic Affairs, London, for a study of these issues.

9 Carter H (2002) Death recording system 'left Shipman free to kill'. *Guardian*. **8 October**. The NHS Chief Medical Officer Sir Liam Donaldson has initiated an audit of Gosport War Memorial Hospital, Hampshire, concerning death rates. The statistical analysis was being conducted by Professor Richard Baker, Professor of Clinical Governance, Leicester University, who analysed Dr Shipman's practice. Rogers L (2002) *Sunday Times (news section)*. **15 September**: 5. Horsnell M, Jenkins R (2002) Shipman experts aid inquiry into 50 hospital deaths. *The Times*. **7 November**; Jenkins R (2002) Doctors failed to act on Shipman's fatal slip-up. *The Times*. **10 December**. Dr Geraint Day has pointed out that mortality data which could have detected Shipman early in his career were neither looked at systematically nor analysed, and this is typical of the NHS attitude to management problems. Day G (2000) *Management, Mutuality and Risk: better ways to run the National Health Service*. Institute of Directors Research Paper, London, October, p.17. See also Robinson G (2000) Bad administration costs lives. *British Journal of Administrative Management*. **March/April**: 4.

10 Bristol Royal Infirmary Inquiry (2001) *Learning from Bristol: the report of the public inquiry into children's heart surgery at the Bristol Royal Infirmary 1984–1995*. Stationery Office, London.

11 House of Commons (2002) Opposition Day. Care homes. *Hansard*. **8 July**: cols 660–712.

12 Pickering WG (2002) Clinical quality should be put at the centre of care. *BMJ*. **324**: 1398. See also Pickering WG (2000) An independent medical inspectorate. In: D Gladstone (ed.) *Regulating Doctors*. Institute for The Study of Civil Society, London. Pickering WG (1996) How to control the misuse of the health services. *BMJ*. **313**: 1408–9. Compare with the uncritical and unfocused approach of the House of Commons, Committee of Public Accounts (2002) *Handling Clinical Negligence Claims in England. Thirty-Seventh Report of Session 2001–02, HC 280*. The Stationery Office, London. Also, the naif approach in Coulter A (2002) After Bristol: putting patients in the centre. *BMJ*. **324**: 648–51.

13 Pickering WG, letter to author, 9 July 2002.

14 Pickering WG, ibid.

15 Pickering WG (2000) An independent medical inspectorate. In: D Gladstone (ed.) *Regulating Doctors*. Institute for The Study of Civil Society, London. Pickering WG (2002) Clinical quality should be put at the centre of care. *BMJ*. **324**: 1398. See also the following informative comment by a doctor on the power of mystery: Daniels A (2002) I have felt the seductive power that corrupted Shipman. *Sunday Telegraph*. **21 July**: 21.

16 Macneile Dixon W (1938) *The Human Situation. The Gifford Lectures delivered in The University of Glasgow 1935–1937*. Longmans Green, New York, p.93.

17 The issues of funding and capacity – and thus of access and of professional training, morale and performance – will, too, grow more challenging, not less. For example, in 2004 the European Working Time Directive for junior doctors (which is obligatory) will require many medium-size hospitals to introduce full shift systems. This will necessarily reduce the time available for formal education, and exposure to clinics and operating lists. At present there are no proposals to increase the length of training to compensate, and the impact on the quality and competence of new graduates is likely to be significant. John Keegan, in his study of Churchill, speaks of professionals who used to enjoy 'the satisfaction of an

insider's life, financially ill rewarded but locally esteemed and emotionally secure'. This situation has much changed. The losses cannot, in my view, be counter-balanced by increasing central control, yet professionals cannot either escape appraisal by the consumer co-operative, on behalf of the individual receiving care.

Chapter 19

With eyes to see: one people, one market, one service

I am impressed with the fact that the greatest thing a human soul ever does in this world is to see something, and tell what it saw in a plain way. Hundreds of people can talk for one who can see. To see clearly is poetry, philosophy and religion all in one.

(Ralph Waldo Emerson)

I have been asked, 'Where is there an example of what you propose?' Do not look abroad. It lies here in our own high streets, with the revolution in optical care in the past 20 years.

The proof of the validity of the patient fundholding concept can be seen in every high street. For in the revolution in ophthalmology in recent years we have all seen for ourselves in our own locality the consequences of the consumer-focused revolution of financially empowered choice in eye care. And, as I urged in the introduction, the change wrought in eye care has been achieved on the foundations of equity and fairness, social justice and equality of access, with everyone being in one market together, and with the poor being protected and ensured of entitlement through the NHS voucher scheme.[1]

This change through deregulation has freed us all from the immoral two-tier market – sorted by income – which we still see in the wider NHS itself, and which persists in dentistry, too. This revolution in optics is the clearest possible demonstration of the benefits of dynamism compared with those of centralism, of choice and competition in place of statism, of consumerism rather than of control from above, and of how progress really occurs in an adaptive market of self-responsibility and voluntary exchange.

The revolution in eye care manifests the truth that, comes the opportunity, comes the investment, comes the provider, comes consumer satisfaction. Indeed, it offers an optimal social and business model for change throughout UK health-care (including dentistry and such areas as hearing aids, which are poorly served) – for all to be in one market, and with tax transfers to the poor in order to equip them as equal purchasers. It shows us that unplanned, trial-and-error, open-ended endeavour works – and much better than conformity to a central vision of 'experts knowing best'. This has been a real example of testing proposals against the public's own dreams. And it has not been a temporary, fly-by-night change. Nor have the poor, the disadvantaged and the unlucky been victimised. On the contrary, they too have benefited. There is special provision for customers on supplementary benefit, as well as for children, pensioners and customers with special health difficulties. Here we have come far from the normal NHS world of 'one size fits nobody' – if only, as yet, in optics, important as that is. This has been achieved without a blueprint, a master-plan or a future which asked permission to become. And it remains an example of continuous improvement, which NHS managers read about when taking MBAs, but find so difficult to achieve in practice.

This is a classic demonstration of how progress really occurs in an economy. It shows the results if we welcome the future and believe that this evolves from the spontaneity generated by an ever-shifting pattern created from the necessary fluidities of life, in which millions of individuals make unco-ordinated and independent decisions for the common good. The optics market has shown once again that this generates large-scale benefits, from the expression of dispersed, diverse and often tacit knowledge. As Postrel puts this:

> *Stasists seek specifics to govern each new situation and keep things under control. Dynamists want to limit universal rule making to broadly applicable and rarely changed principles, within which people can create and test countless combinations. Stasists want their rules to apply to everyone; dynamists prefer competing, nested rule sets.*[2]

The following important points can be made here.

- Financially empowered choice works.
- There can be one market in which all are empowered.
- Everyone is guaranteed service.
- The poor are paid for by the better off, receiving vouchers.
- Competition improves access both to excellent *clinical quality* and to *non-clinical choices*.
- In a single market for all, no one needs to spend time and resources seeking better *clinical quality*. This, by contrast with the NHS itself, where there remains a two-tier system – one for the middle class and one for the poor.
- The changes have not been the thin end of the wedge for the poor.
- Optics is a *public* service, but it is managed privately, within the Government's framework of rules concerning registration, training, quality, and so on.
- Those who want to spend extra money (for example, on fashion frames) can do so. This in no way undermines the higher standards and equal access which have been achieved, and which are maintained by Government setting the rules.
- The protection of competition, choice and financial leverage for the poor is fundamental to the success of the reformed structure.
- The changes suit and benefit from modern technology. For example, you can book your eye examination on the Internet and buy products online.
- Quality products fall in price and increase in value over time.
- There are, too, consumer gains from consistent healthcare screening done by the optician, based on frequent two-year checks, and full computerisation across a national group allows lifetime records to be available.

The cultural argument that is being presented is summarised as follows by Postrel in *The Future and Its Enemies*:

> *Like the present, the future is not a single, uniform state, but an ongoing process that reflects the plenitude of human life. There is in fact no single future; 'the' future encompasses the many microfutures of individuals and their associations. It includes all the things we learn about ourselves and the world, all the new ways we express and recombine them. As a system, the future is natural, out of anyone's control.... This open-ended future can't be contained in the vision of a single person or an organisation. And, as Judith Adams says of technology, it is something we can never be caught up with.*[3]

The UK optical model is essentially a much flatter structure than the centrally planned NHS model. This ensures entrepreneurial leadership, with fast and cost-effective solutions to changing demand. It demonstrates, too, that the staff of the NHS must change what they are doing. Instead of waiting for the public to come to the NHS, the NHS must go to the public, and give people what they want and are prepared to pay for.

The major lesson from change in the UK optics market is that we can have one evolving market for all in the whole NHS. This is shown by the fact that in optics services there is one market and one experience for all. There is no two-tier market. No penny plain and tuppence coloured, save in terms of extras such as fashion items. No poor left with a residue. Everyone served the same, and by a private provider in a public market. People can buy different fashion items (which are lifestyle choices), but they do not purchase any different levels of *clinical* care. The optometrist also meets everyone with the same attitude. They are not more or less polite to some individuals than others. It is not that some have to wait and others don't. No one is 'private', and everyone gets one thing. That is in good part why it is successful – everyone goes through the same door. It is a *public* service, but it is managed privately within the Government's framework of rules – in which all are empowered.

We have exited from the public/private contradiction, and from the moral difficulties which remain the daily reality of the broader NHS/private duality. This, too, demonstrates that public service is offered by private bodies – both non-profit (e.g. the hospices) and for profit (e.g. the large optics providers). The key is that no one goes separately to a private facility on the basis of class, income or connections while others go to a poorer NHS facility. Nor is the optometrist merely a merchant, although the successful managements have the qualities of the successful entrepreneurs while successfully employing clinical professionals. The optometrist does not see different patients differently. Nor behave differently, greet anyone differently, prescribe differently. And so one of the most important achievements is that there is precisely the moral commitment and the practical equal access which people say they want from the NHS itself: equity, fairness, equality. But this equity has not been created by reducing the service to the lowest common denominator, with everybody joining hands to cross the finishing line joint last together. Nor by insisting on uniform treatment for all and disregarding local knowledge, circumstances and potential for adaptation. This evolution shows the commercial organisation with management skills responding to the health-care opportunity and demand to ensure high standards.

Of course, we should ask how different the optics sector is from the rest of healthcare, and to what extent its lessons are applicable or non-applicable. I shall come to that question in a few moments.

As we consider the potential for change in the NHS, let's look at the history of this change in optics, and the nature of the changes. Look at *then* – prior to 1985 and the deregulation of advertising – and look at *now*.

Then: until 1985, the ophthalmic world had largely revolved around standard NHS psychology, to ration allocative resources. Thus there was a restricted service, no choice, high costs, inconvenient access. The emblem of attitudes towards the individual was indeed the standard NHS specs – with the unfortunate child ('four-eyes') wearing uniform ugly NHS glasses (with the usual weak hinges, often repaired with masking tape) familiar in every school playground, the wearer bullied by the rest. The image was a stock-in-trade of Pinewood Studios. The optician was only open from Monday to Friday, 9.00am to 5pm. Closed for lunch – just when the office worker could go in for a consultation. No prescriptions were issued, and so no documentation was made of problems for the patient to see. There was no transparency of prices for customers to compare. There were no performance tables, or transparent data on outcomes or comparative competence. There was no effective complaints handling procedure. Patient expectations were low, as were those of the staff. The patient had to buy glasses at the place where the test was done (whereas now the patient takes the results of an eye test done by one provider to whichever supplier they decide they prefer). If the test revealed that glasses were needed, the design was sent away and the patient had to wait for 2 to 3 weeks.

Now: an entirely different psychological and service world. Optics is indeed a leading part of the modernised services that we expect in the wider economy. Providers are open 7 days a week and in the evenings. Staff evidently enjoy their work, in attractive premises, and are well motivated. A choice of employers who want their skills. With sufficient capacity in the industry to ensure choice and to reduce destructive stresses on both staff and customers. The customer can shop around. There is price competition, as well as competition on location and on styles. There is often same-day service for equipment when laboratories are on site (as increasingly they are) – this prompted by competitive pressures and a genuine focus on satisfying the customer.

There are just over 6900 opticians' premises in the UK. These differ in size from large optical superstores to small practices in local shopping parades or private houses. They comprise about 9000 consulting rooms, all of which are equipped to enable the full eye examination to be carried out as well as the diagnosis and monitoring work involved in NHS co-management arrangements with a GP or hospital eye department. The cost of equipping consulting rooms and providing premises is borne by the optician, and there is too, significant investment by many companies in continuing education.[4]

The role of preventive care is significant. The Department of Health estimates the total number of sight tests to be 16.6 million, with one-third of tests paid for privately. This figure did not change in the year ending 31 March 2001, the latest reported by the Federation of Ophthalmic and Dispensing Opticians (FODO). FODO commented on some changes in what is an adaptive market during the year.

> *This indicates that after 2 years, the extension of eligibility for an NHS sight test (to those over 60 and over) has not had the desired effect of significantly increasing the number of people having their sight tested. It is estimated that more than 2 million people were switched from paying privately to the lower NHS fee arrangements, with a resulting loss in fee income for opticians estimated at over £8 million in the current year.*[5]

In addition, there was a reduction of referrals from 4% to 3% in the year, which was thought to be likely to be a consequence of the change in regulation which allows optometrists to monitor some conditions rather than automatically refer those cases.

FODO recorded 3.5 million spectacles dispensed in the year, 23% of these being purchased using an NHS voucher to pay for all or part of the cost of the spectacles. This reflected a slight decrease in purchases using an NHS voucher:

> 'For 15 years, DoH surveys have indicated a trend for a declining proportion of spectacles to be bought with a voucher.' This reflects two factors, one of which FODO mentions, one of which it does not. First, rising incomes and prosperity. People pay more for themselves, by choice, or are earning more than NHS qualifying levels. Second, FODO's point: 'This [change in voucher purchases] reflects the erosion of voucher values in relation to the cost of spectacles since the voucher scheme was introduced.'

It appears that better use is now being made of optometrists, and that this is starting to reduce pressures both on the NHS and on waiting lists. NHS hospitals find it difficult to retain optometrists, as they offer only half to two-thirds of the pay an optometrist can earn in private practice. And so better use is now being made of optometrists in private practice, which impacts on quality. For example, in diabetic screening and in post-cataract care.

This is one of the consequential primary care benefits which the evolution of the dynamic market in eye care has had for NHS and other patients. Most notably, the expanded role in primary care for optometrists has effectively reduced pressures on the NHS and on waiting lists by managing the referrals of people with cataract, glaucoma and diabetic eye disease. And it is hoped eventually by reducing pressure on GPs by therapeutically managing minor eye conditions.[6]

Another major impact has been on the previously slow and tangled NHS procedures.[7] For example, in some areas, hospital ophthalmology services have streamlined cataract practices – enabling patients to be offered a booked appointment, cataract removal with implant, and then be referred back to an accredited optometrist of their choice before turning to their preferred supplier for final dispensing of spectacles. Some hospitals now enable optometrists to refer patients directly for assessment for cataract surgery. And so the general change in attitudes is gradually shifting professional barriers and NHS management practice.

However, many other hospitals and local optometry committees still require the optometrist to continue to send the necessary completed forms to a GP, who then sends them on to the hospital, from whom the patient awaits a call to tell him or her that the GP has sent the referral onward. The hospital then arranges the appointment. Situations occur where GPs wait for patients to attend their practice before referring them onward. This is a cumbersome loop which patients find confusing.[8] It is a survival from the 'old' NHS.

However, the opening up of the optics market has helped the NHS patient considerably – although some practitioners also complain of over-regulation.[9] You can, if you are eligible, have an eye test on the NHS, or you can have an eye test privately and cheaply. If a patient qualifies for help with the cost of new spectacles or contact lenses, the practitioner will issue the appropriate voucher, which the patient is free to use as a contribution towards the total cost of any spectacles or contact lenses they may choose. Department of Health surveys have indicated that about half of the optical practices surveyed sell spectacles within voucher values.[10]

In the private market, single-vision lenses cost from £30, and frames from £20. Some independent opticians (and many multiples) give free spectacles with vouchers, too. You can purchase fully privately fashion frames and lenses, including professional charges and advice. For those who qualify for vouchers, these are fully exchangeable for a whole range of fashion frames, with no further charge. There is also no distinction made by staff between the vouchered and the private consumer. In addition, special upgrading offers are made to NHS customers.[11]

This situation of choice, competition and improvement has been in place at least since 1984. It offers a proven body of knowledge on which we can draw for more extensive changes. It presents the model of a powerful instrument of cohesive, socially solid, dynamic change. Thus the patient fundholder can be forwarded, not feared.

The NHS is plagued by low morale – demonstrated by high levels of sickness absence and unofficial holiday. This is no longer the case in eye care. As Ian Hunter, Chief Executive of the Association of Optometrists recently wrote:

> *The focus on the healthcare role of optometrists over the last decade has trans-*
> *formed how the profession sees itself. What has been highlighted is the ability*
> *of optometrists to potentiate [sic] the delivery of eye healthcare by working co-*
> *operatively with general medical practitioners, ophthalmologists and diabetologists.*
> *In retrospect, the most remarkable feature of this development is that it took*
> *place outside GOS [NHS General Ophthalmic Services].... Even 20 years*
> *ago, the profession was largely providing sight-testing and spectacles; today, the*
> *emphasis is increasingly on providing primary healthcare. Viewed from the*
> *outside this is an incredible transformation in the role of optometry, which has*
> *taken place only in the last decade and with little help from Government. We*
> *did it ourselves, largely though local initiatives.*[12]

Another optometrist recently told me of the case of a 22-year-old woman who came in to see her early this year, reporting headaches and eye strain. An examination in the practice revealed a tumour, which required immediate action.

She was referred instantly and operated on promptly, and her life was saved. She had walked into a convenient high-street practice that she passed on her way while shopping, whereas she might not have gone to a crowded GP's surgery, and she could not refer herself directly to a hospital surgeon. This type of case is highly motivating to the optometrist, and it saves lives. Indeed, it is likely that under present reviews of the medical professions, optometrists will be considered for prescribing rights.[13]

Clearly, morale, commitment and reward matter to the quality of the services, for these are delivered by individuals, not by systems. The NHS suffers from low recruitment, expensive re-recruitment, serious problems caused by an inadequate medical workforce, and low morale – notably among middle managers, many of whom bear the strain and have nowhere else to go. By contrast, optics shows us the opposite situation. Excellent young and well-qualified graduates (from courses at Cardiff, UMIST, Aston and elsewhere) are being attracted and retained because of better conditions, friendlier environments, good relationships with satisfied customers, and greater rewards. There are flexible employment practices, too, and these help the customer. Trained staff are not lost to the services when they have children, as flexible employment practices are the norm. There has been a revolution in patients' expectations. Patients are much better informed by the media and by their advisers about advances in technology. They expect satisfaction, or else they will go to an alternative provider.

The key change was in advertising and deregulation. As Lord (Geoffrey) Howe has written, 'in 1984 opticians were allowed to advertise, and customers to go where they liked for their glasses. The result is to be seen on every high street today.'[14] Free eye tests are offered by many high-street practitioners to all of their clients, so every supplier makes a loss on this service.

Pensioners, children, the poor and those on income support remain protected. They receive free eye tests as NHS patients. As the former Chancellor of the Exchequer notes, 'These people are also eligible for NHS vouchers' – patient fund-holders! – 'and at Specsavers, for example, NHS customers can have unlimited choice for just a few pounds more. Every patient remains free to resort – even if after a privately financed eye test – to the more specialist services available through the NHS.' Voucher values start at £30.50 for single-vision lenses and £52.80 for bifocals.[15]

There are also clinical benefits for those who take their eye care seriously. The eyes, of course, are the mirror to the soul, and reveal much more to the specialist in the high street. Indeed, optometrists do much more than test for glasses. They catch problems early and have a salient role in preventive care. They advise patients of additional clinical procedures that they believe, in their best judgement, should be applied for the patient's benefit. They are notable as practitioners who discover the unexpected and save lives. They are crucial to early diagnosis in cases of incipient eye disease. And the recent changes, including the attractive surroundings, attitudes among staff to customers who have a real choice, and the huge variety of choice available, encourages people to come in, and serious problems can be detected during an otherwise routinely unthreatening eye test. This is indelible, real, contemporary, current, non-theoretical, practical, non-politicised and local evidence that choice works, and it is legitimised by practice. That the patient can be trusted with choice. And that dynamism and development depend on empowered choice. As Geoffrey Howe has said, 'Is this not a striking demonstration of consumer (and supplier) willingness to share directly in financing at least a part of the market in health care?'[16]

Choice has widened to a hitherto unimagined extent. Competition from attractive premises in prime locations is the norm. All this is real in ordinary lives. The key change was to permit advertising in optical care. There has also been much technical innovation, which was formerly almost impossible. Previously, provision was hog-tied by regulation, and specialists were bureaucratically limited on the care that they could give. Competition and choice encourage innovation and value. Prices have fallen dramatically – for example, in the cost of contact lenses, which has fallen to around 10% of the 1970s' price, solely due to advertising and competition, and to subsequent growth in volume.[17] And contact lenses which may be safely worn for months are the newest innovation to go on trial. They have a special coating that kills bacteria which cause eye infections, which it is hoped will improve on extended-wear contact lenses made from silicon hydrogel.[18] Postrel also notes, too, that innovation in the quality and user-friendliness of contact lenses – hard to soft, and so forth – has been entirely due to dynamism in competition.

The consequences of deregulation have been wholly positive for the consumer, and for the quality of preventive healthcare and hospital referral (where necessary) that consumers have experienced. This is also the case in the deregulation of other non-health services, such as telephone services, gas and electricity – all these services were travellers with the same NHS mind-set of regarding the customer as a burden rather than as an opportunity; all were previously poor performers, inflexible in their attitudes to consumers, all unwilling to change how things must be done, all refusing to offer timed appointments, all working within bureaucracies elusive to the consumer. Meanwhile, the necessity for diversity and extending healthcare funding is a continuing issue. The NHS spends almost £200 million a year on its General Ophthalmic Services (GOS). If there was patient fundholding, there would be a powerful case to re-examine this figure, as many for whom free eye tests are provided may be in a position to fund this service themselves by cash payment. For example, many individuals who have free sight tests do not go to purchase fashion frames. The money spent on free sight tests might be better spent on core services.

The key change in the UK was the advertising deregulation of 1984, and the subsequent evolution of the 'premium' segment of optical care. There are many publicly quoted, responsible, innovative companies who could participate in a new and competitive environment for the wider NHS services, if given direct access to patient fundholders. This model has been driven by customers shopping around, by marketing and information, by competition in a high-volume business, by freedom for opticians to combine with managers in new corporate bodies (including many successful joint venture projects with Specsavers, Vision Express, etc.) to provide new competition, and by freedom to advertise all aspects of products and services, especially 'soft' comparative advertising.

Revenues are a great transformer if the holder of the cash (or NHS credit, or social insurance contract) is free to migrate to the better service. With choice in place, new providers came into the NHS optics market, seeking willing revenues, and unfolding new ways to satisfy the wary and the willing alike. Customers, too – allegedly too ignorant or untrustworthy to make choices – rapidly showed that they were underestimated in their ability to canvas alternatives.

The service providers are a significant presence throughout the UK and Ireland. By 31 March 2002, Vision Express/Optical Lab had 107 stores and 89 Vision Express/Joint Venture stores. Dolland & Aitchison, which is 250 years old, and is now part of the De Rigo company which manufactures and distributes eyewear, has a UK network of 400 branches.[19] Specsavers, founded in 1983 by optometrists Doug and Mary Perkins, has around 450 UK outlets (and is also opening stores rapidly in The Netherlands).[20] The firm has been one of those that have transformed the market.

The success of developments in the eye care market, too, tells us something important about the inherited post-1948 division between public and private care in acute care (and in dentistry). Here the private market is marked by high prices but low volume, whereas the NHS has high volume but no measure of profit (by which I mean a necessary surplus, for investment and innovation, itself genuinely earned from the satisfied consumer). There is insufficient incentive either to NHS providers and purchasers or to private providers to innovate imaginatively. For the NHS funds are 'found money', or merely granted from above by the Treasury. For the private providers are shut out from seeking the huge revenues committed by political allocation to the NHS. There is only marginal competition between the two, much of it generated on the morally improper basis that the inadequacies of the NHS lever people out into the private sector, often in despair – this being the only strategy for accessing services (such as a new hip, or a cataract operation) which they thought they had already paid for by taxation. Patients thus pay privately for an operation performed by the same consultant whom they expected to see in the NHS, and often indeed in the 'private' wing of an NHS trust. This is, too, an exit with a class basis. It worsens the situation of the poor. And, worse still, the inadequacies of the NHS monopoly structure impose a price on both rich and poor, since many die from otherwise treatable diseases while on waiting lists, because neither the NHS nor the private sector has the incentives, revenues and capacity to offer optimal services.

For example, consider the denial of modern drugs for cancer care (which the NHS cannot afford, and which it will not permit willing patients to purchase). Or the insufficient numbers of trained radiographers, resulting in several dozen hospitals turning off linear accelerators (cancer-fighting radiotherapy machines) because there are too few staff to run them. Since survival chances improve with speedy treatment, this is costing lives. The UK has about half the number of radiotherapy machines per million people as France or Germany, and one-third the number of those in the USA. One-third of those who are trained as radiographers never enter the profession, deterred by low status and low pay. A recent Royal College of Radiologists study suggested that, contrary to Government targets, the average waiting time for radiotherapy has risen from 5.1 weeks in 1999 to

6 weeks in 2002. For example, at hospitals in Brighton and Hammersmith patients can wait up to 3 months for treatment. A World Health Organization study showed that English women with breast cancer have a 67% chance of living for 5 years, compared with a greater than 80% chance in France or Sweden. All this is the result of cumulative errors in politics.[21] Hospices are in financial crisis, as Government funding for the terminally ill has fallen. And the 'giving culture' has also been undermined by the expectation of State funding.[22]

Fewer than 50% of patients with treated heart failure are currently prescribed angiotensin-converting enzyme (ACE) inhibitors, drugs which have proved effective in reducing mortality and hospitalisation. Only about one in ten patients being treated for heart failure is prescribed beta-blockers – drugs which have been shown to increase the length and quality of life, according to the British Heart Foundation. In the UK, heart failure has a poor prognosis, and nearly 40% of those diagnosed with the condition die within a year.[23]

This NHS system can *never* provide customer satisfaction in the mainstream acute, chronic and mental care fields. This will remain so no matter how many patient 'consultation' bodies are established – alongside targets, edicts, commands, new codes of conduct setting out 'values', watchdogs, performance action teams, conditional grants and funding increases. For NHS care institutions do not have to focus on the customer's preferences. This system will always embody disincentives, triggers for low morale, professional dissatisfaction, early professional retirement, and difficulties in recruitment to general practice and clinical specialisation. It is shaped by low salaries, inadequate provision and access, the inadequacy of investment and innovation, and the denial of choice and of new treatments that are otherwise available in European service economies.

The division between the NHS and private sectors is a duality of denials which has itself made customer satisfaction impossible to achieve. This division is a perennially unsatisfactory solution to the problems of healthcare provision. The quality of services can only deteriorate, and rationing can only increase. For the NHS has no incentive to seek to satisfy the customer – save for the moral commitment of hard-working professionals. And the private sector has no opportunity to satisfy the customer in huge areas that are blocked to it by walls fabricated by politics. Strikingly, too, there is no such division in the major European systems of social insurance. It pays no one to seek to provide privately for better clinical care, since there is no waiting list for good clinical care in the open-access system available to all (e.g. in France, Germany, The Netherlands, Switzerland) on a routine and legally guaranteed basis.

However, we have to have some understanding of the cultural inheritance which has produced our difficulties, in order to see the ways out. Crucially, though, we have a clear answer to the sceptical question that is often put: 'Show me some examples of where what you want works.' That answer is Europe, of course, and in our own high streets, too!

The history of eyewear itself demonstrates the value of the dynamist approach. For the patient is an opportunity, not a nuisance. The service is rewarding to all concerned, not an act of politics. And innovation leads to renewal and further invention in order to improve the improved, with manufacturers under competitive pressure to discover incremental advantages preferred by consumers, who test these and encourage better combinations in supply.

Eye glasses for correcting near-sightedness were invented around the year 1500, about 200 years after reading glasses. The concept has had a history of innovation, feedback, invention and adoption, leading to a succession of new ideas. The credit for the idea of contact lenses belongs to the late nineteenth-century Swiss physician A Eugen Fick. Practical wearable lenses were created in the 1950s by the Czech, Otto Wichterie, and they are now worn by 4 million people in the UK. Hard lenses were subsequently replaced by 'gas-permeable' lenses, which allowed the user to wear them for many hours. Then came disposable lenses, in 'off-the-shelf' sizes, which could be quickly and cheaply replaced. These, too, could be worn for extended periods. And the history of the product demonstrates the evolutionary power of dynamism and its approach to an open-ended future, with consumer choice a vital cog in progressive change. This history is a paradigm of demand-led progress, of innovation, improvement and the renewal of the search for the better. Eye specialists, polymer scientists and consumers experimented with lens materials, sizes, wetting solutions, ways of matching impressions of the eye to provide appropriate individual correction of vision, and style as well. The process continues, and costs continue to fall. Now there are lenses available that change colour, carry motifs and logos, protect against ultraviolet radiation, correct astigmatism, which are more durable, can be slept in, and so on. The future may hold contact lenses as computer screens or navigation guides, or to enhance night vision. The problem solving that optics has demonstrated is the root of all innovation, and such progress is infinitely assisted by demand-led consumption. As the social historian of engineering, Henry Petroski, put this:

> *Form follows failure: the form of made things is always subject to change in response to their real or perceived shortcomings, their failures to function properly. This principle governs all invention, innovation, and ingenuity ... the future perfect can only be a tense, not a thing.*[24]

If we are to benefit to the full from all these insights, there is no room for snobbery or the closed mind. Indeed there is everything to learn from those who have proved by results that they know how to focus on customers and their costed wants. Alan Tinger, Managing Director of Galaxy Optical Services, optical consultants and suppliers to Tesco Opticians, recently wrote (and he could be speaking for any one of the providers who have come into the market from standing start):

> *According to some in the profession, the world as we know it is coming to an end because supermarkets have become involved [in eye care]. Why was Tesco Opticians set up? The answer is very simple – it is what Tesco customers asked for (and many thousands of them visit a typical Tesco Extra store each week where the non-food space is greater than the food space). Tesco has built its total business to the scale it is today by meeting customer demands (identified by extensive and ongoing customer research) and having a total focus on*

customer service…. At the end of the day, the patients will decide who they want to visit and who provides the quality of care, value and service they demand. There is room in the market for all who are rising to the challenge of meeting patients' requirements.[25]

Finally, let us consider dentistry and what we can learn from change in the optics market. There are no exact parallels between the situation of patients seeking optical services in the 1980s and the dental services now, although there are some uncomfortable coincidences with regard to the restrictions on competition. Clearly the benefits of open markets, transparent information and accountability to the consumer in effective competition would make a significant difference to access, price, quality, accountability and choice. Dental services could be offered on the same basis as eye care, with us all in one market. The Office of Fair Trading (OFT) is currently enquiring into dentistry. This investigation was precipitated by research undertaken by the Consumers' Association, and published in *Which?* and *Health Which?* in September and October 2001. The Consumers' Association made a 'super-complaint' on 25 October 2001 to the OFT 'alleging that competition in this sector was ineffective and identifying a number of core problems worthy of further investigation'. It did so under procedures which the Government proposes to establish in statute under the Enterprise Bill which is currently before the House of Commons.[26]

Clearly the impact of change in the optics market will have an influence on how dentistry is organised, purchased and provided – and indeed on the whole NHS. Dynamism and dentistry could achieve millions of smiles.

This *dynamist* development is a settlement without the necessity of constant 'consultation', voting, political organisation and activism. It is of a positive kind. It shows us that unplanned, trial-and-error, open-ended endeavour works. It gives precedence to concrete reality and detail over abstract ideology. It offers openness, not closure. It binds people loosely together in a moral community. This contributes significantly to the nation in which we are both part of 'a people' and 'a person'. It enables individuals to reach within themselves for an acceptable compromise between risk and benefit, cost and advantage, price and performance. It offers lower costs, higher quality, greater access, more choice and a greater sense of a fulfilled self. Instead of absolutes, it offers negotiation. Instead of the test of an individual in terms of adherence to a set of political beliefs, it offers the test of an individual in their own terms. It sanctions empiricist philosophy, common-sense reasoning, and action in voluntary communities within the rule of law. There is no element of 'beggar-my-neighbour', since the decision of one consumer takes nothing away from another – in the NHS where there is competition for artificially scarce resources, and where my hip replacement is probably at the cost of your wait for a cataract operation. Where NHS denial divides, one market welds us together. No one need jockey to nudge another on to the rails. By organic growth access is ensured for all. There is a shared experience, with all of its moral gains – genuine equity, improved outcome, and an open door to new ideas.

I suggest that this dynamist proof in the evolving market in eye care has been shown to be much better as a model than *stasism* and conformity to a central statist vision of 'knowing best'. It does more to promote a culture of service – which could be revived in wider healthcare in the quiet co-operation of patient-guaranteed care, Patient Guaranteed Care Associations, and patient fund-holding. This does not mean that there will be *no* planning. Of course, a specific provider (Vision Express, Specsavers, Boots Opticians, Asda's vision centres, Batemans, Dollond & Aitchison, Tesco Opticians, Optical Express, and a host of independents with perhaps one to ten shops, such as David H Myers of Southport or Richard C Arnold in Hampshire) must have a plan to provide specific services. And this will contribute to the evolving system. However, this is a different claim to that of the goal-directed 'progressive' overall planner who seeks to control the whole and intrude into every detail.

These recent English changes do not require us to go to Europe – they are different, in any case, 'abroad, aren't they? Scruton has written of '"abroad", to which the English ventured and from which they returned in mild surprise at their good fortune'.[27] However, in eye care at home we persuasively demonstrate the benefits of creativity and enterprise, generating progress in an evolutionary form, where business plans have been undertaken by specific providers. This has necessarily required a detailed and attentive consumer focus, scientific enquiry, market competition, creative development, technological invention, adaptation, comparison, criticism and reinvestment – all of this within a framework of rules set by Government, with the poor given tax transfers, thus ensuring that everyone is in one market. No penny plain and tuppence coloured, no one rule for the rich and one for the poor, no Jaguar on the private consulting room drive at Hove and a broken-down bus at the back door of the District General Hospital.

This is a dynamist paradigm for the whole of UK healthcare – and its impact is likely to spread rapidly.[28] As Detective Inspector Appleby showed – with his creator's gift for lively language – 'England in all its venerable and grotesque stratifications had crept under a single blanket.'[29]

Notes

1 NHS entitlements for eye care are as follows: sight tests for those aged 60 years or over, for children under 16 years or for those under 19 years in full-time education, benefit claimants (Income Support, income-based Jobseekers Allowance, Working Families Tax Credit or Disabled Persons Tax Credit – both with less than £71 withdrawn); for those with diabetes, glaucoma sufferers (and close relatives aged 40 years or over), for those registered blind or partially sighted or needing complex lens vouchers, and for those on a low income (NHS Low Income Scheme). For vouchers, those who qualify are children under 16 years of age (under 19 years in full-time education), benefit claimants (Income Support, income-based Jobseekers Allowance, or in receipt of Working Families Tax Credit or Disabled Persons Tax Credit, both with less than £71 withdrawn), those on a low income, voucher reduced by any amount that the claimant is assessed by the Benefits Agency as being liable to pay. With regard to complex lenses, a registered optician can advise on entitlement. Federation of Ophthalmic and Dispensing Opticians (2001) *Optics at a Glance for the year to 31st March 2001*, p.2. The General Ophthalmic Service in Scotland is almost identical to that in

England and Wales. The services are evolving to suit local conditions, subject to the powers of the Scottish Parliament and Executive and of the Welsh Assembly.

2 Postrel V (1998) *The Future and Its Enemies. The Growing Conflict Over Creativity, Enterprise and Progress*. The Free Press, New York, p.xvi.

3 Postrel, ibid., p.xiv.

4 Like the medical profession as a whole internationally, practitioners have succeeded in exerting significant control over registration and entry, limiting aspects of competition. The three types of registered practitioners are: *optometrists* (also known as ophthalmic opticians), who test sight and prescribe and dispense spectacles and contact lenses; *dispensing opticians*, who dispense, fit and supply spectacles, and must be specially certified to fit contact lenses; and *ophthalmic medical practitioners* – that is, doctors who specialise in eyes and eye care. There were 774 ophthalmic medical practitioners under contract to health authorities in England and Wales by 31 March 2001. In total, 8646 optometrists in the UK were registered with the General Optical Council, with an estimated 6325 whole-time equivalents. There were 4488 registered dispensing opticians. Federation of Ophthalmic and Dispensing Opticians, op. cit., p.2. But see the discussion of how occupational licensure is a Government-created and Government-supported restriction on competition in Friedman M (1962) *Capitalism and Freedom*. Chicago University Press, Chicago, 1962; new edition 1982, ch. IX.

5 Federation of Ophthalmic and Dispensing Opticians (2001) (FODO) *Optics at a Glance for the Year to 31st March 2001*. Federation of Ophthalmic and Dispensing Opticians, London, p.1.

6 The field offers many innovations! Romina, a large female Western lowland gorilla at Bristol Zoo Gardens, can now see for the first time in her life after successfully undergoing pioneering surgery to restore her sight. The 21-year-old had been born with cataracts, but was operated on at the University of Bristol's Veterinary Hospital in March 2002 – the first ever cataract operation to be performed in Europe on an adult gorilla. Top banana! *Optometry Today*. **19 April**: 7.

7 See the 'Fast Track Cataract Scheme' at The Royal Preston and Chorley Hospitals (ref. BJ/02/L0107/AccOpt.doc, 1 July 2002). Email: B.Johnson@PrestonPCT.nhs.uk. Their leaflet is entitled *Direct Cataract Referral Scheme*. See also the following letter: Broadhurst M (Secretary, North West Lancashire Local Optometric Committee) (2002) Direct referral to ophthalmologists. **April issue**.

8 Morris M (2002) In my view. *Optometry Today*. **3 May**: 24. An optometrist recently told me that: 'Usually an ophthalmologist checks a cataract Px after 1 day and after 3 weeks, post-operatively. By training optometrists in practice to do the 3-week check and only refer back to the surgeon where necessary, this makes more capacity available. The surgeon has more time to do more operations and reduce waiting lists – which are currently plus or minus 9 months in the NHS in most areas (per eye!). I only know of two local optometric committees implementing this in Lancashire – for example – in Preston and in Stockport. The optometrist gets paid £31.25 per patient for doing the 3-week check-up. This is more than we get paid for an eye examination (which takes about the same amount of time), but considerably less than the value of an ophthalmologist's time. So this saves the NHS money' (personal communication, 17 July 2002).

9 Federation of Ophthalmic and Dispensing Opticians (FODO), op. cit., p.2.

10 These values currently range from £30.00 to £140.30 for single-vision spectacles and from £51.80 to £154.30 for bifocals, with additional amounts available for prisms

and tints where clinically necessary. For sight fees, the NHS fee paid to optometrists and to ophthalmic medical practitioners is negotiated jointly. The current fee for an NHS sight test is £15.52, with a new settlement to be effected from April 2001 still outstanding. The average charge for a private sight test in the FODO survey was £19.18, compared with £17.96 for the previous year. However, it seems that no industry is without its difficulties. There has been an allegation that opticians are prepared to prescribe glasses to customers who may not need them, according to a report in July 2002. Parry R (2002) High-street opticians fail eye tests. *Sunday Telegraph.* **21 July**: 3. Clearly there is a risk. However, in optics a consumer can seek a second or even a third opinion. Some assessments about vision are also a matter of judgement.

11 Hunter I (2002) Patients need priority. *Optometry Today.* **19 April**: 4. For example, in August 2002 Specsavers was offering an upgrade to frames and lenses priced at £9 for no further charge, and to a £75 pair for £10. Designer-range frames and lenses priced at £129 were available for £40. Above and beyond the regulation sight test there are offers for an extended eye examination. For example, Eyesite offered this service to private patients for £26.50, but for an additional fee of £9.78 over and above the NHS fee of £16.72 to NHS adults, and free of charge to children under 16 years of age.

12 Crown J (2002) College of Optometrists AGM Charter Lecture, 2002. *Optometry Today.* **3 May**: 12.

13 Howe G (2002) Take spectacles and see the answer for the health service. *Daily Telegraph*, 16 April – a hugely prescient and far-seeing article on which I have drawn significantly.

14 In December 1981, Sally Oppenheim, Minister for Consumer Affairs, asked the Director General of Fair Trading, Sir Gordon (now Lord) Borrie, to undertake a review of the effects of certain sections of the Opticians Act of 1958 on competition in the supply of opticians' services and optical appliances. The Director General's report, *Opticians and Competition*, was published in November 1982. The report reviewed the monopoly to dispense and sell glasses held by opticians, and the restrictions preventing advertising by them, made under rules determined by the General Optical Council. The Secretary of State for Social Services, Mr Norman (now Lord) Fowler, set out the Government's response in a statement to the House of Commons on 28 November 1983 (HC *Hansard*, cols.655–60). The Health and Social Security Act 1984 included provisions that ended the monopoly on optical services and lifted the restrictions on advertising. See also speech by the Secretary of State during the Bill's second reading in the Commons, 20 November 1983 (HC *Hansard*, cols.294–98). The optical professions are regulated by the Opticians Act 1989, and by orders, rules and regulations made under powers granted by the Act. See General Optical Council website: www.optical.org.

15 Howe, ibid. The current NHS sight-test fee is £16.08. The real cost of an eye test in August 2002 was about £50. High-street practice overheads run at around £150 an hour. This makes the point about social solidarity in practice. For, based on three NHS tests being undertaken in an hour, if every patient has a basic voucher the maximum revenue from the NHS would be £139 an hour for the practice. As one optometrist said to me, 'If we did NHS work only we would make a loss of £10.26 an hour, or some £21 350 a year! And so private patients are therefore subsidising the NHS ones.'

16 The UK contact lens market grew by 8% last year. The Association of Contact Lens Manufacturers reported that 217 million lenses were sold in the UK in 2000,

representing a 30% increase in volume and a 7.2% increase in value. The market was changing rather than growing, the increase being largely due to wearers switching to more frequently replaced lenses. A later report stated that almost 269 million lenses were sold in the UK in 2001, with a value of over £110 million. These include disposable, multi-use, single-use and continuous-wear lenses, with sales of 'traditional' soft lenses declining in favour of these frequent-replacement alternatives – all evidence of the benefits of dynamism and continuous innovation and consumer feedback. Contact lenses which may be safely worn for months are the newest innovation to go on trial. They have a special coating that kills bacteria which cause eye infections, and it is hoped that they will be an improvement on extended-wear contact lenses made from silicon hydrogel.

17 Henderson M (2002) Bacteria-busting contact lens to end daily chore. *The Times*. **22 August**: 10.
18 Federation of Ophthalmic and Dispensing Opticians (FODO), op. cit., p.2; (2002) Contact lens market continues to grow in UK (figures from Association of Contact Lens Manufacturers). *Optometry Today*. **17 May**: 6; (2002) Fashion and style drive UK sunglasses market. *Optometry Today*. **17 May**: 8.
19 www.danda.co.uk.
20 The firm is run on a joint-venture basis, each practice being a separate business owned jointly by the practitioner and Specsavers. When the firm was founded, Doug and Mary Perkins say that 'patients' confidence in optical care was low and many opticians were dissatisfied, having no role in the ownership or management'. Company information, www.specsavers.com.
21 Wright O and Studd H (2002) Cancer care hit by lack of trained radiographers. *The Times*. **20 July**; Brownlee S and Brevis K, op. cit. See also Capocaccia R, Colonna M, Corazziari I *et al.* (2002) Measuring cancer prevalence in Europe: the EUROPREVAL project. *Ann Oncol*. **13 June**. Micheli A, Mugno E, Krogh V *et al.* and the EUROPREVAL Working Group (2002) Cancer prevalence in European registry areas. *Ann Oncol*. **13 June**: 840–65.
22 Paveley R and Marsh B (2002) Dying patients turned away as £50m promise to hospices is broken. *Daily Mail*. **17 June**.
23 Prentice E-A (2002) A misunderstood killer. *The Times*. **18 June**.
24 Petroski H (1992) *The Evolution of Useful Things*. Alfred Knopf, New York. I am indebted to Postrel, op. cit., for her account of the history of optics in her chapter on 'The Infinite Series'.
25 Tinger A (2002) Providing what customers want. *Optometry Today*. **17 May**: 4.
26 Press release, Consumers' Association/Office of Fair Trading (2002) *Consumers' Association Makes First Supercomplaint to OFT and OFT Launches Major Investigation into Private Dentistry*: super-complaint on private dentistry – preliminary findings on the issues raised by the Consumers' Association. Office of Fair Trading, London. See also Department of Health (2002) *NHS Dentistry: options for change*. Department of Health, London (concerned with payment systems). Extracting your cash. *Which?* **September 2001**: 6. Mouthing off. *Health Which?* **October 2001**: 10. Complaining about dentistry. *Which?* **January 2002**: 8–11. Department of Health (2000) *Modernising NHS Dentistry: implementing the NHS Plan*. Department of Health, London. Buck P and Newton JT (2001) The privatisation of NHS dentistry? A national snapshot of general dental practitioners. *Eng Dent J*. **190**: 115–18.
27 Scruton, op. cit., p.6.

28 The lessons are relevant across the entire NHS. And, indeed, innovative companies like Specsavers are seeking to extend consumer-focused innovation in other areas. In November 2002 the firm announced a medium-sized acquisition in hearing aids, believing that this is an area of healthcare crying out for exactly the same revolution as has taken place in optics. Mr Doug JD Perkins, Managing Director, told me: 'At the moment, the overwhelming majority of patients are relying on the hearing aid services under the NHS. Currently the NHS is unable to cope with demand from the identified list of two million patients who would benefit from the supply of a hearing aid. There is a developed private sector that could easily supply this need (with the appropriate regulation and controls). However, a registered Hearing Aid Dispenser operating on the patient-friendly, easily accessible High Street is not permitted to supply hearing aid services under the NHS – with the resultant waiting list. The misery and frustration that currently exists among this deserving patient group could easily be resolved with the introduction of a voucher system analogous to that currently used in the general ophthalmic service. This would enable a hearing aid patient to take their voucher to any qualified supplier on the High Street (and in the process deciding for themselves whether they wish to pay extra for additional features and benefits). Market forces would bring about improvement in accessibility, speed and quality of service, enhanced patient choice and the desirable eradication of a two-tier NHS/private service'. (Private communication, 15 November 2002). The NHS should form alliances with firms like Specsavers, and others who take the same approach. There are other relevant areas, notably dentistry. See Audit Commission, *Primary Dental Care Services in England and Wales* (London, Audit Commission, September 2002) for a picture of the present unsatisfactory two-tier structure and the potential for change; also, *Healthcare Market News*. Laing & Buisson, London, October 2002, pp.12–14.

29 Innes M (1946) *Appleby's End*. Penguin Books, Harmondsworth.

Part 2

Power and responsibility: some policy in practice

Chapter 20

Order in a self-organised system

[There is] convincing proof that a competitive system of markets and prices ... is not a system of chaos and anarchy. There is in it a certain order and orderliness. It works. It functions. Without intelligence it solves one of the most complex problems imaginable, involving thousands of unknown variables and relations. Nobody designed it. Like Topsy, it just growed ...

(Paul Samuelson)

We need to consider some concrete ideas about policy in practice. But first, something more on the concepts of order which underpin these. The issues concerning the two contrasting concepts of order – control and hierarchy, or evolutionary community – are impossible to stress sufficiently. We need to emphasise that the lack of a hierarchy and a master-plan controlled by central Government does not imply dis-order. Adaptive evolution, as contrasted to the imposed and restrictive order of hierarchical insistence – that is the order that arises from the evolutionary co-ordination of the factors of production we see all around us in everyday living. Price and its companion – competition – offer the infusion of energy which all systems need from outside themselves. Price offers order, too. Indeed it guarantees it. Price relates to one another those countless different enterprises and individuals that are active in a non-hierarchical but nevertheless self-organised system.

If the system is not to be held together by central controls, it can only be integrated by a framework of rules and by price and competition. Price will be the coherent adhesive which integrates a diversity of providers – which Government says it intends – in a successful, evolving system. In the words of the novelist Sebastian Faulks in his novel *Charlotte Gray*, 'A market is made at the price that someone will pay; to some extent you are what other people think you are.'[1] Portia tells us, too, in *The Merchant of Venice*:

> *The quality of mercy is not strained,*
> *It droppeth as the gentle rain from heaven*
> *Upon the place beneath: it is twice blessed;*
> *It blesseth him that gives and him that takes.*

In markets this is the best test of mutual satisfaction, for markets are the most reliable 'windows into men's souls'. Of course, no market can be made without prices. And price offers *an objective, non-political measure of subjective relative value*. It shows how much people value a thing, to whom they will voluntarily give the value accumulated in money, and on what grounds. Thus people's actions on both sides of the client/service line can be freely expressed with regard to the content of the service itself – and not with regard to some separate *political* goal such as equality of outcome.

William Blake told us to beware tigers. But does price take us into the jungle? I suggest not. One of the necessary co-pilots of individual financial empowerment is the recognition of the importance – *and desirability* – of prices. The moment price and price-conscious choice are mentioned many people bridle. In 1946, with Bevan's National Health Service Act, Britain made the error of eliminating price in most health services. It thus eliminated cost constraints on demand.

Promptly and unsurprisingly, however, Ministers found that they could not meet the apparently unlimited demand with sufficient supply. Worse still, with no transparent prices and thus no relative choices having to be made by consumers, the situation encouraged demands for 'rights'. Demand, too, was encouraged by providers ('producer–capture'). Impossible expectations have remained the result. Governments have responded by strictly rationing services by political means – delay, denial and dilution. In doing so, they have depressed innovation and investment. Ultimately they have reduced ambition. English politicians can claim – apparently triumphantly – that waiting lists are *only* 15 months, when there are *virtually none* in France or Germany. The system lowered the definition of what was an acceptable standard. Almost at once money problems threatened to overwhelm the system. The initial 1944 estimate of £132 million had reached £230 million by 1948, and the actual spend in 1949–50 was £305 million. And so it has gone on ever since, with allocative rationing being the fundamental pathology of the system.

However, there is no escape from affordability. Without price, any increase in funding will uncover new unmet demand. This will stretch the gap once more. Price is a signal and an incentive, or disincentive, in the unique discovery process of the market.

So, as I said at the beginning, one key question for *any* healthcare system is, where do you place price in the system? This is an absolutely fundamental question. Do you place it in the system as a general tax? Or at the point of entry into a legally enforceable health plan for the future, by compulsory insurance with some co-payment? Or at the point of use? We shall have to face this question. For price is the only known mechanism for matching demand with supply. And the only known mechanism for setting prices efficiently is a market. However, this idea does not necessarily mean payment for critical illness interventions (or for Accident and Emergency services) at the time of use, although it cannot exclude (save in dreamland) prepayment of some kind, either by taxation or by insurance.

We need to grow up, too, with regard to 'profit'. The issue concerning profit in healthcare is not that it must not exist. For even non-profit organisations must recover their costs, pay for their capital and invest for development. The issue concerning profit is not that we do not want it, but who gets it and why. In healthcare it should go to reward good providers, encourage investment, lower costs to consumers and improve services. 'Profit' (or surplus, if you like) is essential if we are to see investment and the survival of the best provider. Profit should be used for investment, the improvement of services to subscribers and the reduction of costs. We could notice, too, that those who can charge what the market will bear – demonstrating that they give customers satisfaction – have fewer money worries than those dependent on Government for tax allocations.

We should also appreciate that the only alternative to State care is not necessarily for-profit care. Indeed, much voluntary charitable and not-for-profit care is typical throughout Europe (and more so, too, in the USA than is commonly credited). The hospice movement in the UK is a powerful example. This also highlights the truth that public service is not only or necessarily delivered by organisations that are dominated by so-called 'public service trade unions'.

Price raises the issue of the ways in which 'local knowledge' is empowered. This captures those nuances which are difficult for individuals to articulate. Those 'I don't know why, but I just feel ...' points, which an individual should be able to register but which, as tastes and values differ so widely, are very difficult to capture and express as one 'public policy'. This is another reason why price is so helpful. It permits the expression of understandings which the individual may find it difficult to articulate. This frees the individual from having to devote their time to politics, to consultations and to giving 'good reasons why' (a middle-class attribute and way of seeing the world) for their choices to a 'citizens' jury' or an official. These 'public policy' models enforce a particular perspective on articulateness, and limit the information available to that which can be easily (and, in terms of the values and priorities of planners, convincingly) presented by the individual – or, more usually, by the pressure group and vested interest.[2]

These models also expect everyone to have the time and inclination to be active citizens. The former Labour leader Hugh Gaitskell said in 1955:

> *I get impatient with those who think that everybody must continually be taking an active part in politics or community affairs. The vast majority find their happiness in the family or personal relations, and why on earth shouldn't they?*[3]

Individual discretion about our own lives is helped by price, not hindered by its presence – provided that we beef up the purchasing power of the poor, the unlucky and the disadvantaged as I have proposed with patient fundholding. Price admits the complexities of individuals to a richer picture of the potentials that services could accommodate, given the fuller power of choice which is as yet unfulfilled.

Prices provide information about wants and relative values, and are the only way to discover the value at which goods will be exchanged. The alternative is to fix prices by central policy, which usually also means concealing them entirely – from staff, from patients, from voters. And this has been the case for most of the history of the NHS. This cuts us all off from this basic information. Scruton states this succinctly: 'however rational the planned economy may seem, it will never be reasonable, for it destroys the information without which it cannot respond coherently to changes caused by itself'.[4] This is one of the reasons why evolving, adaptive, responsive economies rely instead on price and on the web of economic and social connections through which its unique signals are gathered.

Instead of removing the local knowledge from the situation, it specifically locates it within the most local of all situations – the decision by the individual about what happens to their body. And from the individual expression of these local understandings, new ways of doing things can be prompted, new experiments tried, new ways to organise and improve services can be supported by the investment which follows the patient's individual decision.

We have much evidence of what happens when you pretend that there are no prices, or when you falsify prices (or costs). Subsidies falsify both costs and prices. Tax policies can falsify prices by deploying tariffs, and there are other ways to conceal or falsify honest costs, much of which concerns inappropriate Government manipulation. For most of its life the NHS has existed – like the Soviet system – with the costs of most of its production and services unknown to those delivering the services, and indeed often of no interest to them. Costs have only aggregated in central budgets. Hospital managers, doctors, nurses and those who committed funds literally did not know what the costs were of what they were doing. Endemic waste is one considerable consequence. Budgets have been allocations for expenses, confused by subsidy, and have borne little or no relation to costs or to consumer satisfaction.

The reforms of the early 1990s did something to open these boxes. But in any system where prices are fixed by political regulation, cost accounting is unreal. Where market feedback in cost-conscious choice does not exist, price cannot function creatively. Institutional falsification of prices has deluded many into thinking that there could not nor should not be price in healthcare decision making. Instead, political and 'population' analysis has taken the place of individual preference to command a specific, timely service. The Soviet economic system was but an extreme example of the marginalisation of costs, price and thus quality. Nationalised industry in the UK was another. Yet price is the vital feedback and guidance if anyone is to be able to know what they are doing well and what they are doing badly, and if the continuous, subtle, swift corrections in production and services that we desire are to occur.

It needs to be stressed that the lack of a hierarchy and a master-plan controlled by central Government does not imply dis-order. On the contrary. Price and its companion – competition – offer the infusion of energy which all systems need from outside themselves. Price also offers order. Not the order of hierarchical imposition, but the order that arises from evolution in the co-ordination of the factors of production. Price relates to one another those countless different enterprises and individuals in a non-hierarchical but nevertheless self-organised system. Price offers an objective, non-political measure of subjective relative value. It shows how much people value a thing, to whom they will voluntarily give the value accumulated in money, and on what grounds. Thus people's actions on both sides of the client/service line can be freely expressed with regard to the content of the service itself – and not with regard to some separate *political* goal such as equality of outcome. However, this is a perspective which many health service professionals find very difficult to countenance.

Hayek argued that, under capitalism, distribution is generally in accordance with perceived service to others. That is, what they are prepared to pay for. The major portion of efficient distribution in a free society does not come about through the action of Government, but through localised, individual exchanges and the cumulative power of personal choices.[5] The idea that this approach could be a positive gain in healthcare asks us to accept what comes out from a system which evolves in response to consumers' price-conscious wishes. It does so because of this pedigree of principles. This approach requires loyalty to an ongoing process without fixing *in advance* how it must come out, except to meet those principles of assured and just access which I have outlined, and which we will explore shortly. These principles, of course, concern fundamentals about our attitudes to ourselves and towards others. And they contradict the idea that we should require people to accord to a particular conception of 'fulfilled' humanity.

To build public support for this approach, we need to clarify what goes on when someone expresses a free and cost-conscious preference. And we need to realise how very different this is from when 'experts' second-guess what people ought to want, and why they find this so hard to do. The essence of free expression of this kind is that an exchange occurs in which each participant believes the transaction will benefit both, as it does. Neither necessarily loses. An exchange advantageously takes place which suits both sides. One good is transformed into another. In the case of the provider, a service is exchanged for revenues, which fund investment, while in turn the recipient obtains a desired service and hopefully (subject to the uncertainties of medicine itself) a preferred outcome. This is not a zero-sum game, although many working within the NHS assume that it must be so on the basis of theoretical preconceptions of how society and the individual *ought* to be. However, the introduction of price – I suggest at the point of entry into an insurance contract, but with some co-payment for minor services – is not exploitative. Indeed it is fulfilling.

What *is* exploitative, however, is the deliberate encouragement of a lack of understanding of the truths about economics, and the triggers which can genuinely empower the individual and improve care. A recent flagrant example of this deception was Chancellor of the Exchequer Gordon Brown's insistence to a national audience on the BBC Radio 4 programme *The World at One* on 20 March 2002 that the only kind of insurance to be discussed – and dismissed – is private insurance funded by tax relief to aid the rich. This takes no account of the variety of approaches which are possible and which are seen to be effective elsewhere (and which I shall explore). Mr Brown considered more carefully the continental approaches in his speech on 'Economic Stability and Strong Public Services' to the Social Market Foundation later that day, although he still sought to unbalance the debate by misrepresenting the position of access to services by the poor under European funding systems. He also did this in his recent *Sunday Times* 'op.-ed.' piece on 24 March 2002, stating that 'Taxes are the best way to pay for the NHS'. He did so again in a speech to a debate organised by Unison, drawing attention to the problems of the US system, which no one in the UK has proposed as the basis for reform in the UK, as well as dismissing social insurance, whose investment pattern he distorted.[6]

Mr Brown has otherwise gone out of his way to stress that New Labour is creating an environment in which enterprise can flourish. He made the competition authorities independent of political control. He has recently announced new tax measures to help business, and parts of the new Enterprise bill are positive for business. He has allocated £60 million to a scheme to introduce children as young as 4 years to the virtues of business and enterprise. He is said to have been much impressed by the success of the Young Enterprise charity, which seeks to inspire and equip the young to learn and achieve success through enterprise. He has insisted that Labour has to be the real party of enterprise: 'the priority for our second term, based on fiscal discipline and tough choices to maintain economic stability, is to foster a new culture of enterprise, which is pro-competition and anti-corporatism'. However, his ideas concerning the funding and management of the NHS contradict this view of a radical pro-enterprise and pro-competition agenda which does not protect vested interests or stifle economic dynamism.[7]

Incentive is an aspect of price, and the essential ingredient in the optimal use of the scarcest resources. These are human capital, skills, cultivated human potentials, information, commitment and experience. They are the most important qualitative elements in provision. To release these successfully, the regulated market *environment* is one that must be realised *first* if progress is to be made in improving healthcare. Here the necessary trade-offs will be made by the self-responsible individual. But the market pre-conditions must be constructed before this can work.

Is this just another Utopia? No. It is not. Nor should we want to impose any kind of Utopian vision. We want the very opposite. We seek the evolution of the unexpected. This values the *filter device* of experience, rather than the *design device* of ideology. It privileges the novelist's description of the realities of diverse human desires, aspirations, talents, preferences, values, valuations and intertwined relationships, by contrast to the imposed design of the social scientist and the Utopian thinker.

Given that we all differ about values, it is obvious that a diverse range of opportunities will enable more people – all very different and complex – to come closer to how they wish to live than if there is one monopoly structure. This approach, of course, depends on us accepting the moral arguments for individual liberty, which are well rehearsed by Mill and others. And it relies on extreme suspicion of the idea that there is one best society for everyone to live in, one monopoly structure which is right for us all, and that we (or an 'expert' planner) can know what that might be.

Here, my assumption is that reason, knowledge and determination make it possible for human beings to circumvent the difficulties and resolve the conflicts in modern healthcare – that is, that private concerns and public action can coincide.

Some analysts stress 'the freedom from payment' which was achieved by the establishment of the NHS in 1948.[8] But was this a freedom, or the loss of liberty? An advantage, or an imposition? I suggest that it is the illusion of 'free' care itself which has had long-term damaging effects, and which today is a major force in making it so difficult for politicians to offer arguments to make a persuasive case to change the structure of funding and of provision. Instead of abolishing price – with the inevitable loss of the key signals it uniquely offers – the right course would have been to beef up demand, by ensuring that the poor, the disadvantaged and the unlucky would instead enjoy the buying power that the middle classes have always had.

No other country has copied the NHS. If we made the right decision concerning price and the provision of monopoly services in 1948, every other country must have made the wrong decision. But the Organisation for Economic Co-operation and Development data on 29 countries, including our nearest neighbours, show that they have much better results to show for their errors. And where people in Europe have been left free to spend more of their own income on health services (or on other goods and services, as they wish), they have chosen to spend more on health services than the Treasury has allowed in the UK.

Why is it a problem if costs rise, if this reflects the self-responsible choice of the individual who is prepared to pay for additional services? Government does not discipline our expenditure on food, which is the most fundamental of all, or on housing, holidays, clothing or other leisure items and activities. Why should it do so on healthcare, if people wish to consume more of it and are willing to pay to do so?[9]

A better course than abolishing the customer and prices would have been to beef up purchasing power, especially among the poor. That is, if what we want is to enable individuals *in reality* to get better care, rather than to dream and demand this in the abstract, and in terms of an ideology concerning political structures. This is particularly so for the poor, who have done least well from a priceless system. One of the fundamental tests of any health system is whether policy improves the standard of care and access for the poorest in society. Indeed, in the UK this is commonly accepted as one definition of social justice – of the kind of society in which most people apparently prefer to live. There is not much sympathy for an unpatterned distribution of healthcare benefits, or a distribution that is perceived as unjust. People want society to look, feel and *be* just. However, the issue, as Nozick says, is 'must the look of justice reside in a resulting pattern rather than in the underlying generating principles?'[10] My own belief is that we should seek a system based in principle, which secures a guaranteed minimum level of care for all, but that justice does not require us to seek to achieve the impossible – that is, of a specific pattern which somehow seeks to deliver equality of care (outcome?) rather than equality of access.

There is, too, the question of whether care can in any sense be 'free'. There is a real sense in which people have voted themselves poor healthcare, by clinging to the idea that it can somehow be 'free'. We are the creators of the limitations of the organisation that we have formed. In this sense, time has opened rather than healed wounds – for example, for those cancer patients who would still have been living if they had been treated differently, as European evidence suggests they could have been.[11] And there is now no compensation that can be offered for the losses, risk and insecurity experienced by so many as a direct result of this public wrong (or Government failure, as opposed to market failure) and misdirected activity. Yet many have been worse off than they otherwise would have been, if European evidence is any guide. This is probably true not only of the poor, but also of the middle class – even though they have done relatively better than the poor, they have done less well than their European counterparts.

Services paid for by taxes are not free. John Marenbon has pointed out that this money is, indeed, our own.[12] We are taxed so that we can be offered a service by the State in and on its terms. Umberto Eco says that 'the fundamental question of philosophy (like that of psychoanalysis) is the same as the question of the detective novel: who is guilty?'[13] The answer is, of course, that we all are so. We have robbed ourselves of our self-reliance. We have set aside our ability to learn to choose in this vital area of our lives. We have stolen from ourselves, by self-deception, our own potential common wealth. To this extent the NHS was not a good idea that went awry, but a bad idea that prevented us getting access to the benefits of demand-led care. However, this does not stop even Conservative commentators accepting that the NHS was formerly a world-beating British institution.[14] On the evidence of the results, this seems doubtful in the extreme.

So we can see that it is an error on several grounds to falsify or conceal price, or to pretend that price does not exist and/or is unnecessary. Services have to come from somewhere, and they involve the actions of individuals who have an entitlement over those actions. They bring costs with them, too. Meanwhile, the social costs of this error concerning the suppression of price are borne by patients – because of the provision of poorer services than there might be, because of the lost investment in new technologies, because of the deficits in new opportunities and the diffusion of innovation, and because of less efficient performance than is otherwise possible. And the costs are also borne by staff, who have had less opportunity than they might have had to exercise their talents and capacities, to face challenges, to take independent initiatives, to enjoy self-direction, to feel the greater value of their work, to understand and play a greater role in the achievement of individual and common goals, and to be properly rewarded, both psychologically and financially, for dedication and competence.

Earnings have been relatively depressed because there is no open expression of value. One result is the problem of affordable housing, recruitment and retention in public services, particularly in the south east. Working conditions are also unnecessarily pressurised and much of the environment is threadbare.

We come then to the value of trade, which price reflects and permits as service users signal their wishes. No magic wand has been found by which politics – centralised or decentralised – can enable an individual to signal their wishes. The economist Jane Jacobs reminds us that Old English had a verb meaning 'to trade', which meant literally 'to give with worth' – that is, to give for a price. 'Our word *sell* comes from a truncated portion of that phrase for trading, the part literally meaning "give"', as she says.[15] Price differentiates trading from sharing and seizing, and separates a service from politics. Price is crucial to constructing a credible answer to the problems of modern healthcare. Trading has been a prolific source of economic differentiations in transport, communication, finance, markets, contracts, ownership and liabilities, co-operation and long-distance relationships with strangers. These have carried civilisation forward *from* the jungle, rather than plunging us into its darkness. The power of trial-and-error evolution, of a creative process which yields benefits from the work of economically creative people, has been positive in encouraging new provision, higher standards and greater diversity. It has been done by evolution, in response to priced choices. As Jacobs says:

> *Economic development isn't a matter of imitating nature. Rather, economic development is a matter of using the same universal principles that the rest of nature uses. The alternative isn't to develop some other way. Some other way doesn't exist.... Economic development is a version of natural development.*[16]

Development (and diversity) concerns qualitative change. Expansion concerns quantitative change. They are inter-linked. The practical link is price. The several consequences include diversity, and services evolving in response to the expression of consumer wishes.

But is this merely a right-wing rant? Consider what Karl Marx wrote: 'For the labour spent on them (commodities) counts effectively only insofar as it is spent in a form that is useful to others.' And 'Whether that labour is useful for others, and its product consequently capable of satisfying the wants of others, can be proved only by the act of exchange.' *By the act of exchange* – which means prices and markets. That is, that the measure of what is socially necessary, and how much it is, is determined by what happens in the *competitive marketplace*! And this is the only place where prices can be set, signalled and discovered. Crucially, too, it is in the marketplace that the financially empowered individual – including the vulnerable and the disadvantaged – can make the greatest gains. Indeed, this point will have to be made especially powerfully and persuasively by those advocating change in the NHS as a means of assisting the disadvantaged.[17]

In the wider economy of our daily lives we all know that individual payment, in a priced system, offers the most persuasive feedback about whether a service is wanted or not, whether it meets the wishes of service users, which providers will flourish and which will fade away. Price corrects imbalances between supply and demand, by triggering changes in provision. It encourages a closer correspondence between wishes and wares, through a process of continual adjustment. This is something which politics cannot achieve so effectively.

Some modern Marxist theorists understand this well. For example, Ernest Mandel has written:

> *It is precisely through competition that it is discovered whether the amount of labor embodied in a commodity constitutes a socially necessary amount or not.... When the supply of a certain commodity exceeds the demand for it, that means that more human labor has been spent altogether on producing this commodity than was socially necessary at the given period.... When, however, supply is less than demand, that means that less human labor has been expended on producing the commodity in question than was socially necessary.*

We thus have some initial guidance – and from sources that those opposed to markets recognise – on what the word 'price' means, and what its expression – *payment* – represents.[18]

In the NHS, however, there remains a third-party payer structure. Patients look to the Government (the taxpayer) to pay for their healthcare. Oddly, both Government and patient, treat this money as the Government's, by contrast with individual funds that are voluntarily subscribed to social insurance schemes on the continent where the money is considered (by the patient and by Government and providers) to be the patient's, who then secures a legally enforceable contract for services. The UK structure, by contrast, relies on disempowering, hierarchical assumptions about who should control resources, in a system of 'public ownership'. The individual pays the taxes but does not in fact control resources, despite being one of millions of 'owners'. There is, too, in this system the tendency of individuals to pass responsibility to others. You can pursue an unhealthy lifestyle and pass the bills to others – although, of course, you ultimately may pay the worst bill of all, which is early death or a long period of painful chronic illness.

The third-party payer approach is another example of how the suppression of price limits the responsibility of the individual. This approach carries with it, too, a specific assumption about the competence and responsibility of the individual, about property and ownership, about the right to control resources, and about who should make which decisions, and on what grounds.

The provision of 'free' healthcare has also misled people so that they have no idea what good services cost. Meanwhile, with regard to price, Government pays – but with our money. This does not mean that services are 'free'.

However, competition would provide better benefits for all. And the resulting prices would be lower than the highest price that the recipient would be willing to pay. This price, as we have seen, cannot be discovered except by free negotiation. 'Expert' selection to determine who will receive which benefit and who will be denied a benefit is neither a morally nor an operationally efficient substitute for the signal which price represents as the full payback for benefits delivered and the full receipt of benefits received.

The alternative is some great system – some imposed political and social ordering – such as the NHS. This exists in part to achieve political purposes which have nothing to do with healthcare. Notably, the attempt to use State power to respond politically to the cumulative and historical distribution of income and wealth which has arisen over time. Thus, the attitude that people should not be able to use their own resources to buy more healthcare than the treasury determines they should have. Yet such accumulations of capital have been the result in part of natural talents and abilities and their *development* over time. And society develops when people work to develop themselves and their talents. It is a characteristic of theories which embody a presumption in favour of political equality (often rooted in envy, among other emotions) that the contribution of individual effort to development is disregarded. This attitude itself helps to block support for the expression of a person's autonomous choices and actions. It does so in part because such prejudices attribute much that is individual about the person to external, prior factors and social circumstances such as inheritance, which it wishes to nullify. Curiously, this denial of a person's autonomy and prime responsibility for their actions arises from a theory (Marxism) that apparently emphasises human dignity.

The majority of developed countries have social insurance schemes which guarantee access for all. They combine this with some kind of price mechanism which permits choice to influence the flow of funds. They pay more, but they get more. They are expected to exercise personal responsibility. Voluntary and not-for-profit provision predominates. Tax and insurance collected is specifically guaranteed as health expenditure. There is an important link between behaviour and consequences. In France and in Germany, for example, standards seem higher. There is equality of access. Everyone is covered. Treatment is prompt. Costs are generally lower than ours. There is solidarity, cohesion, differentiation and ethical competition. The UK, however, is unusual in its dependence on public provision.

Notes

1 Faulks S (1998) *Charlotte Gray*; Vintage ed., 1999, p.424.
2 For the wider results, see Olson M (1982) *The Rise and Decline of Nations. Economic growth, stagflation, and social rigidities.* Yale University Press, New Haven, CT.
3 Quoted by Williams P (1979) *Hugh Gaitskell: a political biography.* J Cape, London. However, Gaitskell thought that the minority who were interested in being activists should get on with the job, a sentiment with which I demur.
4 Scruton R (2000) *England, A Eulogy.* Chatto & Windus, London, p.180; Friedman M (1962) *Capitalisation and Freedom.* Chicago University Press, Chicago, 1962; revised edition, 1982, p.25.
5 Hayek FA (1960) *The Constitution of Liberty.* Chicago University Press, Chicago.
6 Interview with James Naughtie and Gordon Brown on the *Today* programme on BBC Radio 4, on 20 March 2002. Brown G (2002) Labour has to be the real party of enterprise. *The Times.* **8 March**. Webster P (2002) Taxation is only course prescribed by Brown. *The Times.* **21 March**. Brown G (2002) Taxes are the best way to pay for the NHS. *Sunday Times (news section).* **24 March**. See also Wanless D (2001) *Securing Our Future Health. Taking a long-term view. Interim Report.* Health Trends Team, London, and among much press comment, the following articles: Webster P and Paterson L (2001) Brown will raise taxes to revive the NHS. *The Times.* **28 November**; Kaletsky A (2001) Confident strategy may yet come unstuck. *The Times.* **28 November**; Sylvester R (2001) Health may prove more explosive than row over Euro [and] How Brown got the answer he wanted on the NHS. *Daily Telegraph.* **29 November**; First leader (2001) Within Wanless. The report is more like a charge sheet than a whitewash. *The Times.* **29 November**; Leader (2001) An expensive prescription. *Daily Telegraph.* **29 November**; McSmith A (2001) Value for money NHS dismissed as 'fantasy'. *Daily Telegraph.* **30 November**; Sylvester R (2001) Wanless denies rejecting other forms of health service finance. *Daily Telegraph.* **30 November**; Baldwin T and O'Leary J (2001) Brown forces Blair to retreat on NHS. *The Times.* **3 December**; Leader (2001) Unhealthy taxes. *Sunday Times.* **2 December**; Webster P (2001) Milburn protests over Brown. *The Times.* **4 December**; Kellner P (2001) Taxing question for Brown on NHS cash. *Evening Standard.* **17 December**; Field F (2002) The great Labour tax con. *The Spectator.* **2 March**. Mr Brown's statement is given in full online at www.thetimes.co.uk/prebudget and edited in 'The Chancellor's speech. Decisive action in uncertain times' and first leader 'Brown's battleground. A political strategy behind an economic statement', both published in 2001 in *The Times.* **28 November**; Brown G (2002) A question of values as well as health. *The Independent.* **26 April**.

7   Smith D and Cracknell D (2002) Brown gives millions to school entrepreneurs. *Sunday Times.* **7 July**: 2.

8   Anderson W and Gillam S (2001) The elusive NHS consumer: 1948 to the NHS Plan. *Econ Affairs.* **21**: 14–18.

9   Dearlove J and Saunders P (1991) *Introduction to British Politics. Analysing a Capitalist Democracy.* Politz Press, Cambridge; second revised edition.

10 Nozick R (1974) *Anarchy, State and Utopia.* Basil Blackwell, Oxford, pp.158–9.

11 World Health Organization (1999) *Eurocare 2 Report.* World Health Organization, Geneva. Sikora K (2002) It's not just cash, we must have a revolution in thinking. *Observer.* **3 March**. Browne A (2002) Deadly rise in wait for cancer care [and] How thousands of cancer patients and doctors have been betrayed. *Observer.* **3 March**. Rumbelow H (2002) Cancer patients 'wait eight months for treatment'. *The Times.* **4 March**. See also World Health Organization (2002) *National Cancer Control Programmes: policies and managerial guidelines.* World Health Organization, Geneva.

12 Letwin O and Marenbon J (1999) *Civilised Conservation [and] Little Platoons or a Free Society.* Politiea, London, p.34.

13 Eco U (1985) *Reflections on the Name of the Rose* (trans. W Weaver). Martin Secker & Warburg, London, p.54.

14 Virginia Bottomley often said this when she was Secretary of State for Health (April 1992–July 1995). See Bottomley V (1995) *Lessons, Challenges and Opportunities of Health Reform.* Lecture given at Harvard Medical School on 31 May 1995, and published as a booklet by the NHS Executive, Leeds. But for a contrasting impression, see Hughes-Onslow J (2002) French break. *Spectator.* **3 August**: 22.

15 Jacobs J (2000) *The Nature of Economies.* Modern Library, New York, p.27.

16 Jacobs, ibid., p.31.

17 Marx K (no date given) *Das Capital*, vol.1. Modern Library, New York, pp.97–8. Quoted by Nozick, op. cit., pp.259–60.

18 Mandel E (1969) *Marxist Economic Theory*, vol.1. Monthly Review Press, New York, p.161. Quoted by Nozick, ibid., p.349.

Chapter 21

Getting it done 1

Patient guaranteed care – the patient fundholder
– social insurance – co-operative buying –
patient-guaranteed care providers – the impact of patient guaranteed
care on general practice and on hospitals.

... whether we do little or much we are sure to discontent everybody ... and we had better satisfy our consciences by doing what is just and right between the contending parties.

(Lord Clarendon)

We have seen the governing axioms and outlined an institutional framework for their realisation. But *the thing still has to be done.* It not only has to be made to *happen*. It has to be made to *work*. This then requires something particular in the process – something beyond 'leadership', something beyond the dramatic political expression of the popular will represented in one political figure or another, or one vote or another. This something, as I have argued, is a revolution in thinking. It is not all about money – as limiting the intrusion of medicalisation and enhancing self-reliance exemplify. However, we do need specific economic devices for change, in the hands of the patient. Crucially, the individual has to have economic power. And the individual member of staff has to want to achieve changes, and to focus their own attention on changing how *they* do things.

This shift requires the liberating force of both imagination and competition. It is a revolution both in thinking and in approaches. Incentive *and* invention.

I have proposed a new structure of institutions, focused on *patient-guaranteed care* – a guaranteed core of PGC, or *pretty good care*. The emphasis is on the guarantee of the core package of care for all, on competitive insurance, purchasing and provision – and with the *patient* sovereign as *fundholder*.

Patient-guaranteed care

Government will guarantee that everyone can purchase a core package of care.

There will be a State guarantee of universal access for all, irrespective of class, income, parentage, ethnic origin and previous history. The coverage will be set at a high level – certainly at a higher level than the present generality of NHS services, and much more like the coverage expected in major European countries.

This proposal pivots on legally enforceable and guaranteed access for all, using a tax credit to buy social insurance which will cover the costs. It will give security, affirm, safeguard, promise and secure the core package of *patient-guaranteed care*. Here Government would clarify – in a wide public debate – what it can realistically fund, and what will not be included. This will remove uncertainty and provide incentives for people to make further financial provision for themselves when they are able to do so.

An independent Commission with a lay chairman and a board of predominantly lay voices would ensure that Government may not change the rules to permit the exclusion of the poor, and that insurers, purchasers and providers must be registered with it. This is an unavoidably interventionist initiative, but it would be at arm's length from Ministers and subject to challenge in the courts.

Ruth Lea's Institute of Directors study and the Centre for Policy Studies pamphlet by Lord Blackwell and Daniel Kruger[1] rehearse the difficulties of selecting and endorsing a package. What is in and what is out? And how to decide? Every patient group will want to shift the axis, and every professional will want to have a pennyworth. The guarantee should include primary care, hospital care and surgical expenses, elderly care for the frail and dependent, mental healthcare, Accident and Emergency care, and access to modern drugs.

Coverage would be for primary and acute care. The emphasis would be on choices concerning efficient, effective, compassionate care. Health and social care would be part of one system. There are essentials which must either be included in the core package or provided by supplementary personal insurance, for which tax incentives and imaginative 'financial products' must be developed. These essentials include residential and personal care, nursing care, dementia care and specialist care. For example, such care is needed for diseases like Parkinson's disease – for which most patients with the disease have no regular contact at present with a consultant specialist – or Huntington's disease – for which patients require specially trained staff and adapted facilities, respite care, convalescent and postoperative care, hospice, palliative and terminal care. Active and compassionate care would be directed towards improving the quality of remaining life. Hospital care and drugs, which are often the high-cost items, would always be covered. So too would mental healthcare. Dentistry could be included, and separately remodelled in one market, with vouchers for the poor along the lines of recent reform in the optical market.

There would be some distinctions depending on income. Where people can afford to pay more for themselves, they would be expected to do so. Those who could not would not be asked to do so. In elderly care, where at present the worst off 70% of the population are paid for by the State, the State would continue to pay. For the poor, cover would include major and minor expenses. For others, additional expenses beyond the 'core' package would be met out of supplementary insurance or cash in pocket. For minor expenses, consumers would negotiate an 'excess' when agreeing their insurance premium with a patient-guaranteed care insurer.

The list of the core contents certainly begs as many questions as it answers. There will be many borderline arguments and costly mainstream innovations to consider, especially with regard to new cancer drugs. However, a phrase such as 'necessary care' is not dynamite with a short fuse. For the UK tradition is to test cases in the courts, to ensure that justice is done in particular cases, and to test abstract principles in this way so that they gain authority. Thus rules will arise from cases, by development and not by prior design. So we need not be fearful that a phrase like 'patient-centred decisions' is an invitation to meet the patient's family at the High Court. Choices here will, of course, be difficult, but cases tried in law will prove to be a more flexible approach than a 'definitive' Act of Parliament. Indeed we should welcome these tests which examine the boundaries and verges of decisions as a reflection of a dynamist, open approach to choices. This process is itself healing, and it protects freedom, reinforces duty and gives rights roots.

The case of Miss B, tried by Dame Butler-Sloss, makes this point. That case also demonstrated that this dynamist process can of course never diminish the necessary costs of choices, all of which involve losses and gains, trade-offs and compromises. This is Berlin's 'incommensurables' again – you cannot have everything, but who is to decide what you cannot have? This will be a permanent revisionary process, and it will never be beyond cultural, social, political and personal dispute. This is itself a process of discovery, which is superior to stasism and diktat.

The promise of an autonomous, non-political instrument of relief to the injured subject from a judge above politics and power is an individual solace and a national comfort, with the potential for the individual to petition to correct perceived wrongs, and thus for society to moderate conflict by peaceful resolution, and to grant relief to the individual in the event of the abuse of powers by institutions or managers. As Scruton argues, English law is 'the common property of the subject, rather than the private possession of the sovereign power'. And it is concerned both with duties and rights.[2] But I think we need, too, a cluster of explicit promises which the public will recognise as comprising what I shall call PGC – *pretty good care* or *patient-guaranteed care*. This is what Government must ensure is delivered, and which the courts would reinforce via the law of contract which will bind Government as well as insurers, purchasers and providers (and patients).

PGC reflects the truth that to be persuasive in a democracy we must begin with absolute reassurance. We must use language which draws on the loyalty to the NHS despite its faults, and use a vocabulary which captures the idea that Government will guarantee cover and provision of all necessary care. It is fundamental to reassure people that they will continue to receive good care. And especially that the poor and disadvantaged will do better. We hear a lot of talk about achieving 'optimal care'. But what is that? It is subjective. However, we need to establish a core of guaranteed services. We need a debate about who will specify this 'needed care' and how this will be done. It is controversial territory – because there seems to be no way in which an 'adequate service' can be objectively defined, as the Viagra debate demonstrated. Every modern new drug will raise the same spectre.

At present the services offered and the standards achieved by the NHS – with no agreed package or guarantee – are politically determined. The guaranteed package will itself ultimately be politically determined too, and so we must debate an agreed definition of what this package would be if the solidarity principle is to be maintained. Those who require additional benefits will have that choice, but they will be expected to have access to these by supplementary insurance or from cash out of pocket. This works well in Switzerland, where patients have the legal incentive to add further investment if they so wish. Tax incentives are the answer here. And if it is legal, there is no bar to such additional consumption of healthcare services.

We need to examine overseas experience of defining a package. For example, since 1971 Canada has defined and used a health insurance plan covering all necessary medical and hospital services, without financial barriers to utilisation. It must be clearly defined what benefits the package includes and excludes, and what must be covered by supplementary insurance.[3] Social insurance, complemented with co-payment and private supplementary insurance – and with tax transfers to the poor – can ensure access to quality care for all, and we need explicit and specific studies of how this can work within the UK culture.

Over and above the core package, competing providers will make other offers to consumers. Then, as Dr DS Lees has said:

> *In a market there would be numerous and competing standards, as there are for other commodities, reflecting individual incomes, choice and other circumstances. The fundamental weakness of a single standard is that there is nothing to compare it with. Progress to better standards is impeded and a range of possible choices is closed.*[4]

Individual financial leverage will encourage a greater variety of services, as there are in the essential markets of food, shelter and clothing. And people will be enabled to spend rising incomes on more consumption of healthcare. Once the guarantee of good care for all is in place, we should not deny anyone the opportunity to consume more healthcare if they wish to spend their own money on this – rather than on other forms of consumption such as second or third holidays, new cars, hi-tech equipment, alcohol, further education, and so on. It also seems likely that many people will want to spend more on healthcare than seems possible in a system which is over-reliant on a limited funding base dependent on taxation, and which denies them information.

Patient-guaranteed social insurance

The requirement for insurers and purchasers will be that they must accept any applicant. There will be open enrolment and community rating of basic premiums, so that all members of the community would pay the same and receive the Government's guaranteed package of services. The State would specify that there will be no exclusions for pre-existing conditions, no selection of subscribers to avoid those likely to make significant claims, and no 'adverse' selection. Alternatively, insurers would be free to compete on these issues. However, it will probably be politically necessary to impose a framework.

Every individual will be protected by compulsory social insurance, guaranteed by the State. In addition, there will be a diversity of additional and optional funding arrangements, including extras insurance and cash top-ups for additional services. The evident and considerable willingness of individuals (including large numbers of trade unionists) to pay for satisfying services – evidenced by many paying by private medical insurance, in health cash schemes like Medicash and HAS, in co-operatives like BUPA, in self-funded surgery, over-the-counter medicines and alternative therapies – tells us something important which we need to re-integrate into the basic framework of the health system.

We would all be covered by an 'NHS credit' from general taxation, including the poor. This would fund the core package, with competing insurers offering competing policies and alternative premium packages. The insurance will be a per capita figure, and will be based on the core package of guaranteed care.[5] There will be 'catastrophic cover' within the basic insurance, or as a special ring-fenced additional compulsory insurance. This would probably have to be compulsory on the individual to insure, with the requirement on all registered insurers and purchasers to accept any applicant for catastrophic cover. Government will manage a pool mechanism to ensure that lower-income, higher-risk groups are not disadvantaged, and that risks are fully covered. Libertarians, of course, have difficulty with compulsion. I appreciate this concern. However, Mill believed that Government might resort to compulsory universal insurance (although he doubted its expediency: he also favoured compulsory – but not state – education).[6] Politically, it may be necessary to compel in order to persuade the voter to endorse a new system. I appreciate the argument that this paternalist compulsion violates the rights of the individual, that it is geared to nullify supposed defects in people's decision-making processes, and that it exceeds the range of the minimal State for which Nozick (notably in recent years) has argued. It is a genuine quandary.

This returns us to the discussion of price and cost. For the only real test of the relative value that people put on consumption of healthcare, and of their willingness to pay more for health services, comes from how they respond to price. An explicit understanding of price and costs – prompted by an element of co-payment in all transactions, with the poor receiving exemptions – will be one consequence of this new structure. It will offer as much incentive as possible to prompt individuals to influence the cash-flow (and cash-ebb) of insurers, purchasers and providers – directly rewarding the preferred supplier. This, in contrast to the present global Treasury funding mechanisms. This approach has the dual benefit of encouraging self-responsibility and also encouraging the demanding, insistent customer who wants quality and a good outcome, who knows who is paying the bills, and who has an awareness of value for money. As Enthoven has pointed out, too, the price that counts is not the cost of a specific procedure, but the annual insurance premium, with a compulsory co-payment excess or deductible (as in car insurance) which encourages consumers to think about total costs and seek to minimise them.[7]

This excess could be negotiated within a statutory band, to enable individuals to bargain concerning premiums and concerning partial costs which they agree to bear as a co-payment – in theory as a deterrent to maximising consumption after paying the insurance premium. (The problem of 'moral hazard' discussed by health economists.) Co-payment may not be popular. But it would encourage people to make price comparisons when they matter – that is, at the time when the consumer bargains and subscribes initially. The essential of cost control is thus achieved not by exclusions, as people often fear, but by management managing costs, including direct financial incentives to consumers to do so, too.

The policy objective in funding (as with diversity of provision) should be an increasing convergence and collaboration between the public and the private funding systems. The two must function alongside one another, to fund access to quality care and to sustain a demand-led system. If we cannot rely on taxation alone – if we should not do so on moral grounds – a broader funding base is necessary if we are to maintain public services and to improve them.

A diverse funding base would correct the extraordinary disparity in the UK between public and private funding, which has so restricted capacity, access and outcomes due to the UK depending on funding by taxation almost in its entirety. The NHS is 80% funded by general taxation, which has meant very significant under-funding by comparison with other more successful systems with a mixed funding base, including user charges, social insurance (e.g in the French or German model) and additional optional supplementary private insurance. Those who wish to opt out entirely from any calls on public provision would have to make entirely private health insurance provision. The level of funding would be based on sound actuarial rules, current knowledge of funding levels in existing European systems, and a national pool of risk.

We would expect the market to evolve in response to consumer's wishes, and to provide innovative ways to provide cover. As Dr Philip Booth has pointed out, 'In particular, we would expect innovative ways of mixing primary care, hospital-based care and preventative medicine to develop in the private sector. The private sector has a long-term interest in reducing healthcare costs by providing proper preventative primary care and advice. The nationalised service has no such incentive (hence its development of what is often called a "sickness service").'

Dr Booth urged a rebate system of financing choice, and his comments are directly relevant to my own proposal: 'It is important for the Government to be protected from the risk that individuals may be under-insured and therefore not be able to obtain the healthcare that they need through the private insurer. However, at the same time, it is important that the market is allowed to develop appropriate risk-sharing arrangements with the insured in order to reduce overall costs by reducing moral hazard. Minimum contract standards would need to be defined. However, there would be complete freedom for consumers to "migrate up the menu" of choices available and obtain better services without the double payment that is required at the moment.'[8]

Patient fundholding

Each individual will hold a personal fund sufficient to buy social insurance which will cover and secure the core package of guaranteed care, with the poor placed by law on the same basis as the better off through tax transfers to their personal and inalienable fund. However, there should be direct incentives to encourage individuals to be sensitive to price – for example, for a significant proportion of unspent funds to be carried forward into an individual's long-term care insurance. Or, as in Singapore, for the fund to be an equity, and also inheritable.

There will be a fund specified for every individual with which to purchase social insurance. This is the indispensable lever to unlock the potentials of the entire system and of us all. User empowerment to command a specific service turns on giving individuals command over a personal care fund. By expressing *costed* preferences, *financially empowered* individuals test out specific adaptations against *competition*. And it is by the expression of preferences that successful and timely adaptations spread because their possessors spread, or are emulated in timely fashion. You are not a customer unless you pay. You have a direct impact on the lives and incomes of managers and professionals if you can go round the corner with your money to another provider.

Patient fundholding is thus the key driver – the vital step to make it clear who is in control, while maintaining social solidarity and the 'pool' concepts of insurance and guaranteed cover. Greater and more diverse provision cannot occur until there are more revenues and individual choice. Providers will only seek revenues and insist on freedoms to do so, and they will only manage assets in the interests of users, when patients control the funding.

The fund will be portable throughout the UK. The dependent will thus have all of the benefits of the independent, and the working class will be enabled to attain the standards expected by many in the middle class, when they are using their own money (and when they don't, but still insist upon and receive better care by the NHS).

This approach also places *consequences* in the forefront of responsibility. An important element in an effective working system is a wider awareness among service users of affordability, costs and the necessary price and benefits (not only financial, but also in terms of personal effort) of good care.

The closest we have come to moving decision making close to the patient was with general practice fundholding in the reforms of the early and mid-1990s.

General practice fundholding was indeed the most useful testing ground for the argument. This showed that money talks and preference walks. Patients had *more* influence. But they did not have *the ultimate say*. We were close, here, to making the next move. This was to give the individual patient the control of money. However, this opportunity was lost, and it is not now being rediscovered by the transfer of budgets into 320 large primary care trusts. These control massive budgets, but there is no more individual patient leverage. There is much talk of placing decisions 'closer to the patient'. There is nothing closer than holding the money – as a social insurance NHS credit, a Health Passport, a voucher, or crispy notes.

With GP fundholding the doctor had to look the patient in the eye in the consulting room. Both knew that the doctor controlled the money. There was often a long-term relationship between patient and doctor. This was a very different relationship to that of District Health Authorities placing contracts on behalf of local 'populations'. There were many individual doctor–patient discussions about risks, benefits, choices, possible outcomes and what the patient would like to happen next. Many services woke up under the pressure of GP fundholding, when doctors shifted contracts, insisted upon access or else, and demurred from having a patient seen by a particular consultant.[9]

Even though there were no measures of outcomes, service quality or of patient satisfaction, this initiative began to change perceptions within and outside the neighbourhood of the practice. It offered a potential model to achieve feedback and adaptation in an open-ended future. To this extent – although unfulfilled – it offered an optimistic model compared with the controlling, hierarchical and static ideas of centralism, suspicious of change.

The innovation of patient fundholding will also acknowledge that in a pluralist society there is no one right way to live. If we are to enable individuals to choose how they will live, we need to find ways to make differences between people count and be legitimate. Healthcare systems must privilege this approach if they are to deliver access to high-quality care for all. We need to support people to articulate their differences legitimately in ways that they understand and by which they can directly influence personal service, while also influencing for the better services that can be secured by others. Individuals need to expect to be capable of drawing distinctions, making personal assessments, and differentially and legitimately acting upon them. None of us do so without advice, and there is every prospect of this being available to us. So we can seek the justice of access to good care for all without seeking to impose one way of living, by the protection of individual choice for its own sake.

It is patient fundholding which will offer 'ordinary' people a genuine pathway to optimal care, and to preventive care.

Patients need direct incentives. First, there will be the regular review of the individual insurance contract, and of the basic 'excess' to influence the premium and thus behaviour. Secondly, in terms of preventive care, there will be the potential of a loading charge for lack of participation in an agreed health-improvement programme – a principle that is understood by every motorist. It is in the insurer's interest to pay bonuses to reduce future costs, too, and it should be in the patient's interest to reduce premiums.

The act of the patient fundholder voluntarily selecting a purchaser from among competing co-operatives will be a very significant change. For it will underline the rediscovery of the notion of acting independently of the State, on behalf of one's family and oneself. The alternative to being paternalistically regulated is to contract independently with a co-operative purchasing organisation – even when this itself involves limitations on one's own behaviour when appointing a supervisory body over oneself. Here each individual would be on a par with others, each an equal in the endeavour, having an equal say with the others. Co-ordinated and self-organised actions in co-operative purchasing, for example, would achieve certain results without any violation of the rights of others.

A central aspect of this approach to purchasing is the ability voluntarily to join (and leave) a purchaser. The purchaser should thus be seen as *a community* which must win and hold the voluntary adherence of its members. This also demonstrates the general virtues of filter processes (in markets) over design devices (such as the centrally controlled NHS triple monopoly). The re-adoption of mutual-aid is itself an example of the argument – for evolution enables us to reconsider and retry old ideas in new conditions. This approach empowers consumers because each person's contribution will have a separate effect as well as a cumulative one. And the mobility of the individual fund will ensure that the subscriber has the choice of staying or going to another competing purchaser. Thus each of us would be enabled voluntarily to join organisations with which we want to be associated. And this approach minimises the 'free rider' problem, as each individual's fund has an individual effect. It is also an approach which responds to the difficulty of being unable to formulate in a planning or political policy all of the complex situations and choices that diverse individuals might want to make. This becomes a matter of direct market responses. It changes the nature of assumptions about what people 'need'. Instead, it is the individual who makes the appeal to values *within themselves*, including deciding on the (politically hazardous and unguessable) 'right' level of investment on healthcare, over and above the core package funded by taxation. We thus make new room for individual trade-offs and people's judgements. We do so within a framework of general rules set by Government.

Such an approach supports the idea that anyone may attempt to unite kindred spirits – by attracting their business – but without having the right to impose their vision upon others. This approach equips every individual with the ability to express their picture of preferred services, compatible with the agreed general framework.

The freedom to move one's business should be compared with the present situation of the NHS service user served by a primary care trust, which will usually be a regional monopoly. The NHS service user has the statutory right to move to another with identical characteristics. However, in the alternative model I have sketched, the individual would help to sustain the legitimacy of the patient-guaranteed care system by the impact of their decision making. The issue, of course, is not to try to discover which one single approach is best for everyone. It is to enable individuals to find this approach for themselves. And so the inevitable trade-offs made by the individual would themselves add legitimacy to the structure. Individuals would also put their interests and those of their families first – and stop relying on politicians to do so on their behalf. And they would do this in a cost-conscious environment which nevertheless guaranteed them and their families core care at a high level of quality.

Patient-Guaranteed Care Associations

All registered purchasers will be member-owned co-operatives concerned with competitive purchasing for specified outcomes. The Patient-Guaranteed Care Association (PGCA) will be large enough to undertake purchasing efficiently – probably evolving from primary care trusts (which typically cover 100 000 people), which will federate and merge to make competing regional bodies, and possibly national bodies with members in every region. All applicants will be accepted on a 'community-rated' basis, with no juggling by purchasers to exclude expensive patients or higher risks. They will buy the core guaranteed package on behalf of members. They will compete for subscriptions (via the insurance contract) from patient fundholders. It seems likely that, at least initially, primary care trusts would evolve as the PGCAs, but with others able to apply to Government to be registered as purchasers. Primary care trusts would thus shift from their schizo-phrenic role as agents of Government, rationers of allocated resources, and rep-resentative of the user as an 'expert' adviser. Necessary closures of poor facilities – or their active improvement – would be legitimised by consumer co-operative decisions, which would be a different context to the usual 'acute service review' which creates local political tumult. To survive, primary care trusts would have to manage their funds so that new money did not all disappear into salaries or debts.

All PGCAs will be voluntary, non-profit, mutual-aid or for-profit organisa-tions, each being devoted to the interests of its subscribing members. Just as in the development in the optical market we have seen – and as in dentistry if the same model was adopted – a volume market would yield volume services, but tailored to individuals and at lower prices. Professionals and managers would form new corporate bodies, generating efficient competition. These would be non-profit mutuals, public service companies, or large public limited companies. The assurance of momentum, and of customer satisfaction, would come from the creativity of competitive choice, liberalisation of advertising, transparent pricing, and new market entrants with new ideas within the regulated framework. PGCAs would have full access to existing NHS revenues and to existing private markets. The size of the challenge itself would facilitate a national business roll-out and high-technology investment, training and management. It is likely that as standards rise dramatically, the volume market will also be one of quality and of low prices. Value for money will combine with secure access, which the NHS promised but failed to furnish. Professionals will always enter manage-ment, but the hope is that management itself will improve so that professionals can spend much more time doing the clinical work for which they were trained, and which most of them wish to do. Clinical leaders in management will be essential.

Group membership (with the Government guarantee of a 'moral minimum' of quality and access) would protect the interests and cope with the apparent problem of the isolated, apparently uninformed, inexpert and occasional con-sumer whose ghost walks the battlements of this debate.

Every purchaser would be encouraged to negotiate a new kind of contract with the provider, linking payment to outcome and to quality of treatment, including the patient's own report of the results. The purchasing of volume at a set cost would not be the model. However, at present – and despite a continuing flow of national 'frameworks' – there is no incentive for purchasers to buy 'quality' nor for providers to deliver it. For it does not get any more numbers treated. For example, when a child is anaesthetised before an operation, a special cream should be applied to each hand, in case the anaesthetic is difficult to introduce into the first hand chosen. This is not always provided for in contracts. Similarly, with patient-controlled anaesthesia in gynaecology, which no-one wants to pay for. There are myriad examples like this. All purchasers and providers would work to develop skills, methods and information sources on behalf of the consumer. In addition, PGCAs would be required to offer incentives to subscribers who take preventive care seriously.

There would be much to learn in particular from US Health Maintenance Organisations to ensure that the initiative was truly with the purchasers, rather than with the presently dominant providers – who throw political clout. Purchasers would use protocols that offered fixed guidance on what providers could deliver, and which required prior approval by the purchaser before providers could diverge from the agreement. This will help to achieve two things: evidence-based medicine, and some control of costs. It would be backed up by practice guidelines set by the continuing National Institute for Clinical Excellence (although this would no longer have a 'rationing' role).

Clinicians would be an important part of the leadership and management of purchasing organisations, to ensure that the system functioned as it was intended. Purchasers would identify poor performers and cease to buy from them.

Changes in the profile of care can be expected. There will certainly be less emphasis on institutional care, and a new insistence on integrated care. Purchasers should continue to direct investment away from institutional care and towards the community, with an increased emphasis on the shift in care settings, including the family home. Here, too, very substantial tax incentives for caring for the elderly at home are one factor in the necessary reconstruction of long-term elderly care.

Professor Enthoven's 'Consumer Choice Health Plan' – first proposed in the USA in the late 1970s – offers an attractive model for a PGCA. His plan for universal health insurance was based on regulated competition in the private sector. It offered beneficiaries a wide choice of health insurance plans, including traditional fee for service and Prepaid Group Practice. Prepaid Group Practice would offer a model in which rights reflect responsibilities, and the discharge of duty justified authority. Here, large multi-specialty group practices in the USA contracted to provide comprehensive health services for a fixed per capita payment, that were set in advance and instead of fee for service, offered advantages, and were provided at lower cost. The approach offered doctors the opportunity to practise in teams, gave patients good access to primary care, matched resources used to the demand by patients, and achieved early diagnosis and treatment, disease prevention and management.[10]

Under Enthoven's proposal, Government contributed a fixed amount, based on a formula related to the premiums of the largest plans. The individual patient then made a choice, and paid any difference. This offered an incentive, both personally and financially, to choose the economical healthcare plan, given that none could be registered unless it offered good care. Where such Prepaid Group Practices operated, they secured a large share of the market. If such an approach were taken, it would be important for Government – as rule maker – to ensure that there is no adverse risk selection, which is a common form of 'market failure'.

As Enthoven says:

> *The key idea of my plan was to expose traditional free choice fee-for-service to economic competition from Prepaid Group Practices and other innovative arrangements that we now call Individual Practice Associations, Preferred Provider Organisations, Point of Service Plans and the like, let people make their choices, and see the health care system transformed, gradually and voluntarily, from inflationary fee-for-service to economical plans that reflected people's preferences and willingness to pay. The government's financial contribution could be keyed to the lowest cost plans in each region, the least inflationary component of the health care system.*[11]

Consider a specific group of patients. For example, the mentally ill. These would be members of a Patient Guaranteed Care Association, to which they take their insured fund. Their co-operative would then be responsible for making sure that they were heard in every context, to enable them to receive the most appropriate treatment. The PGCA, for example, would ensure that their case was reviewed regularly if they were in a high-security hospital. And that they were treated without prejudice or stigmatism in every setting, including Accident and Emergency. They would be enabled to make decisions about their care, including the right to refuse treatment. No PGCA would permit subscribers to accept forcible treatment. It would insist on appropriate acute inpatient care, and half-way houses for those moving between an acute care setting and the community, all reflecting a sense of concern, care, acceptance, support and the safety both of the individual and of the community (where necessary).

There is also the possibility of service users themselves forming and registering a PGCA, and running a purchasing organisation for themselves, as well as the possibility of a providers' organisation being established by an organisation of mental healthcare users – as is the case in Sweden, with the RSMH organisation.[12]

These examples show that it is not sufficient just to be told what is available. For a short walk on a map can be a harsh struggle through bramble. And when the gates are closed against you, your dignity, calm and self-respect are damaged. The contract that the patient fundholder could negotiate would seek improved, more flexible, more accessible services, including the provision of mentors, sheltered homes and other facilities that would be attractive to service users of all kinds. If these were not provided, the co-operative would buy from elsewhere, and new entrants would come in to offer such services. The very significant revenues available would be a magnetic pull. For the mentally ill this approach would be the key (in contrast to throwing away the key), instead of just accepting what is given to you.

Indeed, I expect that most PGCAs will be formed by GPs, and that by this means we shall at last move the pivot of care to general practice. This is where the investment is most needed, too. In the PGCA structure, patients would also have to take responsibility for their own decisions. Most GPs battle against the self-neglect of patients. They are exercising personal rights, but the system takes the strain and meets the costs, which is no incentive to consider the consequences of one's behaviour, or its costs.[12] The PGCA would take a role in how people live, by negotiating premiums accordingly as incentives to change.

These initiatives would also focus on the deepest concerns of the individual, and would be set in place by contract by the co-operative. For example, they could ensure that we have such a simple but innovative thing as a 'patient's page' inserted into the clinical notes. This was proposed by Dr Jacqueline S Maxmin, a GP, writing in the *British Medical Journal* recently after the death of her partner, Geoff, an acute care patient.[13] It could be introduced for every kind of patient, including the mentally ill. This patient's page would help professionals to understand what the patient and relatives are really concerned about. It would also help them to understand how the patient was feeling. And if the patient deteriorated, the relatives would not feel – as they can do now – that their feelings and fears were ignored.

Dr Maxmin said of her partner:

> *He told me how important he felt it was for the patient's views to be heard. He suggested that a patient's page be inserted into the clinical notes. On this page patients could write their agenda of ideas, concerns and suggestions. The process of working out this agenda with them could develop doctors' communication skills – which too often remain doctor-centred rather than patient-centred – and promote understanding so that problems could be openly discussed. Maybe this could promote a more patient-centred approach – doctors could address the patient's written agenda at the same time as the traditional medical agenda .... Talk of tasks, tests and discharge dates is no longer enough.*[14]

The Nurse's Care Plan should help, but this is a nurse's interpretation of a patient's wishes, and written by the nurse after talking to the patient. The PGCA could insist, and in view of the disinterest of senior house officers reported by Dr Maxmin, it should do so.

The PGCA will thus seek on behalf of its subscribers to achieve integrated care, quality, good outcomes and patient choice. The NHS increasingly insists that patient's 'representatives' must be 'consulted'. If patients are to be represented – which makes sense in terms of collective buying, provided that it is always tailored to the unique situation and perspectives of the individual when it comes to treatments – then they had best be represented strongly, effectively and with sanctions. They require representation both to Government (but not by a vested interest with no competition) and to professionals and providers. A consumer co-operative of the kind I have outlined could do all of this well. It would also refocus services, attitudes, behaviours and treatments, and not only increase volume and access, important as these are. For example, it would encourage the necessary shifts in attitudes towards older people, and to specific diseases such as the dementias (if they continue to be called diseases, a view which itself is controversial).[15] They would encourage the recognition of patient concerns about coping strategies and the quality of life.

Such an imperative list will require many changes, not least much better NHS data and management systems. The PGCA will be equipped to assist patients to make choices, and it will do many of the things on their behalf which are difficult for individuals to do. For in making choices we must learn how to appraise information critically, to determine its relevance and validity to our context, and compare various sources of information. If purchasers have high ethical standards and employ key appraisal skills, they can assist patients to learn. They will also each have incentives to do so. This is of particular concern with regard to long-term elderly care. Here the elderly – whether cared for at home, in very sheltered accommodation or in nursing and residential care – should determine what matters most, and this must be a key factor in standards and in funding to purchase high-quality care. Clearly this will be of particular relevance to recruiting the right kinds of people with appropriate attitudes, and to training and rewards.

If the service user is empowered, too, providers will then be required to take quality seriously and to invest in it. The insistence of the purchasing co-operative will reinforce the calls for quality already discussed in accreditation, certification and regulation programmes. The context will be one of partnership, and of the integration of services, with the emphasis on flexibility. And they will have to maintain the commitment over time.

The PGCA would be much concerned with the integration of care. It would also look hard at the relationship between general practice and hospital medicine. It would make full and skilful use of performance data and, if it can obtain it, of data concerning individual incidents. It would do so fully informed by medical expertise – no doubt also noting that when doctors and nurses experience NHS care for themselves, they often report very distressing experiences.[16] The PGCA would employ data and statistical specialists and clinicians – to search out and purchase optimal providers, individual performers and quality outcomes. These would seek to make good use of numerical probability information, which many doctors misinterpret or do not understand.[17] In addition, individual consumers do not make use of all the available performance data, but a competing purchaser would do so.

A PGCA will, too, necessarily seek to impact on such common and seemingly intractable weaknesses as poor productivity, weak (and/or unused) management information, and failure of the NHS to reconstruct historical patterns of work – notably by giving nurses and pharmacists much more responsibility. In addition, it will seek to tackle such issues as the often chaotic organisation of operating-theatre time and its efficient use.[18] A co-operative purchasing organisation would also be aware of many issues which do not surface to patients.[19] Less wasteful, less dangerous, less inconvenient locations would be carefully considered. And the money would be there to make decisions click. Intermediate care between primary and secondary care – including pre-admission assessment units, early and supported discharge, community hospitals, domiciliary stroke units, hospitals at home and rehabilitation units, all under-funded – would become a much more important feature. Moreover, intermediate care (although generally un-evaluated) 'can help shift the balance of power from secondary care to primary care and empowered self-care'.[20]

The PGCA would also pay attention to such cultural issues as whether or not a 'representative' organisation should seek to change people's behaviour irrespective of the motivation of individual patients, or instead seek to deploy incentives to prompt change. It would look hard, too, at such 'details' as how and why day surgery practice varies enormously. And why many patients are being denied the opportunity to recover in their own homes rather than in hospital. It would look, too, at poor social service care for recuperating patients, weak co-ordination of services in hospital and poor clinical practices. For example, it is difficult to imagine that a PGCA which had to satisfy its subscribers would have permitted a breast screening service like the West London service to continue for long. This service failed to implement national guidelines, and lacked clear accountability, was pervaded with poor working relationships, and lacked rigorous safeguards and protocols. This situation had continued, with what the Commission on Health Care Improvement called 'unacceptable and avoidable' errors. The service failed to change its policies after previous errors or to learn from similar failures made in Birmingham as long ago as 1994.[21]

The PGCA will thus be asked to manage a constructive patient journey throughout the system, as the US organisation Kaiser Permanente apparently achieves – with improved performance, and at no greater cost. It would seek to work with networks – as in cancer care – as well as with specific hospitals. And the better integration of primary and secondary care, with the whole system managed, can be sustained *because of competition, and emphasising user choice* and better personal management. The people who know how to do all of these things are medical professionals trained in management. These are the people who must be in the lead in partnership with subscribing members in the PGCA.

Finally, the PGCA will be a multiple-class body, and contribute to harmonising social relationships in community service through individual service. It would distinctly not be an instrument or a unit of collectivist local government – unlike Liberal Democratic proposals for relocating authority.[22] Indeed, far from being the site of massive apathy – as local government is – the PGCA would be the focus of lively personal interest.

Patient-guaranteed care providers

These will be registered providers who will have to seek willing purchasers, and who will be motivated to genuinely manage their resources and respond to market forces. These could develop from Foundation Hospitals and PCTs.[23]

A diversity of competing registered providers will be encouraged. All providers will make contracts with Patient-Guaranteed Care Associations. Providers will be registered as patient-guaranteed care providers (PGCPs), and they will compete for funds. With the *actualité* of provision tested in the market. With unsatisfactory providers improving or removing. This will encourage improvement in existing provider units and promote some new entrants to seek these very substantial revenues. This will help to achieve the renewal and renovation of existing provision by indirect incentives for innovation and emulation of the best in the market.

More diverse and competing provision will arise from diverse sources – from the State, and from independent, voluntary, charitable, not-for-profit and for-profit organisations. The selection and endorsement of a provider of care will be a matter for the autonomous and empowered consumer, instead of the approach of the present system, where individual wishes are subsumed in a political agenda concerning 'equality' or 'redistribution of wealth'. There will be freedom to bargain as a means of sorting out the inevitable conflicts of daily life. And freedom to move voluntarily between competing social insurers and competing mutual purchasers of care. In addition, the real costs should be visible. In France and in Germany they are shown on pay slips. And a pay slip is the one piece of paper that everyone reads. We need an equivalent document to be given to every user for every episode of care.

Existing NHS providers will be mutualised. We need careful enquiry as to how to transfer NHS facilities from State ownership. And to be conscious that a transfer of assets to a local charity or community body will *not* by itself empower the individual consumer. Hospitals (and other service providers, too) could be established as charitable bodies independent of Government, as not-for-profit and for-profit organisations (although of course each must operate responsively and competitively in the market). A more modest view sees at least a proportion of NHS hospitals as being independent of Government, as in Germany (where just over half are independent), a third in France and some 80% in The Netherlands.

NHS hospitals could be reorganised on the model of the old UK voluntary hospitals, with elected local boards, and function as not for profit or for profit as local management determines. The State will end public sector quasi-monopoly in provision and the imposition of uniformity. All state healthcare institutions will become independent, non-profit private corporations, in a similar position to universities.

Direct incentives and competitive choices, I suggest, are the only way to achieve these essentials, and to change the mentalities and behaviours of managers and professionals so that we get these desirable changes throughout the healthcare system on a routine basis.

The owners and managers will have a direct incentive to serve every individual represented by PGCA co-operatives – and with more clarity and more user leverage than we can hope for as our money goes into the Treasury pot.

There should also be representation of consumers at board level in mutual-aid organisations, and direct election of the board by the subscribers. Certainly some token system of consumer 'consultation' – some mutual-aid version of 'citizen juries' offered symbolically – is no substitute for a direct consumer voice concerning the make-up of the board itself. Such an approach has the potential to enable the disadvantaged and those who are on low incomes, or unemployed and on benefit, to have the same level of care as the middle class.

Local institutions of healthcare (like the Victorian railway station) reaffirm the spirit and sense of place. Now they need to be renewed voluntarily by the patient fundholder (gathered voluntarily in co-operatives as purchasers). Then services could be improved by local liberty (and necessity!) to experiment, and to seek local solutions with local leadership legitimised by local loyalties. Such bodies would have two kinds of fundraising powers. They could go to capital markets, and they could earn revenues. This would increase responsibility and genuine sharing. It would help to rebuild an awareness of neighbours and their lives and concerns.

The impact of patient-guaranteed care on general practice and hospitals

First of all, patient-guaranteed care would be likely to shift spending from hospitals to primary care. It would diminish the political authority of hospital consultants. It would also ensure that GPs were paid for the many non-medical things they now do, and those who were unwilling to pay would be deterred from crowding the surgery. If the patient, via the PGCA, had to make choices conscious of what things cost and with an awareness, too, that we are responsible for the consequences of our own actions, it would be a different world. Certainly it would be one in which 15.5 million patients would not miss appointments with their GP in a year, in part because the service is *un*-priced. One in which GPs did not have to refuse to take on new patients because of shortages. One where new patients – with an NHS credit and with supplementary personal insurance and other funding – would be an opportunity instead of a tiresome extra burden.

It would be a world in which primary care practice staff were provided and funded to help undertake the many new social roles as 'vicars in society' which have been pressed on to the shoulders of GPs by individuals who have not been encouraged to take responsibility for themselves. These demands go well beyond medical decision making, and far beyond the accepted ritual of bringing illness to a shaman in society.[24]

If people want this service, and if doctors or others are ready to provide it, we should recognise it, organise for it, staff it and expect to pay for it. Meanwhile, society unreasonably looks to the GP to accept the burden (to adapt words by Lewis Mumford) to serve as 'a seat of government, a court of justice, a parliament, a marketplace, a police station, a telephone exchange, a temple, an art gallery, a library, an observatory, a central filing system and a computer'.[25]

We should reconstruct our culture within which medicine nestles, so that many social, personal and organisational issues in ordinary lives are no longer thrust upon GPs. This particularly concerns the shift away from a biomedical life where we are dependent on medicine and on medical advice for non-medical issues. An amended structure would be one in which the treatment would be less based on drug prescription, and instead focused on having time to understand the clinical difficulties of the patient.

A new structure of relationships between doctors and patients, and between patients and their selves, would offer hope of such a world developing. It would raise the morale of doctors – among whom 25% of GPs in the UK plan to take early retirement because of NHS reforms and increased patient demands.[26] It could also shift us from a medicalising model to a personal structure of thought, consideration and self-responsibility in a necessarily risky (but therefore exciting, challenging and worthwhile) world.

The institutional model that I have outlined offers a positive, optimistic, creative approach to the individual coping with illness while pursuing a full life. It privileges and encourages self-reliance. It respects professionalism. It recognises risk and the inevitable costs of choices. It offers a basis of incentive for more funding, more efficiency, lower costs, higher productivity and more satisfaction, both at work and in the outmodes that individual patients decide and prefer. This, by contrast to the medicalised model, of which Misselbrook says that 'Yesterday's fit and healthy elder is today's hypersensitive patient, processed, medicated and monitored.'[27] He points to this expansionist, medicalising challenge 'within the context of our beliefs about a healthy society'. And as Armstrong has put this, we should ask whether we really want the 'new public health dream of surveillance in which everyone is brought into the vision of the benevolent eye of medicine through the medicalisation of everyday life'.[28] Or do we want the alternative of a more self-responsible, risk-accepting, creative society in which the individual is valued (and values him- or herself) and is enabled to express values, beliefs and preferences in their unique, lived-only-once life? If we do want this, we should seek what Toon has advocated (and to which Misselbrook draws proper attention), which is a healthcare system that serves the patient's own values and their life narrative, and which encompasses and enlarges their understandings.[29]

So, too, we need dynamist reform of social work, probation services and other such 'client' services. We need to have much more respect for arts education – which looks at the individual, and at idiosyncrasy – as well as for medical science, which looks at the pathology, not the person. Family breakdown must be addressed, and also single parenthood, as Murray has shown.[30] Housing, income, nutrition, preventive care and anti-smoking measures have much more impact than does medicine itself on the pool of ill health. Here we need dynamist rather than stasist answers.

I shall now turn to the questions concerning the Government as rule maker, open information and direct incentives.

Notes

1 Lea R (2000) *Health Care in the UK: the need for reform.* Policy Paper. Institute of Directors, London. The problem was addressed very early in the history of the NHS. It was admitted that 'there is no objective and attainable standard of "adequacy" in the health field'. Committee of Enquiry into the Cost of the National Health Service (1956) *Report of the Committee of Enquiry into the Cost of the National Health Service.* HMSO, London. See also Blackwell N and Kruger D (2002) *Better Healthcare for All. Replacing the NHS monopoly.* Centre for Policy Studies, London.
2 Scruton R (2001) *England: an elegy.* Pimlico, London, p.121.
3 Evans RG, Lomas J, Barer ML *et al.* (1989) Controlling health expenditures. The Canadian reality. *NEJM.* **320**: 571–7. Coyte P (2001) Current trends and future directions for the Canadian health care system. *Econ Affairs.* **21**: 24–7. Redwood H (2000) *Why Ration Healthcare? An International Study of the United Kingdom, France, Germany and Public Sector Healthcare in the USA.* Civitas, London, pp.117–18.
4 Lees DS (1961) *Health Through Choice. An Economic Study of the English National Health Service.* Institute of Economic Affairs, London, p.9.
5 This should not be employment based (which Dr Liam Fox, Shadow Secretary of State for Health, has been thought to be considering), for this approach has many known disadvantages from US experience. It encourages fee for service and reduces

discrimination between providers. It does not offer consumers multiple choice, because many plans are too small and the administrative costs too high and complex. There tends to be one insurer with a monopoly in each employment group, and no good alternatives offered to consumers. It also denies choice to those who would prefer less costly care if they could keep the savings. This is an inflationary model, especially if trade unions bargain for greater benefits in health plans and if employers paid the entire premium. See Enthoven A (2002) *Introducing market forces into healthcare: a tale of two countries*. Paper delivered to 4th European Conference Health Economics, Paris. 10th July, for a description of informative USA experience.

6 Mill JS (1910) *Letters* (edited by HSR Elliott). Longmans, London. *Hansard.* **191**: col.1860, 5 May 1968, cited by Vincent JR (1966, revised edition 1976) *The Making of the English Liberal Party, 1857–1868*. Constable, London (revised edition published by The Harvester Press, Brighton).

7 Enthoven A. Paris, op. cit.

8 Booth P (2002) *Getting Back Your Health. Rebate Financing for Medical Care.* Adam Smith Institute, London.

9 Audit Commission (1996) *What the Doctor Ordered: a study of GP fundholders in England and Wales.* Audit Commission, London. Le Grand J, Mays N, Mulligan JA *et al.* (1997) *Models of Purchasing and Commissioning: review of research evidence. A report to the Department of Health.* London School of Economics/King's Fund, London. Enthoven AC (1999) *In Pursuit of an Improving National Health Service.* Nuffield Trust, London.

10 Luft HS (1978) How do health maintenance organisations achieve their 'savings'? *NEJM.* **198**: 1336–43. Manning WA, Liebowitz G, Newhouse G *et al.* (1984) A controlled trial of the effect of a prepaid group practice on the use of services. *NEJM.* **310**: 1505–10, both cited by Enthoven, Paris, 2002, op. cit.

11 Enthoven, Paris, 2002, ibid.

12 Fox L (2002) Speech to the Second Conservative Mental Health Summit. Conservative Party press release, 25 June 2002.

13 I am indebted to Dr R Lefever for our discussions. See also Hattersley R (2002) Obscure charm of the inner city. *Guardian.* **20 August**: 20.

14 Maxmin JS (2002) Do we hear our patients? And would a patient's page help? *BMJ.* **324**: 684.

15 Payer L (1992) *Disease-Mongers. How doctors, drug companies and insurers are making you feel sick.* John Wiley & Sons, New York. Moynihan R, Heath I and Henry D (2002) Selling sickness: the pharmaceutical industry and disease mongering. *BMJ.* **324**: 886–90. Gotzsche PC (2002) Commentary: medicalisation of risk factors. *BMJ.* **324**: 890–1.

16 Anon. (2002) Daughter and doctor: two conflicting roles. *BMJ.* **324**: 1530. La Combe M (ed.) (2000) *On Being a Doctor. 'Voices of physicians and patients'.* American College of Physicians, Philadelphia, PA.

17 Fuller R (2002) Are choices irrational or doctors and patients misinformed (letter)? *BMJ.* **324**: 215. Ashworth J (1997) *Science, Policy and Risk.* Royal Society, London. See review of league tables and alternatives in Adab P, Rouse AM, Mohammed MA and Marshall T (2002) Performance league tables: the NHS deserves better. *BMJ.* **324**: 95–8.

18 Audit Commission (2002) *Operating Theatres: a bulletin for health bodies.* Audit Commission, London.

19 Marteau TM (1989) Psychological costs of screening. *BMJ.* **229**: 527. Stoate H (1989) Can health screening damage your health? *J R Coll Pract.* **39**: 193–5. Marteau TM (1990) Reducing the psychological costs. *BMJ.* **301**: 26–8. Marteau TM and Kinmonth AL (2002) Screening for cardiovascular risk: public health imperatives do matter for individual informed choice?. *BMJ.* **325**: 78–80. See also discussion in Misselbrook D (2002) *Thinking About Patients.* Petroc Press, Newbury, pp.136–9.

20 Pencheon D (2002) Intermediate care. Appealing and logical, but still in need of evaluation. *BMJ.* **324**: 1347–8.

21 Commission on Health Care Improvement (2002) *CHI Investigation Into the West of London Breast Cancer Screening Service at Hammersmith Hospitals NHS Trust.* Commission on Health Care Improvement, London. Rumbelow H (2002) Breast cancer inquiry a 'wake-up call for NHS'. *The Times.* **16 April**. Department of Health (2002) *National Survey of Cancer Patients.* Department of Health, London. See also www.gov.uk/nhspatients/cancersurvey.

22 Liberal Democrat Party (2002) *Quality, Innovation, Choice.* Liberal Democrat Party, London.

23 Mr A Milburn, speech to NHS top managers and overseas visitors, London, entitled 'NHS Foundation Hospitals to be freed from Whitehall control'. Department of Health press release 2002/0240, 22 May 2002; www.doh.gov.uk/speeches/may2002/milburnnhsfdn.htm]. NHS Foundation Hospitals (modelled on the idea of 'public interest companies', or non-profit bodies with a 'public service' ethos, and protected from private-sector take-over – championed by Mr Milburn's Special Adviser, Professor Paul Corrigan, with borrowings from Scandinavia) offer more freedom from centralised control. It is a start on liberating provision, since Foundation Hospitals would be held to account 'through agreements and cash for performance contracts they negotiate with primary care trusts and other commissioners'. Like PGCAs? Not quite, for these do not yet have to earn their revenues from the ultimate consumer of their services. And so this is still not a sufficient means to differentiate quality. Nor does the failing hospital, which most needs the stimulus and the opportunity of freedoms to improve, figure – at least initially – in the plan. Hospitals have been reluctant to apply so far, because of Treasury controls over financial freedoms. Cracknell D and Rogers L (2002) NHS chiefs snub super hospital plan. *Sunday Times (news section).* **4 August**: 1. Also see Milburn A (2002) We have to give the voters more than this. *The Times.* **7 August**: 18. First leader (2002) Right idea. An efficacious prescription for the Labour Party. *The Times.* **7 August**: 19. Miles A (2002) Labour duel threatens revival of ailing NHS. *The Times.* **8 August**: 18. Eames L (2002) Foundation trusts: the European perspective. *NHS Magazine.* **July/August**: 6–7. Four existing three-star trusts expressed a firm interest in foundation status, namely Northumbria Healthcare NHS Trust, Peterborough Hospitals NHS Trust, Norfolk and Norwich University Hospital NHS Trust and Addenbrooke's NHS Trust, Cambridge. The General Healthcare Group in the UK, Kaiser Permanente and United Healthcare in the USA, GerMedic and Medicine Net in Germany, the Swiss Group ONO in Switzerland, Capio in Sweden, and Deluca Medicale and Generale de Sante in France are in discussions concerning management, procurement and delivery – probably initially to design, build and run the network of fast-track diagnostic and treatment centres planned on a public–private basis, with eight under way by the end of 2002, and 20 by the end of 2004 in England. McGauran A (2002) Devil in the detail. *Health Service J.* **9 May**. Charter D (2002) US health firm 'costlier than NHS'. *The Times.*

25 May. Pfeifer S (2002) Europeans bid to run failed NHS hospitals. *Business*. **23 June**. Timmins N (2002) Overseas providers issued with NHS prospectus. *Financial Times*. **25 June**. Lyall J (2002) Bidders for overseas teams named. *Health Service J.* **4 July**. Moore W (2002) Milburn recruits private companies from abroad to increase capacity of the NHS. *BMJ*. **325**: 10. www.doh.gov.uk/internationalestablishment. See also Wintour P (2002) Brown wins battle with Milburn over borrowing for foundation hospitals. *Guardian*. **8 October**. Miles A (2002) Blair outlines radical plan, to be really, really bold. *The Times*. **2 October**. See also, The Queen's Speech (2002) House of Commons. *Hansard*, **13 November**, cols. 3–5; Charter D and Bennett R (2002) Local people to run elite NHS hospitals. *The Times*. **14 November**; Kruger D (2002) Medical negligence. *The Spectator*. **16 November**; Charter D (2002) Milburn to face battle for Labour Party's soul. *The Times*. **11 December**; Charter D and Riddell P (2002) Backtrack over foundation hospitals. *The Times*. **11 December**; Charter D (2002) Foundation plan comes under fire. *The Times*. **12 December**; Charter D (2002) Hospital reforms face fresh attack from within NHS. *The Times*. **23 December**. On European private sector management and franchises to run failing hospitals, see Hawkes N (2002) Sweden may give failing NHS a shot in the arm; and Wright O (2002) Emergency care for England's worst hospitals. *The Times*. **20 December**; Charter D (2002) Overseas firms to compete for surgery centres. *The Times*. **24 December**.

24 See Misselbrook's discussion, op. cit., especially pp.150–63. Also see Balint M (1964) *The Doctor, His Patient and His Illness*. Pitman, London. Belsky MS and Gross L (1975) *Beyond the Medical Mystique. How to choose and use your doctor. The smart patient's way to a longer, healthier life*. Arbor House, New York. Helman C (1990) *Culture, Health and Illness* (2e). Butterworth-Heinemann, London. Dixon M and Sweeney K (2000) *The Human Effect in Medicine*. Radcliffe Medical Press, Oxford. Feinmann J (2002) Power of the placebo. *The Times*. **3 September**: 12.

25 Mumford L, cited in (1967) *The Myth of the Machine. Technics and human development*. Harcourt, New York. Collis JS (1978) *Living With a Stranger. A Discourse on the Human Body*. McDonald and Jones, London, p.76.

26 Sutherland V and Cooper C (1993) Identifying distress among general practitioners: predictors of psychological ill health and job dissatisfaction. *Soc Sci Med*. **37**: 575–81. BMA Working Party (2000) *Work-Related Stress Among Senior Doctors*. BMA, London. Hawkes N (2002) One in 20 misses a GP appointment. *The Times*. **20 August**: 5. Hall C (2002) Doctors bar new patients as crisis deepens. *Daily Telegraph*. **20 August**: 1. Miles A (2002) Reform, not fines, is the solution to 'GP crisis'. *The Times*. **21 August**: 16.

27 Misselbrook, op. cit., p.142.

28 Armstrong, op. cit.

29 Toon P (1999) *Towards a Philosophy of General Practice Study of the Virtuous Practitioner*. Occasional Paper No. 78. Royal College of General Practitioners, London.

30 Murray C (1984) *Living Ground. American social policy 1950–1980*. Basic Books, New York. Murray C (1988) *In Pursuit: of happiness and good government*. Simon & Schuster, New York. Murray C (1997) *What it Means to be a Libertarian. A personal interpretation*. Broadway Books, New York. Also see Institute of Economic Affairs, *Charles Murray and the Underclass. The developing debate*. IEA, London. IEA (1996) *The Emerging British Underclass*. IEA, London. IEA (1994) *The Underclass. The crisis deepens*. IEA, London. ICSC (2001) *Underclass + 10. The British underclass 1990–2000*. Institute for the Study of Civil Society, London.

Chapter 22

Getting it done 2

Government as rule maker – the risks of regulation – open information – direct incentives for preventive care.

The world is full of people who believe that men need masters.

(John Gardner)

The role of Government as rule maker

We have earlier rehearsed the idea that the emphasis should be on the civil association described by Michael Oakeshott, by contrast with intrusive, goal-directed, ideologically derived, managerial government. And such government should be a neutral umpire which administers neutral rules of behaviour, permitting many choices to be co-possible. Within this framework of rules, individuals will themselves 'get it done', pursuing their own goals. And thus the social order will be one of unending adjustments and exchanges – adaptive, dynamic and mutually respecting. There will be no overall master-plan, no one 'system', no 'right' way, save that Government will foster a situation where individuals can exist at civilised levels and work out choices for themselves, both singly and co-operatively.

This is not a ruleless jungle. No one wants the chaos of the entirely unpredictable. None of us can deal with total uncertainty. We do not wish or seek to cope with a ruleless world. And it is a public virtue to maintain a framework of rules which support dynamism, and to ensure appropriate services. Yet we know that regulation tends to spread into areas where it is not justified, and where there is no technical monopoly justifying intervention. We know, too, that it is not more efficient or more economical to have a single supplier rather than many.[1] Government should, as rule maker, rule the roost, but not provide every rooster or egg. And so the issue is which structure of rules does most to promote dynamism and service to the individual, and which can renovate UK health-care.

We begin with the idea that Government must set the rules. As Postrel says:

A dynamic system, whether a single organisation or an entire civilisation, requires rules. But those rules must be compatible with knowledge, with learning, and with surprise. They must allow the tree to grow, not chop it into timbers. Finding those rules is the greatest challenge a dynamic civilisation confronts.[2]

In healthcare the State will set the framework of rules so that consumers make the running. It will do this by three quintessentials – it will guarantee 'core' patient care, it will vigorously protect competition, and it will ensure the prompt, clear and timely publication of relevant information. Its role will be to establish and supervise the rules for an infrastructure within which an evolving system develops in response to consumers' wishes – one in which competing insurers, purchasers and providers function and are regulated by the State. The State will also regulate medical education, registration and other institutional arrangements. If competitive regulation is required, it could establish more than one regulatory body and permit relevant bodies to choose with whom to register.

Government will ensure that the system functions, notably by protecting information, competition and choice, by preventing anti-competitive mergers and anti-social business behaviour. Critically by protecting the effective freedom of 'exchange', voluntary selection of membership of co-operatives and individual choice among competing alternative purchasers and insurers. Otherwise, standing at arm's length from providers. It will not be tempted to protect them for political reasons. Government will guarantee the structure, offer re-insurance, and manage the rules, which will include appropriate pool-risk management, and the existing cross-subsidy of the young/elderly, sick/healthy and able/disadvantaged. Government will also, vitally, protect competition and open information. It will also operate a competitive capital market, to enable providers whose services are in proven demand to secure operating funds to enlarge facilities, improve technologies, etc., and to enable weaker performers to put forward improvement plans for which capital could be subscribed.

And so the specific role of Government should be to seek to guarantee care, rather than to express our unexpressed 'real will'. It should instead protect the soundness of the system without guaranteeing any *specific* individual choice concerning access to a specific service, institution or outcome – save for the fundamental structure of guarantees for enabling the institutions to evolve which offer good care for all. For example, such guarantees will include ensuring the flourishing of *categories* of institution, such as a co-operative purchaser of care acting on behalf of willing, subscribing members. However, they would not include the protection of any specific purchaser or provider which would otherwise seek to be left unchanged over time.

Postrel suggests general principles by which to frame dynamist rules, with Government withdrawing to the ramparts of basic funding and limited regulation. My own adapted formulation of these principles is that the rules should, in the UK context, be set by Government to deliver the structure of patient-guaranteed care that I have outlined.[3]

Government should:

- *Establish a **general** framework of rules within which people can create **specific**, nested, fluid and competing frameworks of more specific rules.* By this we mean rules which permit and encourage what we should call 'voluntary communities'. For example, competing purchasing co-operatives who will buy services on behalf of individuals, and which seek willing adherents. These people can join, choose to accept willingly, and support or not. This is the dynamist objective of order without control. It would set in place simple rules which permit people to build by adaptation on good foundations, rather than being restricted by vastly detailed rules which form an initial master-plan. This would be a flexible framework within which people can create other nested, competing frameworks of more specific rules (for example, different services from different providers). This they would do through trial and error, feedback, adaptation, market testing, and those recombinations which offer further legal choices.

All of this could be achieved under the general umbrella of patient-guaranteed care (the 'core' package guaranteed by Government). Individuals would be allowed to choose the specific voluntary community (or PGCA) within which they would receive services. For example, an individual could choose to take their patient fund to one of many different mutual-aid purchasing co-operatives, formed by charities, voluntary bodies, churches, trade unions, employers, etc. They would offer guaranteed delivery of the core package, but with different emphases, for example appealing to different client groups. Thus there would be nested alternatives within the overall flexible system.

Within this structure, of course, the standards set for professional practice are another set of rules established by Government. However, the particular offers of legally permitted services will be differentiated by different purchasers and providers. The rules will say that people can leave them if they do not like them. No one will set a 'one best way'. No *single standard* of quality, efficiency or responsiveness, no single expression of local knowledge or satisfaction with outcome could survive such a structure. The NHS itself – or rather its constituent institutions – would each become one competing model, one alternative way, one singular prospectus, one specific provider with a set of nested rules. And these would directly compete – insofar as new capacity could be created – with other competing models.

- *Crucially, protect competition, choice and feedback.* Thus there will be no monopoly guarantees of permanence to any provider. Instead there will be a continuing challenge to both established and new ideas. There will be freedom to offer alternatives and to compete for mobile revenues. And there will be no political insulation for winners picked by Government. Government itself will strictly limit its own powers of intervention. This approach institutes a cultural welcome for the challenge of the innovator who can freely enter the market, compete with existing offers and attract willing subscriptions. Thus there would be a genuine system of decentralised expression in which public policy ensures that the individual can regularly appraise all of the competing (and thus constantly improving/reinventing/new thinking) options in healthcare insurance, purchasing and provision. And they would be able to move between them in the self-regulating test of competition, where we learn which are the good ideas, and where discovery (rather than 'democracy') confers provisional authority. As Postrel notes, 'The more that rules must compete for adherents, the more legitimacy they enjoy and the more local knowledge they can incorporate'.[4]
- *Ensure that in healthcare there are credible, understandable, enduring and enforceable commitments.* Thus every single person will be guaranteed the core package of

care. Each will engage in a legally enforceable and mutually binding contract of reciprocal responsibilities, where both the patient and the provider can rely on one another. There will be *reasonable* expectations on both sides concerning future actions. The individual will be self-responsible and concerned, too, with the link between lifestyle and results. The provider will be committed to delivering a quality service where and when it is wanted, and for which the purchaser (in a co-operative) has contracted. Whereas the statist (but in contractual terms, wholly ambiguous) NHS structure offers no means for the patient to enforce what he or she thought was the contract, this dynamist structure embodies both commitment and flexibility. It does so both between strangers and between intimates, for the informed activist and for the person who does not want to think about healthcare planning, but who wants a service when he or she wants it. This approach ensures the certainty of access for the patient, the predictability of revenues for the successful provider, the flexibility of choice between competing providers, incentive and direct reward for successful service, the encouragement of specialisation and niche services, the development of an 'extended order', the renewal of faith from proven outcomes, the protection of reputation in every detail and by every employee, and the injunction that every example of one's work must be able to be held up as the best example – perhaps an actual impossibility, but a reasonable and necessary aspiration.

- *Allow individuals (including groups of individuals) to act on their own knowledge, in a system which welcomes and accommodates the latitude of varied tastes.* Thus we shall recognise that people are more directly in contact with themselves than any planner can be, and that they can responsibly make many different assessments of costs and benefits in terms of personal taste, circumstance and preference. This itself is a theory of dispersed knowledge which respects tacit difficult-to-articulate knowledge.

- *Support and release self-responsibility and the traditional wish for self-improvement by making choices real, genuine and attainable.* More on self-responsibility in a moment.

- *Enable the framework of rules to apply to simple, generic units.* By this we mean a co-operative of patients, a group of doctors in practice, an entrepreneurial provider, a cluster of clinics, and so on. And Government must allow them to combine in many different ways (responding to locality, to form new co-operatives, to take initiatives in mutual-aid, or to offer new services or more convenient access).

- *Empower new groupings to pursue specific goals, subject to competition.* Thus exemplifying dynamic processes, including competing for freed up revenues. Thus, permitting credible, understandable, enduring and enforceable commitments which utilise direct incentives to prompt new services.

- *Free people from the constraints of status, class, gender, ageism, disability, race and geography – and from the necessities of networks and cultural power.* This will enable people, among many gains, to get access. It will enable escape from the immoral two-tier system where the better off can purchase better *clinical care* and not merely shorter waiting times. It will focus on measures of ability to benefit, and on patient wishes to risk it or not, as well as on personal vitality – instead of focusing on age, gender and other markers.

- *Government, will also have to address four further inescapable concerns, which Professor Enthoven has expressed.* The first of these is to allow losers to shrink as they experience cash-ebb from losing support, and not to bail them out 'with "extra contractual payments", inevitably at the expense of winners, thus destroying the incentive to be a winner'. The second is to let go, and resist responding to every problem 'with a blizzard of new directives'. Public employee unions – once again, in September 2002, exercising their muscles – will have to allow genuine free competition from hospitals in the private sector. There is also the risk that primary care trusts (PCTs) will be territorial monopolies, as may any purchasing organisation which evolves from them, and so Government should ensure new entrants. In order for effective incentives to improve service and care, there must be competition among them, as my plan for PGCAs offers. As Enthoven says, 'A pilot project in which people could change PCTs in pursuit of better service would be compatible with Mr Milburn's commitment to consumer choice.' Ministers have said that they will 'pull the plug' on failing universities. This will lead to the inevitable closure of some institutions of higher education. Will this extend to failing hospital units when people have a choice of avoiding being sent to them? The approach to failing councils suggests a discouraging precedent – of wholesale take over from the centre. This takes us in the opposite direction, even if the intention is to improve performance.[5]

These issues are all real. They will not go away. We shall have to make some decisions about them. Action on doctors and incentives will be a matter of political finesse, hard bargaining, leadership, and the appeal by politicians to a much changed context. And action on price and consciousness will necessarily involve some element of compulsion if service users are to face direct financial disciplines, as they should. I argue broadly against coercion on principle in my principles of liberty, but it is a difficulty that without a legal requirement some important actions will not be taken. This is a quandary which runs through the book, and which we cannot escape, just as there is no escape from affordability. And, as Lincoln said, 'extreme tenderness of the citizen's liberty might make the Government itself go to pieces'. It is a difficult question.[6]

Still, with politicians of all three main parties we see a reluctance to consider these questions. They mean, of course, a change in their own predominant role in the healthcare culture. They also mean reversing the new managerial model of Government–doctor relationships. This means giving money to patients and trusting professionals, with whom PGCAs will negotiate. It also means accepting that poor providers will have to re-train, re-tool or re-move. When one looks at the current state of the debate – enriched as it has been by new thinking by Enthoven, Misselbrook and others – the image of politicians which comes to mind is one of reluctant discussants who seem like sea birds – wary of land, and only driven there to nest. Yet a general contextual shift in attitudes *outside* the NHS concerning liberty itself and the responsibilities of the individual may indeed be driving them before the wind of change. This, in education, in family life, in child care, in self-control. This is a necessary condition of an adult society. I suggest that sufficient change within the NHS itself is unlikely to happen without this wider, external cultural shift. But that these contextual changes make a response inevitable and timely.

The risks of regulation

John Blundell and Professor Colin Robinson have recently reviewed such questions raised by rule making and regulation. They argue that 'Government regulation rests on uncertain foundations of principle and leads to practical difficulties'. And that it is not legitimate to assume, as advocates of Government regulation frequently do, that on balance it will be beneficial to that elusive concept, 'the public interest'. They offer a number of arguments which make the dynamist case. These should be considered as we continue to learn from the experience of rule making by Government. David Boaz has offered the point, too, that 'often the real issue at hand is not whether a particular activity will be regulated, but whether it will be regulated coercively, by the State, or voluntarily, through private actions'.[7]

Blundell and Robinson say that rules are an essential part of life, but that making them is not necessarily a Government function. They can be, and usually are, established through voluntary action, and they evolve through experience. The best protector of the integrity of services is the spontaneous rules that are evolved in markets, from the incentive for firms to promote their own credibility by striving to offer value for money and safe services, while seeking competitive advantage among consumers whom we assume have the capacity to make rational decisions. Clearly we need to do all that we can to express the role of Government as rule maker in dynamist terms. And to curtail unnecessary regulation.

Open information

We should break the seal on open information. The imperative is to inform the consumer, and to encourage every individual to be free to make comparisons and reach personal judgements. Every service user will be equipped – by information and advice, and by comparative information on competing insurers, purchasers and providers about quality, performance and price – and will be empowered to make effective and personal choices. This will help to ensure that patients and service users are placed at the centre of the system, where the utmost respect for individual choice and self-responsibility is protected by open information, advice and supportive consultation.

Government will systematically publish up-to-date information in order to educate the market, and to encourage and support open comparisons on performance, price, costs and management. This will include information on risk-adjusted outcomes, waiting times, individual performance records of doctors and clinical teams, and data on patient satisfaction. This information will be produced by Government, and also by independent, charitable, voluntary and patient bodies separately. It will be a requirement of registration in the system that a provider will only be licensed if this information is forthcoming and current. No purchaser would be licensed to buy from a source for which this information was not forthcoming – whether a public, private, UK or European provider. This will require much better information technology and systems management, which is itself a major contributor to better care (as the recent study of Kaiser Permanente demonstrated).[8]

Information must take account of the technological revolution, and must make as much available on websites as possible, with good links. It must be presented in the most digestible format, supported by literature, tapes, video discs and interactive computer programs. Raw data must become 'knowable', usable and relevant to individuals. The risk of 'framing' to manipulate responses is well known. Visual presentations which enable patients to narrate their experiences and their choices are also important, and these should include carers and relatives, too.[9]

This contemporary approach is crucial for effecting the broader adoption of the recent new approach to eye care we have seen in the UK. As I have described previously, the revolution in optics evidences the truth that comes the opportunity, comes the investment. Open information and freedom to advertise all aspects of products and services, including 'soft' comparative advertising, has been the fulcrum, together with vouchered services. This approach offers an optimal social and business model for change throughout UK healthcare. The availability of open information has empowered customers to shop around.

To be able to act reasonably in a social context such as healthcare, we each need information. However, in a State monopoly system all of the incentives are to suppress information. For information generates demand, and informed demand in a rationed and allocative system is a terrible nuisance. Since we cannot discuss every possibility and cost every alternative choice – even in the age of the Internet – with every other person in the community, we need some short-cuts. Every factor and detail changes constantly as each decision is made, each new technology applied, each consequence in turn generating consequences. The actions of the unknown and the unknowable change our situation while we even sit down to consider the matter. We rely on open information advice, counselling and advocacy. Markets generate these. They enable us all to compare.

The necessary context is one of open information, competing advice, and alternative safe provision from competing providers. For the system to work at all, the exchange of appropriate information to inform the consumer is needed. Open information is a key building block in ensuring informed choice by which purchasers can ensure that the worst off can receive service and quality care as good as that which is received by the better off. This should include using the power of information more effectively, by *requiring* purchasers, insurers and providers to advertise specifics, while supporting patients with evaluations (e.g. of the particular results of care team outcomes). Information will be available by law, on quality, access, performance of clinical teams, price and reported consumer commentaries, to ensure all of the above, building on current work pushed forward by Mr Milburn. All participating organisations will be required to publish specific information at fixed intervals.

Government must ensure that information is relevant to the individual, and thus usable for choosing a specific, personal, intimate, evaluated, routine and successful approach to care.

Direct incentives for preventive care

It is *individuals* who respond to incentives and penalties. Only individuals can contribute that vital element in care, which is the practical discipline of self-responsibility. This idea has a practical and philosophical basis. For in Nozick's account, we are the owners of our own selves, and it is individual rights which should set the limits of State action. Equally, individuals should bear the costs of their choices.[10] Preventive care is the true source of most good health, provided that we can avoid the medicalisation of our lives and statist 'coercive healthism'.[11]

Incentives are critical. As Enthoven recently said:

> *People respond to many incentives other than economic ones, especially in healthcare. Yet it is important to get the economic incentives right so that resources will flow to those people and institutions that do the best job. Engineering economic incentives is crucial to good long-term outcomes. In health care, it is not possible to make them perfect, but they can be made roughly right, and that, in turn, can be improved upon. Economists have valuable expertise in this domain.*[12]

If incentive carries strong messages about the rewards of work and of saving – central themes of Government policy – this must also be so for the rewards of changing behaviour and taking direct personal responsibility for preventive action. Incentive is vital, both in terms of the cost of health insurance and in terms of better individual health status. In addition, the technical and organisational system should be designed so that incentives – such as having to earn revenues – prompt providers to respond in their areas of competence. Thus, as the Kaiser Permanente study showed, there must be better integration of care, treatment of patients at the most cost-effective level of care (which users significantly determine), much better information and information technology (the two are different), and protection of competition and choice.[13] We need to do some hard thinking about direct incentives and penalties which – combined with education – may work better than exhortation and putting leaflets among piles of old magazines in GPs' surgeries.

For example, consider smoking. Information and education are key influences. But still some people – distressingly, more young women than ever – prefer risky behaviour even when they are informed about the links between smoking and serious diseases. There are 13 million smokers in the UK. Smoking costs the NHS £1.5 billion a year in related diseases. The question here is twofold. First, which direct incentives can do more to deter smoking? And secondly, who should bear these additional costs, and by which mechanisms? Some argue that as smoking generates around £7.6 billion a year for the Treasury, smokers pay for themselves, and they pay the most dire penalties, too. Others urge that smoking is not an illness, but a lifestyle choice whose risks are well known, and that the health costs that result should be borne by the smoker. Yet early and unnecessary deaths, and spending the last years of life in acute misery, harm the individual, their families and society.[14]

We know that the one thing that can make a huge difference to millions is to encourage people, help people, offer incentives to people to give up smoking, and to help the young not to start it. A Government that is serious about preventive care would tackle smoking, finding a substitute for its tax revenue or seeking fewer taxes, narrow the contexts within which smoking can be done, expand the public safety argument, and integrate incentive into the relationships between the individual and the healthcare system.

It is often assumed that the problem is the State, with the NHS representing archetypically the failings of State enterprises. But both the State and the individual are part of the problem. And the basic source of good individual health is the individual – how we live. We do need to narrow the role of the State and enlarge the role of the individual. More individual choice is needed, of course. But also more individual concern with preventive care, more concern with consequences, and more incentives to be so concerned.

Crucially, personal self-responsibility and the well-being of the individual are within the grasp only of the individual. One's well-being is not the responsibility of the State, and if people leave it to the State they will be disappointed as they cope with the consequences of their own neglect. But self-responsibility can only become real if the individual understands and believes that it is beneficial. That is, that it is worth active participation within a social construct which they regard as significant, worthwhile and individually advantageous in their everyday life. Somehow self-responsibility has to become a personal contact with reality which changes how people think about their own lifestyle and health, and not only about the shape and structure of health services.

There should, I believe, be direct incentives for individuals to take personal responsibility for lifestyle and preventive care. Efforts should be made in three chief areas, using reward and penalty to achieve encouragement and deterrence, to promote changes in behaviour, and to establish personal responsibility and accountability. First, there is a need to encourage and support greater personal responsibility, self-care, and self-awareness of the impact of lifestyle on health status. Certainly there are institutional measures that we can use. There should be a biannual review of health status when the individual and the patient guarantee care insurer discuss the insurance contract. The basic 'excess' would influence the premium, as would a loading charge for lack of participation (or meeting agreed targets) in the individual's planned improvement programme. It is in the insurer's interest to pay bonuses to reduce future costs, and it should be in the patient's interest to reduce premiums. They will be healthier, too, as a result. And if they have a no-claims bonus they should be able to keep part of this gain to save as part of long-term care plans.

In the patient-guaranteed care structure the consumer will be offered tax incentives, which will influence their premium and encourage further savings in private insurance and long-term care plans. The biannual review of their insurance by an individual would include a personal health plan to which the individual signs up, with a 'loading' potential on the premium for specific destructive lifestyles, such as high consumption of alcohol and tobacco, abuse of substances, and lack of exercise. To do these things new and special training for professionals will be necessary. Secondly, social conditions that can be changed, such as bad housing, are a separate but important area for action, to which the redirection of personal resources by the individual could also help significantly. Thirdly, more creative educational work, linked to tax incentives – for joining and using a gym, or for taking reliable steps to take appropriate medication, or for undertaking an agreed health improvement plan and actually doing it – will be needed.

There is another huge sphere which concerns preventive care. This is the cultural error of our over-emphasis on medicine as a solution to self-imposed ills. This, too, needs review. A shift to preventive care would itself be a huge cultural change. The NHS has not proved successful as a preventive agency against illness or as a powerful advocate for positive health. Instead, it is focused on curing disease and illness – inevitably so since it is underpinned by the scientific paradigms and medical models of clinicians who have successfully protected their status as the core practitioners and providers of services, and dominated its politics.

We need radical suggestions for the State to use its powers, especially the creative use of taxation. The State could use our money with more flair, shifting its spend from sickness treatments to disease prevention. Every measure costs money, but I suggest that they have the potential to reduce costs overall. The key is to find ways to appeal to what Misselbrook calls 'the locus of control' – the controlling focus, the motivational force within the individual – and how relevant factors can be within the control of the individual.[15] First, direct incentives are needed to influence the young, and to encourage change in individual behaviour in childhood. Self-responsibility is a characteristic of a *whole* life. Wordsworth's healthcare advice was: 'The child is *father* to the man.' It is a key to the citadel of better individual health status that we all should become more aware of consequences, starting in childhood. With a more conscious link between our individual behaviour, costs and the future. Incentives should begin with the young. The foundations of our attitudes, values, assumptions, expectations, preconceptions, commitments, knowledge and virtues are laid in our childhood. And l'Estrange encapsulated the humanist commonplace that 'The *Principles* that we imbibe in our *Youth* we carry commonly to our graves.'[16] There is a continuous line from infancy to adulthood, and on to old age. And our childhood (and of course our genetic inheritance) circles back on itself. It connects the extremes of youth and old age.

The key is to help people to enhance their personal skills, in order to increase control over their lives. Young people today are also more likely to be motivated by discounts on rock concerts if they meet a healthcare and lifestyle target. And why not? If Government is to continue to tax our incomes, it should spend our money where it does the trick. If disease can be prevented by collaboration in personal health plans, this is certainly better and cheaper than intensive acute and chronic care over an extended period of years for millions. And if there is a focus on choice, informed responsibility and individual incentive, this does not breach a principle of liberty. So we should seek motivations which galvanise the young to go for things that mean something in young lives, and which are linked to better living. These might include much cheaper enrolments in health clubs (with tax incentives), guaranteed tickets to major pop concerts and major sporting events for meeting health targets, and cheaper travel packages to holiday resorts in the sun (screening creams provided!) and to World Cup matches for those showing gains in self-care, in an agreed care programme as part of their biannual insurance contract. We can be much more inventive about persuasive messages and their form in new media and on the Internet. A novel programme, *Journey to the Centre of the Lungs*, that uses virtual reality to teach young people about asthma, offers a way forward. This is a creative example of the best health education. It uses a motion simulator, and helps teenagers to visualise what happens in their lungs.[17]

Modern societies are better at solving some kinds of problem than others. The easy ones are technical and scientific – those with no human element. The difficult ones involve the revision of inherited social structures, challenges to institutions and vested interests, and shifts to behaviour. However, if we want benefits we must take some chances. For example, we should enable children themselves to make videos, using their language, attitudes and cultural styles. This might be persuasive to other children. Children could be funded via schools and police forces to make videos about drug taking, alcohol and smoking, using images and language in the idiom of their contemporaries – in their own style and tone. Role models, peer group influence, and the language and idiom of the young, used by the young to speak to one another, should all be used.

Secondly, there should be direct incentives for adults. These might include tax incentives for people whose lifestyle improves their situation (e.g. vis-à-vis diabetes), or cheaper mortgage loans and tax-funded extra credits in long-term care plans and pensions for improvers (e.g. those individuals who show significant improvements in blood pressure, body weight, or exercise regimes in an agreed health plan on a two-year cycle).

Thirdly, there should be disincentives for large at-risk groups. Disincentives for the obese (more expensive travel is being proposed in the USA).

No provider should be registered unless they offer integrated care, on the Kaiser Permanente model.

GPs and other purchaser and provider institutions should be influenced by direct incentives to promote preventive care and to think of consequences. The patient-guaranteed care provider and the patient-guaranteed care purchaser are almost certainly reliant on the GP. The latter has the key role, as the person who is in regular contact with the patient. When GPs have financial incentives to do things, they do them (e.g. immunisations and health check-ups). A successful incentive would be one in which both the patient and the GP make a gain. GPs have to be able to keep some of the financial benefit. The GP as a provider should be able to earn bonuses. As a provider who improves care, the GP should be able to earn from health gains by contract with purchasers. For example, if a GP gets a patient's diabetes or blood pressure under control (conditions which otherwise go on to cause worse problems) by diet, exercise and lifestyle, and thus reduces the burdens of clinical interventions and drugs, they should have a direct incentive to do so. There should be major tax incentives, and access to cheaper capital, for providers and purchasers who succeed in preventive care measures.

There is also the question of the medical model. A new emphasis on personal responsibility would contribute to moving the emphasis away from the medically determined model of health status to a social model. The impact of such changes would be a move away from relying on curative care, towards disease prevention, and away from the high costs and uncertain outcomes of those disease interventions which are avoidable. The system will be built on more direct financial incentives both for purchasers and for providers to encourage responsive provision, and a more holistic and co-ordinated health system. This will end the situation where professional incomes in the public sector are often unrelated to any assessment of individual activity or of results.

We too easily accept sickness where we could insist upon health by taking serious responsibility for own selves. Here HJ Massingham, Rolf Gardiner, Lionel Picton, Sir Albert Howard and other organisists (or proto-'Greens') in Britain in the 1930s and 1940s have sadly been proved correct – although they were long regarded as marginal, eccentric figures, with slight policy or popular impact. They made the case that 'The desire to take exercise ought to be a consequence of health, not a consciousness of ill health', and that Britain had 'no science of health, only a science of disease'. They warned against the medicalisation of life and society (which the NHS has helped to supervise), and cautioned that the nation had a false sense of the norm, leading to an acceptance of sickness. They argued that health encompassed the mental and spiritual as well as the physical, and was 'a state of balance internal and external, a unity, a wholeness, a power'. Thus their emphasis was on the primacy of physical experience, on diet, and on purity in foodstuffs. This was once – and only recently – all regarded as a dissident diagnosis. It has now become central to our hopes for self-responsibility in personal living, as well as in large-scale changes in production.[18]

Educational change has a part to play in every respect, and much more broadly than in the conventional slots reserved for 'health education'. We need an education system which encourages curiosity, awareness, enthusiasm and the self-responsibility of informed choice. This health issue is not only about the NHS. We should indeed reshape *all* of our institutions so that they encourage learning to choose – and continued learning throughout life, rather than the passivity which leaves people lost when they no longer have instruction. Kierkegaard said that each of us seeks 'a truth that is true for me'. However, this kind of learning cannot occur unless people have genuine choices before them and the hope and confidence of being able to exercise choice in self-education and self-discovery.

Equally, discipline should be internalised if we wish to avoid it being imposed from without. We most of us approve of the idea that the individual has unique worth, and that the idea of individual fulfilment within a framework of moral purpose must be a deep personal and social concern. This implies the idea of individual fulfilment and lifelong learning to make choices in seeking to live a satisfying life. We need the support of education as well as of experience.

We should also recognise that self-responsibility is more likely to occur when people feel that significant consequences can result from what they do. Obviously this is not always the case, but we would live better lives if incentives prompted us to consider consequences both for ourselves and for others. Personal awareness of consequences is crucial in life.

There is a valuable point, too, which is encompassed by the idea that the *whole* is contained in any *part*. Thus, in terms of diet, this contrasts organic practice with mechanistic planning and commercial production. And it highlights the interconnections of issues such as health, disease, politics, the ownership of our bodies, and who lives with which consequences.[19]

Every opportunity for the individual to top up spending

It will be for the individual to decide what they see as the 'right' amount, over and above the core package, which itself will be better than the existing normality of the NHS. For individuals should not be prevented from making an investment (e.g. in extra drugs for cancer care which are denied to them by the NHS) when they are willing to bear the costs, the extra amount that is invested being determined by individual choice and bringing extra resources into the system. We also need a society-wide endeavour to find ways to prevent cancer, and not just to prioritise its management and control.[20]

A presumption within the system against the problemisation of normality, and that the biomedical model will be seriously queried at every stage

I have explored these issues concerning the biomedical model, and Dr Misselbrook is the outstanding guide.

The whole functioning through effective direct incentives and contract

These will strengthen competition (which reduces discrimination against age, colour, gender, disability, or deficiencies in social skills, and separates economic efficiency from such important but often irrelevant characteristics), increase diversity, encourage self-responsibility and self-awareness (of both patients and care staff), and coincide with the necessary redistribution of income to eliminate inappropriate inequalities.

And we should keep in view the comment by Marcus Aurelius: 'The universe is change; life is opinion'.

Notes

1 Friedman M (1962) *Capitalism and Freedom*. Chicago University Press, Chicago, 1982 edition, p.128.
2 Postrel V (1998) *The Future and Its Enemies. The Growing Conflict Over Creativity, Enterprise and Progress*. The Free Press, New York, p.109.
3 This formulation began with Postrel's list, to which I have added. Postrel, op. cit., p.116.
4 Postrel, ibid., p.144.
5 Enthoven A (2002) *Introducing market forces into healthcare: a tale of two countries*. Paper delivered to 4th European Conference on Health Economics, Paris, 10 July. Dillon J (2002) Ministers to pull plug on unpopular universities. *Independent on Sunday*. **11 August**. Sherman J and Fresco A (2002) Hit squads to take over the worst councils and Councils of despair. Voters, not minister, control local Government. *The Times*, first leader. **12 December**.
6 Quoted by Morris J (2002) *Lincoln: a foreigner's quest*. Penguin, Harmondsworth, p.117.
7 Blundell J and Robinson C (2000) Regulation without the State. In: Blundell and Robinson (eds) *Regulation Without the State … the Debate Continues*. Institute of Economic Affairs, London. High J (ed.) (1991) *Regulation. Economic theory and history*. University of Michigan Press, Ann Arbor, MI. Boaz D (2000) Commentary: the benefits of private regulation. In: Blundell and Robinson (eds) *Regulation Without the State … the Debate Continues*. IEA, London.
8 Feachem *et al.* op. cit.
9 Edwards A, Elwyn G and Mulley A (2002) Explaining risks: turning numerical data into meaningful pictures. *BMJ*. **324**: 827–30.
10 Nozick R (1974) *Anarchy, State and Utopia*. Basil Blackwell, Oxford, p.243.
11 Skrabanek P (1994) *The Death of Humane Medicine*. The Social Affairs Unit, London. R Lea challenges the scientific basis of much healthism. See Lea R (2000) *Healthcare in the UK: the need for reform*. Institute of Directors, London. February; revised edition, June 2000.
12 Enthoven, Paris, op. cit.
13 Feachem *et al.*, ibid.
14 Second leader (2002) Not a nice habit. The NHS should not waste money on smokers. *The Times*. **12 April**. Hawkes N (2002) Smokers offered drug treatment on the NHS. *The Times*. **12 April**.
15 Misselbrook D (2002) *Thinking About Patients*. Petroc Press, Newbury, pp.97–9.
16 Cited by Manning, op. cit., p.154.
17 Fricker J (2002) A ride inside the lungs. *The Times*. **1 July**: 11.
18 Matless D (1998) *Landscape and Englishness*. Reaktion Books, London.
19 Matless, ibid., especially chapter 4.

20 Sikora K *et al.* (2002) Should NHS patients be allowed to pay extra for their care? Patient payments bring new resources into system. *BMJ.* **324**: 109–10. Sikora K (1999) Rationing cancer care. In: J Spiers (ed.) *The Realities of Rationing,* Institute of Economic Affairs, London, pp.123–39. New ideas needed to revive the NHS (letter). *The Times.* **20 February**.

Chapter 23

Market mimicry, or the alternatives to the patient fundholder

The law doth punish man or woman that steals the goose from off the common,
But lets the greater felon loose that steals the common from the goose.

(Anon.)

Look, and beware!

We see all around us the immense fecundity of nature. And the protection that imitation brings: the leaf that jumps up and stings; the stone that bites; the flower that closes its jaws over the fly. Butterflies that look like leaves, beetles which simulate moss, insects which live by imitating twigs or stones. Nature is the source of artistry, and of miracles of pretence and persuasion. These miracles of mimicry are to be found in public life, too. Its market mimicry is vivid, and it too carries its stings. Thus centralisation, control 'from above', the suggestion of co-operative and mutual alternatives – but without individual economic autonomy – all these are overlain by market mimicry. The innocent should be wary. For these devices of market mimicry fundamentally deny free will, freedom itself – and the freedom to act or not, to believe or disbelieve, to express self-responsibility, to learn to choose, and to develop those personal decisions from which creative change comes. They offer not an enlightened, rational or 'progressive' but ultimately a narrow view of human nature and capacity. For it is free will in which each of us acts out our particular wishes, passions, interests, characters, talents, hopes, values, and choices. Here, freedom is much more than the freedom to buy or sell. It is a moral and a spiritual condition. And the assumptions of market mimicry contradict this by assuming that people are not competent to understand (or to learn to understand) to protect their own moral, cultural, physical and social interests.

The alternatives to real markets (which use the particular to realise the universal, and which can give the poor the freedoms enjoyed by the middle class) offered are these:

- more provider freedoms (for example, 'Foundation Hospitals') – but without demand-side change by which individuals secure budgetary power
- devolution – decentralisation – but without leveraged individual financial choice
- the transfer of NHS assets to 'the local community' – but what could this mean?

- more accountability through 'local democracy' – but how, in the apathy that surrounds it?
- more political activism and consultation in planning – but this does not equip the individual to command a specific service
- hypothecated taxation – but which offers no individual leverage
- the money to follow the patient – but unless there is direct cash payment there is no individual control or financially empowered choice
- more inspection and regulation – but which brings new costs and uncertainties.

However, as I have suggested, more politics – more health activism – is no solution. We must rely not on politicians but on ourselves. We should encourage politicians to stand aside, save to represent the interests of consumers by protecting competition. Yet paradoxically, in a democracy it is only politicians who can deliver us from politics. They may do so in order to avoid the rage of voters and respond to large cultural shifts in contexts. And we must press politicians to help us make our health safe in our *own* hands.

I have offered an approach which starts with the insistence on patient-guaranteed care for all. A core of certain, specific, legally guaranteed services, and on the patient as the fundholder. As I have suggested, this is an approach which engages co-operative purchasing, mutuality and social solidarity. It is one, too, which builds on our own history – those earlier mutual associations until very recently were often regarded with either bafflement, misunderstanding or even contempt. As I outlined in the introduction, these bodies sought to find genuine solutions to what have been, and remain, intractable and fundamental problems. Or what Noel Coward called 'The delights of equal independence. State controlled'.

We should ask if the solutions offered instead of markets can serve as answers, or no. Each of these is itself a 'cultural' challenge about how much is to be provided, how, by whom, when, how patterned and structured, reflecting which social relations? For nothing 'just is'. Every institution, assumption, expectation, attitude, acceptance and rejection has evolved, and is evolving further. Everything is culturally specific. It is underpinned by ideas. Meanwhile, in the NHS regime many users of services have remained profoundly 'de-skilled', and have then been blamed for their ignorance and incapacity to manage their lives and to make choices. Equally, it is striking that the best efforts to inform choice, and to guide the selection of services, have been private, charitable or co-operative initiatives.[1]

After its return to Government in 1997, it was politics which prevented New Labour from abandoning the anathematised 'internal market'. However, supplemented by inspection and regulation on a large scale (to achieve priorities and targets), this approach has increased 'management' and raised the debate about quality, capacity, cash, access and empowerment. Labour is attempting to deliver ambitions which cannot be achieved except by markets. Thus the Secretary of State for Health has spoken of modernising the NHS to create a 'twenty-first century, consumer-focused service'. This will be 'a personalised service,' with greater choice for consumers.

Mr Milburn is the most creative Secretary of State for Health in modern times. He has shown finesse, in many surprising ways. He has consistently urged that the NHS must focus on the patient; that the NHS must put the patient at the centre; that NHS facilities and staff must be more accountable, to purchasers and to regulators, and that there must be improvements delivered in every locality. He has urged that patients must be 'given a greater say' and more information. He told the New Health Network in January 2002:

> *Patients are disempowered, with little if any choice. The system seems to work for its own convenience, not the patient's – a frustration that is shared by patients and staff alike. The whole thing is monolithic and bureaucratic.... For 50 years, the structure of the NHS meant that governments – both Labour and Conservative – defined the interests of the NHS as a producer of services when they should have been focused on the interests of the patients as the consumers of services.*[2]

But he had in the main offered more consultation rather than individual financial clout. And much of the potential to accomplish optimal healthcare lies in the potential of evolving, non-Governmental institutions. It also depends on a wide variety of non-profit agencies in getting done what has been thought of as public work. These should evolve (rather than be subordinated) in mutually respecting partnerships with consumers, central government and a regulatory system. We need institutions to have adequate autonomy, responsiveness to consumers' wishes and the capacity to utilise appropriate freedoms.

Meanwhile, in a statist approach we see many new institutions created 'from above'. Guidance issued by the Department of Health and the NHS Appointments Commission (which went 'live' in January 2003) for applicants to chair the new Commission for Patient and Public Involvement in Health said some extraordinarily revealing things about the limitations of thinking within the Department of Health and the NHS. The Secretary of State has also supported these initiatives, although I suspect that he has moved on since their inception. But the momentum of the process is carrying forward already outdated ideas. As Douglas Hurd once said, 'inertia has its own momentum'.[3] The documents reveal that, after more than 50 years, the stasist system shows how the patient remains marginalised by process. And that the system can only imagine improvements in processes to offer any answer to how empowerment can occur. Thus patients will now have 'a real say' – but through improved processes, not via prices or markets. Remember the traditional quip about the pig being 'involved' in the bacon sandwich.

The new Commission shows from its guidance document that:

- the NHS solution is more activism – the staff will run events 'about getting [patients] involved and the skills needed to do this'
- it is our 'needs', not our wants, which are to be 'delivered'
- there will be more 'involvement' of patients *as citizens* ('in the decision-making process' and in 'local consultation exercises'), but not as individual consumers with empowered choices
- involvement will mean helping to configure services – which is different from being enabled to command a specific service
- every Patients' Forum will receive the support that it needs 'against a set of agreed standards *the Commission itself will set*' (my italics)

- every Patients' Forum will nominate one of their number to be put forward for appointment to Trust Boards – and 'they will be one of over 600 new voices with direct influence at the heart of the decision-making process', as the UK population approaches 60 million
- every Patient Advice and Liaison Service (now in existence in over 200 NHS trusts) will continue as an early warning and advice system. However, this is an interpretative system, with all the difficulties of class, communication skills, assumptions, expectations and decibel planning
- individuals will be 'placed at the centre of the NHS' to influence its work by communicating views – but with no accountability improved?
- the system will be held 'to account "democratically"'. This does not guarantee individual choice, as my earlier discussion indicates.

This structure is a drawn-out rearguard action. No reader who has stayed with me this far will be surprised if I suggest that all real change is only achievable by prices and market signals. It is these which change attitudes and behaviour, if indeed they can be changed. It is these which genuinely involve every patient as a consumer. It is these which hold a system *and* an individual to account. It is these which apply appropriate pressure from outside. It is these, too, which offer the service user a relationship, which evolve mutual trust, and which also offer the *benefit* of redress by the threat or *actualité* of litigation by due process of law, if this becomes necessary. The most efficient and the most representative national survey of issues of concern to individuals (because it involves and represents *every* consumer) is the market. All these aspects of relationships in markets ensure effective mechanisms of information, communication and 'involvement'. It is price and markets which can *ensure* what a stasist system ever finds so elusive. That is, to match demand to resources and to 'bring about a change in culture in the NHS so that taking account of the individual patient's experience of the NHS becomes the norm'.[4]

The processes of 'market mimicry' are thus all part of the bureaucratic response to the pressures of consumerism, to growing litigation against the NHS, to the activism of Labour local support, and to shock at the denials and deficits of the nationalised system. If you want to run a system of controls from above, but do it more efficiently, this is as good an approach as we have seen. However, it will actually function in parallel rather than as a substitute for revolutionary developments in giving patients direct cash payments, and will ultimately be subsumed (less expensively) in the quality control systems of the provider in an open market.

The system is not actually interested in the empowered consumer. It is interested in 'the informed and trained user' – to whom it offers more local activism, more politicised management for 'equality', fairness, redistribution of wealth, user 'consultation', user 'advocacy', citizens' juries, 'political restructuring' and local authority 'health scrutiny', patient surveys, 'needs-led' commissioning, and health authorities as 'champions of the people'. This is a relentless architecture of anything but money in individual hands – a confetti of advisory and executive bodies, regulatory participation, targets, guidelines, 'internal markets', a panoply and a panjandrum of managed scarcity. This inevitably gathers *some* useful information from consumers. But they have no sanction over its use.

This is, of course, an area with some grey. Of course, some patients and service users *can* influence themes for consideration, and perhaps encourage some detailed changes. There will always be some people locally who will push the boundaries, and help users make gains. Some Community Health Councils showed this. But this is in the main a case of some patients urging reallocation of rationed resources. It is a beggar-my-neighbour system. It takes away from Paul to give to Paulette, or vice versa. It is a bidding process. And it excludes those who are not organised in this way. For example, the Parkinson's Disease Society produced an impressive *Local Guidance* series in 2002, 'helping individuals, groups or alliances' to express their views as individuals, or as representatives of groups, in order to 'achieve the most influence' with NHS Trust Patients' Forums and Patient Advice and Liaison Services (PALS). However, this is very much action by those 'within' the system, replacing Community Health Councils, which were external commentators, however ineffective. And relatively few are involved. The material that the society produced shows the limits of the consultative approach in many respects. For example, Somerset Health Panels meet twice a year in each primary care trust area, and up to 12 members of the public are recruited to attend three panels.[5]

In August 2002, Mr Milburn published an article in *The Times* saying that Labour must seize the policies of diversity and choice, in order to transform State-controlled public services into consumer-driven organisations. He wrote:

> *There is no automatic correlation that tax-funded healthcare has to mean healthcare run simply by central Government.... Existing NHS hospitals should be able to become NHS Foundation Hospitals with more freedom from centralised State control and greater local community ownership.*[6]

This reflected a dispute at the heart of Government over public sector freedoms to borrow and to undertake private sector work. It also underlined Mr Milburn's expressed belief that Foundation Hospitals will empower individuals through 'greater community ownership'. It is not clear what is meant by 'community ownership', but we can recall that when the people 'owned' a sixty-millionth each of every nationalised industry, in practice they owned and controlled nothing. This is the case with the NHS, on which users are being 'consulted' by all manner of new agencies. And, as with nationalised industries of the past, their rights of ownership could not be *realised* in the marketplace, nor could they enable them to command a specific service. These rights of ownership did not correspond to normal rights of property at all. However, the majority remain trapped. Mr Milburn has also offered a few of the best hospitals Foundation status, seeking to liberate provision and to broaden access to a variety of providers. But the majority of patients must go to the remaining hospitals. He has emphasised *redesigning the service* (which is not new – it is more than half a century old) *focused on the patient.* This has raised anew the rigorous questioning of 'how?' The consequences of Mr Milburn's struggle to add a consumer focus to an organisation with no such incentive will, I believe, reveal the contradictions which must ultimately be resolved. And they will push us forward to look at the issues from a different, dynamist perspective.

Now, managers are not answerable to consumers but to Ministers. They have necessarily responded to plans, not to prices, and, if not to peerages, then to perks. And the politics of ministerial life has meant that appointees interfere constantly in management. Indeed, for a while Mr Milburn, while Secretary of State for Health, was also his *own* Chief Executive. Yet as services have worsened, managerial salaries – apparently unconnected to results – have gone up. Many NHS Trust Chief Executives now earn more than £100 000, with generous pensions and benefits, yet with no comeback from the consumer. Such increases in costs, which in industry contribute to rises in prices (and possible consumer rejection), are met by further subsidy from the Treasury, not by more satisfied consumers. As Dominic Hobson noted, 'Nationalised industries neither go bankrupt nor get taken over.'[7]

Where are we to look for better solutions? The solutions concern the freedoms of the informed consumer. This requires a decisive change in mentalities, where the purchaser has to perform in order to retain support. What matters most is competition for customers. Mrs Thatcher admitted in her memoirs: 'Ownership by the State is just that – ownership by an impersonal legal entity: it amounts to control by politicians and civil servants.'[8] Until Mrs Thatcher used State power for non-State purposes, those on the left had not much noticed that the State was not merely a phenomenon but a problem, and a revival of discussion about alternatives – notably associationism and mutual-aid – began.[9]

However, it is notable that neither Mr Blair, Mr Milburn nor Mr Duncan Smith has yet specified what they mean by 'community ownership', or any other mechanisms, incentives and changes which would ensure that *consumers* exercise full and effective personal choice and competition in all public services – although I believe that Mr Milburn has made a beginning with direct cash payments, and that he knows exactly where this can lead us. That is, by having the hands of consumers directly on the money, there can result a concrete programme of action necessary to turn 'a patient-centred NHS' into a realisable policy. These initiatives indeed, I have suggested, will separate political and managerial decision making. They will bring realities to the surface. They will prepare the public for wider market-driven reform, in which value and efficiency, performance and profit coincide. And it is necessary to offer education about specific devices for change. Such a programme can be achieved by stealthy increments. But there will come a point when a real argument breaks out, and then the benefits will need all possible publicity and to be structured so that public opinion can group itself in support.

However, it will be insufficient to show a capacity for seeing small sections of the problem with steadiness, if the issues are not seen whole. A prelude to wider change is to consistently set out first principles by which both to lead debate and to explain events. Thus the systemic sources of the persistent difficulties of the NHS would be shown – why there are shortages, too few medical staff, poor environments, lower-than-possible quality, and why alternative systems do not suffer these inequities. This approach could lead education, build understandings, and widen support for necessary reform.

Genuine decentralisation means redistributing economic power out of the hands of Government and its proxies and into the hands of the individual consumer of services. Otherwise, decentralisation means readjusting the holding of *political* power, but retaining *economic* power in those reshaped hands – whether this is done centrally or locally makes no difference. Friedman put this difficulty with his inimitable clarity as follows:

> *Viewed as a means to the end of political freedom, economic arrangements are important because of their effect on the concentration or dispersion of power. The kind of economic organisation that provides economic freedom directly, namely competitive capitalism, also promotes political freedom because it separates economic power from political power and in this way enables the one to offset the other.*[10]

There is evidently not yet any realisation that the Government's approach remains instead an expert definition of the wants of individuals (which is a contradiction in terms). And that when Government talks of placing decision making as close to the patient as possible, this still does not mean actually enabling decisions to be made *by* the patient. Having decisions made for you, but made *geographically* nearer than Whitehall, does not change the process or the nature of the decision, whether or not it becomes a more approximate guess from above than it has been until now. And, indeed, in a politicised system it seems likely that the local managers will spend much of their time and energy *accounting* to the centre, rather than to the patient. And so discussion of 'a patient-centred service' and 'decentralised decision making' is disabled before it starts. Instead, it emphasises *partnerships with local government.*

It remains to be seen whether at the next general election New Labour will line up on the side of the providers, and the Conservatives on the side of the patient/service user and the individual. The Liberal Democrats have already offered regional health taxation and decentralisation – but with no individual economic power in the hands of consumers. It will be an advance if hospitals and other providers can become mutual companies, as they propose. They can be called 'public benefit organisations', too. However, even if they are owned by staff (and by 'local communities' – but what does that mean?), they must still be required to seek revenues from consumers who have control over where they spend their NHS credit. Otherwise the position is no different from Labour's concept of 'earned autonomy', which means central controls.[11] Without this change there will still be no real choice, if the consumer still has no power of choice, nor will the provider have the direct incentives to offer services. Consumers must control financial clout. What each party leader has said about consumer-led services does not seem to be the same thing as individual consumer empowerment to make costed personal choices.

However, it is impossible to gauge demand and to change supply without a price mechanism. Administrative substitutes cannot capture the essential signals of the evolving market. 'User councils', patient representatives, citizens' juries, lay visitors and patient forums are indeed symptoms of the *lack* of user control. Sainsbury's does not have a customer jury, with the purchaser at the check-out being 'represented' by a consumers' council. And in healthcare such a body, I have suggested, can neither know nor express the wishes of users at the time of private necessity, which is often the only time the user discovers their own values, wants and preferences. However, the NHS continues to insist on user 'involvement' as a substitute for choice. Asda, Safeway, Morrisons, Ford, my local sports centre, British Airways, Lane Cove Sunshine Holidays and Penguin Books do not demand your 'involvement', your time in planning or your collaboration in rationing services. They offer you a service with a choice. And thus standards continue to rise, and prices fall. Innovations offer you new options. These innovations are rapidly diffused. We make our own lifestyle decisions and invest in what matters to us. Surpluses are reinvested and others benefit as well. This does not mean that we do not support the idea that the poor should have much better healthcare. We all certainly want this. But the evidence seems not to suggest that this comes about by people being 'involved' in politics or planning, or in the role of political activist. For everyone to have the same choices as the middle classes, the key is to have money in their hands with which to exercise those choices. Again we come back to patient power and money to transform the services, if significant change is to be achieved *throughout* this vast and complex organisation, and as a matter of everyday routine.

There are significant difficulties with each of the proposed alternatives to individual empowerment.

Let us examine the alternatives.

More provider freedoms (for example, 'Foundation Hospitals'), but without demand-side change

The flagships of this change are the new Foundation Hospitals, to be established 'as free-standing entities', free from direction by the Secretary of State, as public interest companies – in Mr Milburn's words, 'not-for-profit, public service organisations representing a middle ground between State-run public sector and shareholder-led private sector structures'.[12] They will earn their incomes from agreements and cash-for-performance contracts negotiated with primary care trusts and other commissioners. So the money will still ultimately come from the Treasury, if by proxy.

At this point in this book perhaps the problems with this approach hardly need to be argued. For this is the drive for change under the banners of a mix of more money and better management. As I have outlined, this approach takes us further towards real change, but it still does not take direct incentives sufficiently seriously. And to reform a huge and diverse institution like the NHS demands huge, devolved, driving (even enraged) energy from literally hundreds of thousands of people, many of whom remain reluctant to change, and who at present have no incentive to do so. The reform that genuine markets can achieve is not a job which can be done by centralised exhortation, targets and moral campaigns alone, nor by restricting some freedoms to a limited number of hospitals, in a generally failing context. It is direct incentive which is essential to change attitudes and

behaviours towards consumers, as well as to maximise the benefits from investments made by the public and by independent decision makers. If we accept the
importance of incentive, and of price and markets, we gain access to a powerful
body of theory and analysis which can help us to understand the nature of the
challenges and find solutions. However, supply-side shifts without demand-side
changes still shut this out.

Direct incentives are necessary to bring abstractions down to earth. Just as
individuals should bear the costs of their choices, so too individuals should gain
some of the bouquets and prizes of success. It is individuals who respond to
incentives.

However, we should notice that some opportunities arise with Foundation
Hospitals, despite the approach being outweighed by the conceptual limitations.
The Foundation Hospitals widen the debate, and they imply a different kind of
change. They have a major psychological importance, as did the two Concordats
with the private sector.[13] They suggest new possibilities while revealing the limitations of the initiative itself. One significant limitation is that the project is not
proposed as a solution to the failing hospitals, for these are excluded from the
programme. It leaves the least successful in the old mould. This is a two-tier system which does not achieve the model of the optics market, where all are in one
market. Nevertheless, the inception of Foundation Hospitals begins the process
of greater diversification of provision. They may, too, gradually encourage looser
ties with Whitehall, and may even lead to every NHS hospital trust becoming an
independent local charitable body. However, it is difficult to see sufficient benefits
– and certainly not on the vast qualitative and quantitative scale that is required
when comparing the UK system and its performance with, for example, the
Swiss or the Dutch system – without the patient fundholder.

Mr Milburn has questioned how to empower patients, but by preferring
'consultation' to control over cash he has increased the attention that is paid to
the cultural contradictions of the NHS. Mr Milburn may well find that relaxing
controls on an ossified structure as a way of seeking to resolve its internal difficulties
may subvert the whole structure, as Gorbachev found in the former Soviet Union.
For monopoly and central control are of a piece, and will be unable to coexist
with empowered individual choice. In this sense – like Soviet Communism – the
system is unreformable because it is incapable of adjusting to new circumstances.
It is inherently rigid and systemically bureaucratic. For the present reforms
demonstrate that decisions about systems can be taken which reveal but do not
really decide the issues. These concern moral and operational questions which
many wish to evade – notably of power, profit and efficiency. Each is properly the
concern of leadership to open people's minds to evolutionary change, to articulate meaningful goals, to strive towards them and to help to deliver the values
that people respect.

The temporary 'draw' between centralism and dynamism within a public
monopoly – represented by the NHS Reform and Health Care Professions
Act of 2002 – is unsustainable. Indeed this itself will prove a handicap, blocking
development and finally uncovering the alternatives. Instead of correcting the
instabilities of centralised monopoly, the further centralisation of initiatives and

controls will intensify the difficulties. Ultimately, such an approach will prove self-terminating. A negotiated change would be a better means to embrace dynamic alternatives.

Devolution, but without leveraged individual financial choice

We live much of our lives locally. Our community is where much of our life is rooted – composed and organic. Power should be decentralised to 'the community'. But, *there is a fault line here which we should recognise*. Decentralisation without individual financial clout in the hands of consumers will not advance choice. Indeed, decentralisation to local government or local health authorities of Whitehall powers over purchasing merely moves central power and mentalities into a local postal district. It is a managerialist change, and it is merely geographical. It is a change of location rather than of nature. It entirely lacks the imperative that must be placed on competing providers, with consumers in charge of their own destiny. We should be cautious that decentralisation without individual financially equipped patient power is the fatal error of metropolitan urban 'political philanthropy', which leaves control in the hands of the controllers.

This policy of 'democratising decision making' is stasism writ large, even if it is transferred to smaller communities. It is not the incentive to personal responsibility, nor the alternative to control which the patient fundholder offers. It is not Burke's 'small platoon' empowered. It is the regimen of the large regiment moved to a local barracks. We all live in communities, but these are not necessarily coterminous with local boundaries. They are hardly likely to be those which we identify with local government. There is no evidence that we feel that local government responds to our concerns. If local decisions are to be responsive to local circumstances, and to the individual, then it is the individual who must be empowered. As it is, Matthew Parris is correct when he says that 'Halfway between hub and rim, local government is the enemy, not the ally, of the only decentralisation that works – to the very rim.'[14]

By contrast, consumer power offers a major counter-current to control. It depends on radically different assumptions to those of the 'expert' and the centraliser, concerning the nature of knowledge, the potential competence of the individual, and the gains from an evolving, creative, flexible and innovative market. The system has not been able to accommodate any of this, or work out what it would mean in terms of specific devices for change, or adjust to the idea that it would necessarily produce unexpected (and, within existing financing structures, unaffordable?) demands. Such cultural change, too, would undermine the considerable cultural and political power of managers, professionals and politicians. This is both the significance and the limitation of discussion concerning 'decentralisation' as a solution. For this does not imply or include individual financial power and leveraged choice, or the dynamism of evolving markets. Instead of a provider seeking to justify a service to the empowered individual, anyone with a new approach must justify this to a technocratic regulator. Thus, the trinity of licence, subsidy and tax incentive will continue to be the preserve of the powerful lobby in Friedman's 'iron triangle', in which managers, professionals and politicians permit some things to be done and prevent the doing of other things which patients might well prefer if they had the economic power to insist.

Market mimicry may deliver a warm feeling, but it does furnish reality. Here consider an analogy from the land. The soil scientist GT Wrench once said of fertilisation of the land something which summarises this problem. He wrote that 'It does not want *symbols of reality; it needs reality itself.*'[15] So, too, does the user of services, who wants to have a say in what is *specifically* provided to them, when, and with what outcomes.

There is, however, compelling contemporary evidence that when local communities take voluntary work seriously, local energies and aspirations can be harnessed, and this can produce startling results when compared with the failures of big bureaucracies. The voluntary sector now engages 3 million people, accounting for £12 billion of services. Specific initiatives in Tower Hamlets, East London have transformed the lives of many.[16] However, the language of decentralisation itself assumes that the natural place for power to be held and concentrated is at the centre – decentralisation is a permissive process. The test of proposals for decentralisation is this: will the ultimate contracting party be the individual, who is free to enter or not to enter any particular exchange, so that all transactions are voluntary, self-responsible, and price- and cost-conscious? Decentralisation – in Francis Maude's words – may enable 'local units [to be] controlled by local people and local doctors'. But how? And by whom? And with which specific results in terms of the various outcomes of care preferred by diverse individuals? We come to this next.[17]

The transfer of NHS assets to 'the local community'

Under my proposed new structure, existing NHS providers will have many new opportunities to compete for willing custom. But who will own the assets that they presently hold? This needs a great deal of careful study. It is easy to say that they should be mutualised, but what will this mean? Purchasing organisations will be owned by their subscribing members, who can stay or go to another purchaser. But in what sense could patients of a provider own it, or indeed why would they want to do so? If the State is to dispose of these assets, it hardly seems likely that the voter would accept a traditional privatisation model, or a hand-over to existing staff whose performance is already of concern. Nor does it even seem likely that local institutions – universities perhaps? – would accept the responsibility of managing the assets of a hospital which may have an uncertain future. We need careful enquiry as to how to transfer NHS facilities from State ownership. And we also need to be conscious that a transfer of assets to a local charity or community body will not by itself empower the individual consumer.

Hospitals (and other service providers, too) could be established as charitable bodies independent of Government, as not-for-profit and for-profit organisations (although of course each must operate responsively and competitively in the market). Trustees would then have to be appointed, perhaps by an independent appointments commission. A beginning could be made with the Foundation Hospitals, with the objective of learning from the experience and gradually spreading the change. We could see at least a proportion of NHS hospitals becoming independent of Government within five years. There are lessons from Germany, where just over half are independent, as are a third in France, and some 80% in The Netherlands.

NHS hospitals could be reorganised on the model of the old UK voluntary hospitals, with elected local boards responsible to trustees, who would appoint the executive directors. They could function as not-for-profit or for-profit organisations as local management determines. The State would thus end public sector quasi-monopoly in provision and the imposition of uniformity. However, the individual consumer would not own the service in any meaningful sense. The issue is whether the consumer is in charge of choices in any possible location and under any possible owner. It is purchasing power which must be transferred, not geographical emphasis or managerial in-trays. Even so, changes of ownership can encourage a different relationship to the services, and a more flexible and local management.

Mr Maude has urged that hospitals would 'belong to the community'. Certainly we feel more comfortable with local institutions, and with smaller ones, too. And even when complexity and larger size are unavoidable – for example, in a large teaching hospital or a district general hospital with full Accident and Emergency facilities – institutions should still be organised so as to give the individual a sense of identity and control. They should be built and managed so as to enhance the individual experience, and selection and staff training should encourage the attitudes of mind which support free choice.

Of course, it is an important value that people must be able to bind together in a local community (which itself contains overlapping communities). Many of us wish to identify closely with the world we belong to and know best. Meaning in our lives is often deeply associated with particular places, people, institutions and communities. The uncertainties of modern life often encourage a sense of fragility as well as one of opportunity. A sense of identity derived from a coherent community is important, and the existence of a local hospital (even when outcomes are poor, on objective evidence) is something people have wanted to hold on to. This contributes to a visible and familiar social context, as well as one of mutual obligation, of which the individual can feel part.

We each need meaning, spiritual nourishment and a sense of identity in our lives. And so Mr Maude's rhetoric is attractive when he stresses the word 'community', and the idea of institutions belonging to the community. But what would these words ('institutions belonging to the community') *actually mean in practice*? How would *this* make a reality of the often heard aspiration that the system is run in the interests of users rather than of staff and vested interests? In what sense would a hospital *belong to a community*, or to *an individual* or his or her family? And how would that 'ownership' help people? What relationship might this sense of community ownership (whatever that is) have to an individual being directly enabled to exercise a *specific* choice about a necessarily personal, uniquely intimate, separable and timely health treatment in order to achieve a personally preferred outcome? The presence of a hospital may give a sense of identity to a community. Its presence – irrespective of the quality of its work, or lack of it – may be a comfort. But how does this specifically help a service user who wants prompt access, say, to good-quality cancer care services, especially if the hospital has a poor record?

Do Mr Francis Maude and Mr Ian Duncan Smith mean – when they speak of hospitals belonging to a community, and of management being decentralised – that services should be controlled by consumers with individual financial clout? That is, having a direct impact on the revenues and thus on the existence of a specific service, which has to seek and satisfy individual customers? Individuals, too, would be acting not as voters but as local and individual purchasers, probably organised in a voluntary and co-operative purchasing organisation.

What would it mean for doctors – as Mr Maude suggests – to 'control' a local organisation such as a hospital? And why is this a good idea? Mr Duncan Smith spoke to a Birmingham audience of hospitals having more money to spend 'according to *doctors'* priorities'. Would that necessarily be helpful to consumers seeking a specific quality service? We need to do some hard thinking about this. And doctors cannot escape accountability, where the most appropriate form is to the consumer organised in a purchasing co-operative. 'Decision makers' should not retain power over consumers. It is retrograde to suggest that more power should be transferred by Government to professionals as 'decision makers'. For they are advisers, and the service user is the ultimate decision maker.[18]

Mr Duncan Smith's speech – surprisingly, in view of what the rest of the speech said – retained the provider point of view as well as the deference to the medical establishment which is being so widely challenged. The idea of doctors making all of the decisions, and the fear of their political power, still lets this idea slip into speeches – often unnoticed and unchallenged because it is apparently obvious. Mr Duncan Smith, too, still speaks of 'a system based on need' and, like the Labour Party, he shares the idea that it is Government which should work out 'how much more money we need for healthcare'. We have seen that Government can never know the 'right' amount that we should spend. It is the individual who should decide.

More accountability through local democracy

One solution to the question of how to empower the individual is offered as bringing accountability for public spending closer to its consumers through the agencies of local democracy. Leave aside for the moment that very few people vote or take any interest in local government. Accountability in political generality is not sufficient to enable a person to secure a service in particular. If we wish to secure the benefits of voluntary relationships with not-for-profit mutual-aid bodies, then individuals must be enabled to subscribe voluntarily to co-operatives which purchase care on their behalf.

It is not an answer to the problems of personal command over appropriate care to bring 'accountability for public spending closer to its consumers through the agencies of local democracy'. We should therefore be wary of accountability through local democracy, as advocated by Bernard Jenkin in 1982 and by Simon Jenkins in 2002.[19]

Mutuality is indeed not encouraged by transferring accountability to local government. It is undermined. As Marenbon has written:

> *The concentration in regional and local authorities is as much centralisation as the concentration of power nationally – and more so when, because of the closeness of the governed to their governors, the freedoms of individuals and small, intermediate institutions are all the more limited.*[20]

Individuals, small groupings, voluntary associations, local mutual-aid efforts, personal moral responsibility and the institutions of freedom are all undermined by the intrusion of Government – whether central, regional *or* local – in territory which should be the responsibility of the individual.

More political activism and consultation in planning, which does not equip the individual to command a specific service

We have seen that there are two ways in which consumers express preferences: by voting and by spending – as voters, in elections, and as consumers, when holding money. As actions, these are different *in kind* – one being very indirect, one very direct. One being diffuse, the other being specific. One being disconnected from direct results, the other very directly connected. One disempowering the individual (by submerging minorities beneath majorities), the other empowering individuals in concert (by empowering the personal voice without detracting from solidarity). The following exchange (from a Michael Innes novel) makes the point:

> *Mr Hoobin considered. 'Mister', he said heavily, 'did 'ee ever see a saw?'*
> *'Dear me, yes.'*
> *'And would 'ee ask which tooth cut board?'*[21]

Postrel tells us that individual progress has a particular source:

> *We make progress not toward a particular, certain and uniform destination, but toward many different, personally determined and incremental goals. In a global sense 'progress' is the product of those parallel individual searches: the extension of knowledge and the gradual improvement of people's lives – an increase in comfort, in life options, in the opportunity for 'diversified, worthwhile experience'. Progress is neither random Darwinian evolution nor teleological inevitability.*[22]

This approach reflects a significant problem of knowledge, and of the nature of knowledge – of what we can know of ourselves or of others, as discussed earlier. The denial of choice is based on the idea that 'decision makers' can have all of the relevant information about individuals, their values, lifestyles and preferences concerning treatments, practitioners, side-effects, outcomes and what they can and would prefer to live with.

We should note, too, that much NHS consultation is primitive, in its own terms. For example, in mental healthcare, despite many years of 'consultation' with user groups, there is still (in the words of Louis Appleby) no meaningful information on mortality, morbidity, quality of life, or users' and carers' satisfaction with services – which, in a developed market, we should surely possess. There is only throughput measurement. In its 54th year, in his words, 'We need a new system where we measure things that are relevant to the lives of people in mental healthcare.' Only from April 2003 will specialist services start routinely to collect standardised information on every adult whom they treat. At present there is no adequate information on how effectively services are performing, none on how well people recover through treatment and support – and certainly no comparative use of the existing data, poor as it is. No organisation in a market could have survived for five minutes with such an approach, where users had choices. The stoicism that prevails in the UK worsens the situation, as a German doctor newly employed in the NHS noticed with some surprise.[23]

Hypothecated taxation

This device would enable the Treasury to raise more money. And it seems to offer both transparency and simplicity. People would know what is being raised by taxation for healthcare, see openly if anyone tried to change it, and notice whether or not the Treasury actually spent on healthcare. However, the temptation would still be for the fund to be merged with existing aggregated monies. And even if this were not so, sums raised by the tax would not be 'owned' by an individual in a personal care fund. The money would remain managed by politicians or their agents – such as regional officials – on our behalf. It is not a step towards a genuine social insurance structure unless the funds are controlled by each individual, when they are required to use their 'NHS credit' to go to a Patient-Guaranteed Care Association.

Lord Haskins, Chairman of the Government's Better Regulation Task Force, has said that:

> *Insurance can be an effective alternative to State regulation. Indeed, Lloyd George and Beveridge planned to fund the Welfare State through National Insurance, and today's German social security is still effectively funded out of personal and corporate insurance contributions. Its great advantage over funding out of general taxation is that it gives recipients a sense of ownership, and promotes mutuality. One would expect more participation, less abuse of the system, and consequently less regulation. Unfortunately, the principle of insurance has been gradually eroded in Britain's social security system, in favour of funding out of general taxation, resulting in less commitment and more abuses.*[24]

Hypothecated taxation – although possibly assisting Government by helping to legitimise fundraising by Government – does not empower the consumer. Again great weight is being placed by centralisers (and decentralisers) on a framework too fragile to bear their ambitions.

More inspection and regulation

Government policy has significantly enlarged regulation. It has moved away from using markets and competition, from contracting as a lever to manage performance, and from the traditional bureaucracies. It prefers regulation, targets and the overview of what is increasingly seen as a Department of the Prime Minister, where advisers have huge influence but are not accountable to Parliament – unless they become civil servants, when they can be questioned by Commons committees. Walshe has shown that 'the responsibility for problems is shifted to the regulator, but the reach and scope of Governmental control is retained, or even increased'.[25] Healthcare regulators, as he says, 'have little independence, and, taken together, represent a significant strengthening of central Government's control of the NHS'. Indeed, it is difficult to see how this could be otherwise. These regulatory bodies are not the equivalent of 'Offload'. They are part of Government, while serving as a mechanism to distance politicians from blame. Yet they are accountable to Government, rather than to the consumer, and they have little scope to encourage innovation and risk taking from which beneficial change arises.

In general, Government has substituted many new regulatory bodies for the adaptive evolution that we see in markets.[25] These all divert us from the truth that if there is to be decentralisation as a means of achieving optimal healthcare in a society of political freedom, dispersion of power means dispersion of economic clout. For politics and economics are not separate – they are closely connected, if complex. And individual freedom is an economic problem as much as it is a political challenge. The argument is that economic freedom is a means towards political freedom, but that the latter is no substitute for the former. The example of healthcare, and of sure access to safe services irrespective of social class, makes the case. And when politicians speak of making the NHS consumer focused and of decentralising power, this dignifies the argument.

Proxy mechanisms (in 'market mimicry') are philosophically dangerous and also relatively ineffective. And such mechanisms of performance management misunderstand the sources and nature of 'knowledge' – and are also inevitably subverted by other agendas. The methodology is suspect, and the results do not offer individual accountability or specific individual leverage. The Commission for Health Improvement, for example, gives us one of many indications of centralised ideas about 'being patient centred'. CHI has a strategic Patients and Public Project Board and a Head of Patient and Public Involvement. It meets in public and listens 'to many different groups of patients and NHS staff' about 'their needs'.[26] It substitutes 'governance' (which avoids individual accountability) for consumer empowerment and for the investigation of individual competence, performance and incident. It generalises problems, which can of course produce some changes in management and in services. But it does not empower the individual, nor do its inspections clarify the source of suspect medicine where it exists. And, as every GP knows, every hospital has a doctor to whom they would not refer their own daughter.[27] However, from the fables of market mimicry no solutions can be derived. Indeed, one recalls Roy Campbell's famous couplet: They use the bridle and the bit, all right, But where's the bloody horse?[28]

Worse, the creation of tightly accountable management systems – which reflect risk aversion and deny the necessity of experiment – tends to drive out innovation and imagination. It will be a major disaster if regulation generates legally enforced biases against enterprise and experimentation. The present position of elderly care – which is struggling with an enfeebled business model and an administrative financing model – gives us fair warning of these risks. In addition, public regulatory bodies such as the National Care Standards Commission weakly struggle to capture 'key performance indicators' 'to manage the market in the interests of users'[29] and to lever up standards in the absence of consumer power. This is in part because it is the 'soft stuff' of user experience which matters most and which is so hard to measure by proxy. It is, too, because of the lack of direct power in individual hands in effective markets. These could be made real by tax incentives to change the funding model both for institutional care and for home care. And by incentives for support for care of the frail and dependent elderly at home. We should recognise that to use tax incentives is to load the picture in one way or another. It is not a neutral process. But tax incentives could be deployed to encourage self-responsibility on the part of family members towards one another, and they could be used alongside the patient-guaranteed care package of core care.

Meanwhile, remember the stonefish, and its spiky spines. Lethal, and poor eating.

Notes

1 For example, in September 2002 the Elderly Accommodation Counsel (EAC) and Help the Aged are collaborating to establish a comprehensive database of care homes. This will focus on aspects of choice directly related to quality of life within the care home setting, such as ethos, culture, management style, relationship with the outside world and social activities. The free guidance – *Care Options* – will enable people to make informed choices about their future home at a transitional and often frightening period of their lives. This is by contrast with 'regulating with a ruler', and it is an initiative which a charity took. (2002) Charities compile new database of care homes. *Caring Times*. **September issue**.

2 A Milburn, speech to Greater London Association of Community Health Councils, 'Patients must be given greater say', Department of Health press release 98/084, 9 March 1998. The Patient Advice and Liaison Services (PALS) is one result; and his speech to the King's Fund, 'Secretary of State sets out a new programme of modernisation for the NHS', Department of Health press release 2000/0066, 2 February 2000, urging 'a new emphasis on empowered patients', interpreted as more information, but with no specific leverage. 'Radical reform will put patients at centre of NHS', Department of Health press release, 6 December 2000. A Milburn, speech to New Health Network, 'Milburn announces radical decentralisation of NHS control', Department of Health press release 2002/0022, 15 January 2002, proposing Foundation Hospitals. See also A Milburn, speech to Healthcare Financial Management Association, 'Doctors and nurses should be in the driving seat', Department of Health press release 97/372, 3 December 1997.

3 I owe the story to Lord Howe.
4 Department of Health/NHS Appointments Commission (2002) *The Appointment of Chair of the Commission for Patient and Public Involvement in Health. Information for applicants.* Department of Health/NHS Appointments Commission, London. Department of Health (1999) *Patient and Public Involvement in the New NHS.* The Stationery Office, London. See also Spencer A (2002/3) Evolving involvement. *NHS Magazine*, **December/January**, interview with Mrs Sharon Grant, Chair of the organisation. The public is to be 'trained' to see things properly. Mrs Grant said: 'This is not about sending in spies but about enabling the public to be better informed about the challenges facing the NHS, to contribute in a constructive way – as equal partners.' This looks like the old game under a new flag, with experts spinning a double-headed coin. The Commission began work on 1 January 2003: 'The Government said that the Commission would train people in skills needed to be involved in NHS decision making and support them to make sure their voices were heard.'
5 On PALS, see Department of Health (2002) *Involving Patients and the Public in Healthcare: discussion document.* Department of Health, London. Department of Health (2001) *Involving Patients and the Public in Healthcare: response to the listening exercise.* Department of Health, London. Department of Health (2001) *Patient Advice and Liaison Services (PALS).* Department of Health, London. See also National Consumer Council (2001) *Patients and the Public in Healthcare: a discussion document.* National Consumer Council, London. Lewthwaite J and Haffenden S (1997) *Patients Influencing Purchasers.* Long-Term Medical Conditions Alliance/NHS Confederation, Birmingham.

The reports of work with focus groups and patient/carer groups reiterate old themes, and generally demonstrate that the system has not responded, save in the margins, despite consultation. For example, the themes emerging from work done (under the rubric of the Government's new PALS by Mayday Healthcare Trust in Croydon, Surrey, recently) were that patients encounter confusing messages and lack of information, being talked about as if they are not there, professionals failing to recognise patients' and carers' knowledge, problems with cleanliness and the ward environment, brusque attitudes from doctors and nurses, lack of privacy, and delayed discharges because of prolonged waits for drugs or lack of written information. Many detailed changes have been introduced (probably empowering staff to do things they have seen for themselves), but it is an open judgement whether the changes (an information officer, being more welcoming to patients, introducing open-backed hospital night-dresses, etc.) have changed the *cultural fundamentals* of attitude and behaviour. These are all old chestnuts, too – constantly echoed old messages to which managements have not obviously responded throughout the service.

All of these detailed and fundamental changes would easily and quickly have been made years ago if patients had competitive choices among providers. No independent business would stay in business without acting on them immediately. And in a market it is easy to judge what has changed, whereas it is difficult to assess whether or not panel views have had any impact on services. The emphasis of this report – as an exemplar of what we shall see from PALS – also concerns 'involving patients in planning services'. And these pilasters, pedestals and crested balustrades of 'consultation' in the main mean measures of success devised by bureaucrats disconnected from markets. One such initiative is that taken by Louis Appleby, NHS Director of Mental Health

Services. Outside all of this is the so-called 'uninformed user', who is probably just getting on with normal life, and only takes an interest (rationally?) in the health services when the necessity arises.

The circumscribed nature of decentralisation as an answer to the many deficits of the NHS is exemplified by the Government's project to hand over operational management of services in England to 28 new strategic health authorities and to 320 large primary care trusts. This is described in the recent government publication *Shifting the Balance of Power*. The plan does not directly empower one single consumer, even though the reform is intended to give patients more choice. Patients may be offered a wider choice of hospitals, waiting times and specialists, and benefit from new technology links. However, the Government's own pamphlet, *Reforming Our Public Services: principles into practice* (published in March 2002), offered no support for consumers exercising direct choice. Instead, reform continues to be manager driven. In the words of a leading advocate of the project (featured by the *NHS Magazine*), the changes concern 'a service built around patient *needs* with the delegation of decision making and resource allocation to *as near the patient as possible*' (my italics). Note the use of the term 'needs', which 'experts' decide, not 'wants', which individuals express. Note also the phrase 'to as near the patient as possible', which does not mean giving the service user control over money.

See Department of Health (2001) *Shifting The Balance of Power Within the NHS. Creating strategic health authorities.* Department of Health, London. The 28 new strategic health authorities replace the existing 95 authorities. Their main functions include supporting primary care and NHS trusts in delivering care, building capacity, and supporting performance improvement. For a commentary, see interview with N Crisp, NHS Chief Executive, in *NHS Magazine*, February 2002. On the emphasis concerned with local government, see Beecham J (2002) The local angle. *NHS Magazine.* **March**; Carr-Brown J (2002) NHS 'big bang' will give GPs new powers. *Sunday Times.* **31 March**; Hawkes N (2002) New GP trusts could inherit debts of £1.5bn. *The Times.* **1 April**; Riddell P (2002) Consumers will remain low on the public sector's list of priorities. *The Times.* **8 March**; Brown G (2002) Taxes are the best way to pay for the NHS. *Sunday Times.* **24 March**; Williams C (2002) It's good to talk. *Health Service J.* **23 May**.

6 Milburn A (2002) We have to give the voters more than this. *The Times.* **7 August**: 18. Riddell P (2002) The Tories' lack of direction keeps them in the wilderness. *The Times.* **29 July**: 16.

7 Hobson DL (1997) *The National Wealth. Who Gets What in Britain.* Harper Collins, London, p.391, especially chapter 10 on 'The nationalisation of industry'.

8 Thatcher M (1993) *The Downing Street Years.* HarperCollins, London, p.676.

9 Yeo S (1987) in Outhwaite W and Mulkay M (eds), *Social Theory and Social Criticism.* Basil Blackwell, Oxford, p.91.

10 Friedman M (1962) *Capitalism and Freedom.* Chicago University Press, Chicago; revised edition 1982, p.9.

11 Liberal Democrat Party (2002) *Quality, Innovation, Choice.* Liberal Democrat Party, London. Riddell P (2002) Lib Dem assault on Whitehall is weakened by compromise. *The Times.* **17 September**: 12. (2002) Reform. *Bulletin.* **19 September**.

12 Milburn A, speech to NHS top managers and overseas visitors, London, 'NHS Foundation Hospitals to be freed from Whitehall control', Department of Health press release 2002/0240, 22 May 2002.

13 Department of Health (2000) *For the Benefit of Patients. A concordat with the private and voluntary health care provider sectors.* Department of Health, London. Department of Health (2001) *Building Capacity and Partnership in Care. An agreement between the statutory and the independent social care, health care and housing sectors.* Department of Health, London.

14 And, as he says, 'when you have finished proclaiming the caring sensitivity of local government, try getting planning permission for a porch'. Parris M (2002) Small may be beautiful, but in Government big is best. *The Times.* 3 **August**: 24. Otherwise, however, his is a paternalist argument that the expert knows best.

15 Wrench T (1946) *Reconstruction by Way of the Soil.* Faber & Faber, London, p.71.

16 Appleyard B (2002) Will this be Britain's can-do revolution? *Sunday Times.* 3 **February**.

17 Maude F, op. cit.

18 'Duncan Smith: Conservatives will make policy from principle', Conservative Party press release, 17 January 2002; www.conservatives.com. Mr Duncan Smith has not yet specified detailed policies. He makes no mention of choice or empowerment in his latest article, see Duncan Smith I (2003) A national expects ... a lot of waffle from the PM. *The Times.* **22 January**.

19 But see also Simon Jenkins' fascinating article in which he urged that both art and landscape are better protected by the agency of existing owners and occupiers than by the hand of the State, and that tax incentives offer 'an efficient alternative to "crude nationalisation"'. Why not make the same argument for empowering the patient? Jenkins S (2002) For once, taxation can be a thing of beauty. *The Times.* **19 July**.

20 Marenbon J (1997) *The Dominance of Centrism and the Politics of Certainty.* Politica, London.

21 Innes M (1946) *Appleby's End.* Penguin Books, Harmondsworth; 1969 edition, p.137.

22 Postrel V (1998) *The Future and Its Enemies. The growing conflict over creativity, enterprise and progress.* The Free Press, New York, p.57.

23 Steele L (2002) Marked change. *The Guardian.* 3 **July**: 120. Elliott J and Woodhead M (2002) Herr Doktor halves NHS queue in week. *Sunday Times.* **14 July**.

24 Haskins Lord C. 'Commentary: the challenge to State regulation', in J Blundell and F Robinson, *Regulation Without the State ... the debate continues.* Institute of Economic Affairs, London, p.65.

25 Walshe K (2002) The rise of regulation in the NHS. *BMJ.* 324: 967–70. Walshe K (2002) Power with responsibility. *Health Service J.* 7 **June**. Timmins N (2002) Health providers to be inspected by a single body. *Financial Times.* **17 January**. Department of Health. *The NHS Plan: next steps for investment, next steps for reform,* April. See also NHS Reform and Health Care Professions Act, 2002. And see Rogers K (2002) NCSC will be absorbed by 'super regulators'. *Caring Times.* **July/August**: 12–13. Sherman J (2002) Birt wins key role in 'Department of Prime Minister'. *The Times.* **25 June**. Riddell P (2002) Civil service shake-up hands Blair levers to secure swift change. *The Times.* **15 June**. Riddell P (2002) For better or worse, this was the real Tony Blair. *The Times.* **22 July**. Hobson is right to say that 'Doctors know which of their colleagues is a danger to his patients, but professional *omertà* ensured that they were not exposed.'

26 It has already established a host of new bodies, including the National Institute for Clinical Excellence, the Commission for Health Improvement, the Modernisation Agency, the National Patient Safety Agency and the National Clinical Assessment Authority. The Government is now reorganising the Commission for Health

Improvement, the National Care Standards Commission and the Social Services Inspectorate to regulate both public and private sectors. There are also Patient Forums, a Patient Advice and Liaison Service, Independent Complaints Advisory Services, Local Authority Overview and Scrutiny Committees and a Transition Advisory Board.

27 Hobson, op. cit., p.647.
28 Campbell R, cited by Trilling L (1936) *Matthew Arnold*. Unwin University Books edition, 1963, p.155.
29 The changing shape of regulation. *Registered Homes and Services*. November 2002. I draw also on my experience as a Board Member of the National Care Standards Commission since May 2001.

Chapter 24

Conclusion: look, see, choose

If the answer lay in Whitehall, we'd have found it years ago.

(Marjorie Wallace, Senior Civil Servant, Treasury)

I have urged a structure based on practice rooted in first principles in a society of liberty and self-responsibility. The key step is the emphasis on civil association and self-responsibility described by Michael Oakeshott, by contrast with intrusive, goal-directed, ideologically derived, managerial and transformational Government. This accepted, all else follows.

This book has sought to offer an approach to health and social care of adaptation, evolution and self-reliant choice, rather than one 'system' to replace another. The view is that which is generally characterised as 'dynamist', as opposed to 'stasism', and which is brilliantly set out by Virginia Postrel. The general perspective is that of Oakeshott, as I understand his work, and of Robert Nozick. Government will be an umpire, to administer neutral rules of behaviour, and so will permit many choices to be co-possible. Within this framework of rules, individuals will themselves 'get it done', pursuing their own goals. And thus the social order will be one of enduring adjustments and exchanges – adaptive, dynamic and mutually respecting. As I have outlined, there will be no overall master-plan, no one 'system', no ideologically driven approach, save that Government will foster a situation where individuals can exist at civilised levels.

This approach will offer a guarantee of core care; the patient as fundholder, and protection of the poor, the unlucky and the disadvantaged. I have set out the ideas on which the actual practical steps for change should be based, and I have suggested the actual initial steps themselves. All this is a matter of *choice*. It recognises, too, that we cannot divide ethics from economics. It was HJ Massingham who told us – speaking of RH Tawney's *Religion and the Rise of Capitalism* – that 'it was the Puritan party which divided ethics from economics and played a decisive part in the changeover from the conception of society as a spiritual organism to that of society as an economic machine'.[1] We are now holding a ticket for the return journey. And with 'incentive' prominently labelling all of our luggage.

To summarise the ideas:

- Government will function as an umpire to administer neutral rules of behaviour, permitting many choices to be co-possible, in civil association.
- We should renew civil society and mutual-aid organisations, in which everyone has a stake, through the collective character of social insurance and the reciprocity of voluntary association.

- We should protect the idea of private property and private decision making (together with the ability to adapt to realities which its existence uniquely permits). This underpins civil society, and the realisation that individual liberty can only be guaranteed when this is so. The guarantee of private property rights forms the necessary barrier against State encroachment.
- It is 'negative liberty' (in Berlin's phrase) that we must protect – the liberty to live one's own life for oneself, *sto magni nomini umbra*.
- The concept of individual healthcare that we should more fully appreciate is that it is uniquely specific, separable, individual, personal, intimate and timely.
- There is a fundamental distinction between being able *to command a specific service* (by money or social insurance) and being able to *discipline a system* (by occasional voting, or taking part in planning consultations). Having a say in how *a system* is run is different to having a say about *a personal service* that is supplied when you want it.
- Preventive care is vital, and this emphasis on self-reliance should replace the medicalisation of society, for personal responsibility is the key.
- There are two possible concepts of order in a society – one of control, hierarchy and expertise which knows best on our behalf, the other of evolutionary trial and error, deduction and controlled experiment, surprise and dynamism.
- These two concepts of order each imply quite different principles of latency, or the potential of the individual. And of power relationships (in healthcare commonly reflected in the different uses of the mirror words 'needs' and 'wants'). The two concepts encapsulate the confrontation, ultimately, between freedom and slavery (dramatised for us by Herodotus in his *Histories*, and no different today).
- This approach requires Government to enable effective, leveraged, individual choice and to introduce direct incentives which encourage efficiency, responsiveness, effectiveness, innovation, evolution and competitive development.
- It also requires Government to protect competition and choice (and the dissemination of innovation) as a foundation of society.
- The successful revolution in optical care in the UK since 1985 has established a body of knowledge and practice which enables us all to see the commended approach at work in actual local practice for UK healthcare in every aspect, and within the UK culture.
- The present NHS structure relies on disempowering, hierarchical assumptions about who should control resources, in a system of 'public ownership' where public information is restricted. The individual pays the taxes but does not in fact control the resources, despite being one of millions of 'owners'.
- There is also in this system the tendency of individuals to pass on responsibility to others; by contrast, by placing the service user at the centre, we should empower choices made by individuals for themselves, with incentives for self-responsibility. For these have a vital moral value compared with decisions that are made for us from above by 'experts' – they rebuild self-responsibility and self-jurisdiction.
- There must be a core package of guaranteed care for all, and a legally enforceable contract for each individual, set out both in an insurance contract and in

a contract with a purchasing co-operative which buys on behalf of its subscriber members.

- We must ensure that there is an unimpeachable and legally enforceable guarantee that the poorest in society have equal access to essential and high-quality health and social care – thus bridging the gap which the NHS and the present private market have widened.
- We can and should insist upon social solidarity and more fairness in society (by which we mean that the poorest receive quality care, and that those who cannot afford to make contributions have them paid by the better off, from taxation).
- We should absolutely rely on competition and choice to deliver solidarity and enable everyone to enter the quality circle by transferring tax money into a personal healthcare fund for the patient fundholder.
- This approach would fit with the idea of targeting funds to help the weakest, to focus State spending where it is most effective, and to improve the ability of the poor to participate in the economy and in society by giving them financial clout and advisory support. Users standing there, money in hand, asking for service. Individuals with an invested fund to which they made individual contributions, held in individualised accounts that provided cover for 'all necessary healthcare'.
- Those who are able to do more for themselves should be expected and encouraged to do so, by fiscal policy.
- This universalism will run with the grain of human nature, instead of adopting authoritarian structures such as Government monopoly provision, the denial of choice and the suppression of competition.
- We must rigorously protect competition and individual personal choice in insurance, purchaser and provider markets.
- We must radically increase healthcare revenues from diverse sources. However, general taxation will continue to be a very significant part of the total cost of health and social services, not least in ensuring access to high-quality care for the poorest. Co-payment and additional private insurance will be specifically encouraged by direct financial incentives, which would have both moral and practical benefits.
- We must embed direct incentives for purchasers and providers (beginning with choice and the accountability of competition) in order to ensure a continuous improvement in standards, as we stimulate new and more diverse provision, if that is what consumers want. Only in this way can we have a system which is responsive to costed demand.
- We should encourage a much more even balance of provision and collaboration between the public and the private sector in health and social care, and that convergence which is more typical in Europe. Among other benefits this should encourage cost control, which competition uniquely prompts.
- We must abandon the delusion of seeking a comprehensive, all-encompassing plan which will solve all ills, and rely instead on the spontaneous evolution of innovation and emulation in the creative marketplace, once the basic framework is in place.

- Government must set this framework of rules, but withdraw from its monopoly position in being the sole funder and sole payer for care – no longer being the purchaser from itself, and the provider to itself.
- This framework would guarantee good care for all as a *public good*, and a regulatory framework (including the option for institutions to register with one or more competing registered regulators) would be set up.
- Government would be responsible for open, relevant and current public information, training, professional registration, encouragement of financial diversity while providing through taxation financial transfers to the poor (uprated in line with prices but not earnings), protecting competition and choice, and supporting structures which lever up standards.
- We must all be much more aware of explicit price and costs.
- We should endorse the idea that unsatisfactory providers will leave the market and the market, will create new alternatives.[2]
- As some rationing in health and social care is ultimately unavoidable (because of inevitable scarcity even in a much better supplied market, and the need for cost containment), we should each ration for ourselves as we consider our own priorities, and make relative judgements about opportunity costs and our willingness to pay. We should not automatically suffer rationing due to the conceptual framework of the NHS, nor accept the existing situation where rationing imposes the displacement of the interests of one patient by another, one group of patients by others. Much of the rationing that we experience in the UK is due to the refusal to encourage more private revenues in order to support more capacity and access.

It will be seen that the problems are far from being merely technical or managerial. However, we can make progress in applying principles to practice.

First, we can benefit from the recent attainment of less exasperating and limiting discussion than that by which we have been distracted for too long, in the consideration of a social subject of tremendous force. Instead, reference to first principles in all that is done can lead us towards huge advances in care, on a radically revised basis. For example, we could admit that there is no 'right' level of funding, save for what a competitive market and willing purchasers determine. This is not discoverable through political guesswork.

Secondly, we can move towards actually leaving people alone to do what they want, provided that their actions do not interfere with the liberty of others. That is, we should be privileging choice as the foundation of liberty itself, and ensuring that Government vigorously protects competition – which has been shown to improve care.

Thirdly, this means ceasing to distrust the people, and abandoning an approach which substitutes some cultural mythologies about their capacity to choose for other observable realities. We must abandon a view of 'the vulgar', which goes back in European culture at least to Shakespeare's groundlings and also actors (Bottom, Snout, Snug, Starveling), which reappears in Hardy's writing, which we see in George Eliot's novels, and which is expressed by Spinoza (on behalf of many), who said that expert dispensations are 'extremely necessary ... for the

masses, whose wits are not potent enough to perceive things clearly and succinctly'. This attitude – as we have seen, Sidney Webb is its most influential modern
exponent – has run through the NHS and through other areas of life that were
centrally planned under the post-war settlement. Here the suspicion among
'experts' is that people (transgressively and waywardly) will persist in making
'wrong' decisions if they are allowed to decide for themselves. Here we should
compare, for example, the attitude discussed by the radical geographer David
Matless of those 'experts' considering people being allowed to roam and ramble
in the post-war countryside: 'many of them are simple folk with little power
of expressing their opinions, and most of them are more or less lacking in comparative experience, and therefore tend to be unreliable outside the region or
regions in which they have lived and observed'.[3]

Fourthly, we can at last set in place real levers which will at last empower individuals to take self-responsibility, make cost-conscious choices, and command
affordable and appropriate services – which does not necessarily mean the cheap-
est – and to do so within a structure which we would each recognise as fair and
socially just.

Fifthly, we can recognise and replace a cluster of illusions, delusions and self-
deceptions – that the NHS is the best health service in the world; that State monopoly funding, purchasing and provision are appropriate, sufficient and effective;
that health is 'the Government's business' rather than our own self-responsibility;
that Government knows how to run things; that deficits and denial of service are
correctable by making the NHS incrementally more efficient at the margins.

Sixthly, we can do all of this while ensuring that the richer pay for the poorest,
and that we all share the responsibility to help the weak, the unlucky and the
disadvantaged.

Finally, we can at last recover from plodding down superficially attractive
vistas but never actually getting anywhere that we really want to go. Instead of a
conveyor-belt we now require a turntable.

We need to seek a morally sound healthcare structure which guarantees care
for all, by at last giving everyone a legally enforceable contract for routine access
to good-quality services, when they want them. The choices should be those which
individuals wish to make for themselves – and to afford (philosophically, culturally,
and in practical terms which work for them). This should be so, incorrigibly
imperfect as our individual personal judgements may be.

We should also recognise that what we require is evolving knowledge, not
completion, not 'truth' (ideologically discovered for us by 'experts'). And not neat-
ness either. We need to respect diversity, dynamism, trial and error, differentiation
and unexpected developments. What Steve Jones called 'Darwin's great idea – of
life as a series of successful mistakes'.[4]

Meanwhile, the demand for healthcare will continue to increase, as will the
assertiveness of informed consumers and an ageing population. As our population ages we shall feel the keen responsibility to ensure that everyone in their
early and late years has the kinds of experience and control which build the
capacity for self-responsibility and self-renewal. New opportunities will forever
present themselves. Indeed, the scientific advances have hardly begun. There

will be surprises in pharmaceuticals, in technological gizmos, in genomic interventions and in cloning – initially for 'spare parts', but further with the ultimate ethical challenge – and in we-know-not-yet-what. There will be many things which are genuinely essential to many – for whom costs are unlikely to be slight, or necessarily to fall. In addition, growing resistance to antibiotics will remain a serious difficulty, as we seek to find and fund alternatives (which may be more costly). The future may indeed bite back as well as show us unimagined innovation.

However, we live life forward. So we should welcome and embrace innovation and invest in advances. We should do so while rationally seeking to control their costs, and warily eyeing the ethical dilemmas that will arise. We cannot sustain the NHS with its artificially low spend and its atypical dependence on taxation. We cannot go on with a situation where the NHS fears innovation and its diffusion, since this will breach its rationed allocations. The NHS already seeks to deter the application of progress – such as the routine introduction of major new pharmaceutical products of high therapeutic value – within its artificially restricted monopoly budget. It creates the scarcities which it then rations.

Many radical ideas – no doubt including the *patient as fundholder* – are often dismissed by NHS managers along the lines of 'everyone has problems' and we need not change. Or that the meaning of the OECD data can be minimised by urging that all difficulties are relative. Or that none of these approaches suits our culture. But it is difficult to read the long-term OECD data and then to insist that this material is, after all, merely subjective. It seems unquestionably the case that State monopoly has suppressed capacity and reduced access which more diverse funding and a more open market would have provided. Of course, all systems do have problems. This is because there is no escape from costs or affordability in *any* system. However, I have sought to show that a mixed-funding approach with open competition and choice works in all situations.

Trade-offs have to be made – and re-made – whichever system we adopt. The individual should make these for themselves. Of course cultures differ – although there is much global harmonisation (much of which the Left regret).[5] However, we are the authors of many of our own misfortunes. There are many aspects of contemporary British culture which welfarism and the NHS itself have helped to create, including dependency, lack of personal responsibility, aggression, lack of information and some clinically doubtful demand. All this is part of the problem. Much of our current culture is part of the unforeseen difficulties that have arisen from welfarism and the NHS itself. And surely we want to change that culture rather than necessarily accommodate to it. There are many possible lessons which could dramatically improve standards and survival rates from serious diseases, and change the wider culture, too. If we believe in evolutionary change, we have the opportunity to explore carefully the response to change and give ourselves the chance to adapt as we go, which may help us to avoid other unwanted consequences.

Fundamentally, this enters an argument about the nature of society – about how we relate to ourselves, to one another, to Government. The answers I have offered are not wholly novel. But we do need the novelty of *genuinely following through* by ensuring that there are real levers for individual action, and direct incentives too which ensure that all can access best care. By these principles we shall most successfully discover how to navigate the unknowable future, what the opportunities will be, and how best to ensure that all have access to these. We should not deny ourselves these opportunities by retaining in place a structure of control, rationing and denial which cuts us all off from the benefits of spontaneous evolution, investment and improvement.

Mr Milburn has achieved much more in the past three years than the accumulated efforts of several of his predecessors added together. And I suspect his has been a journey, too, of personal surprises. The Government continues to edge towards a genuine revolution in UK arrangements, if by stealth and self-surprise. My hope is that the analysis of first principles and of actions for change offered in this book will assist this steady process, help to open out thinking about the true meaning of events as they occur, link the story and its sequel, and move us through a new understanding to a firmer footing for improved care for all.

An understanding, too, around which we can organise both sentiment and specifics in a coherent and capacious (rather than finalised) design. One which will achieve honour and quality for patients *and* professionals. The kind of equality (of access) which matters to the individual – the old theological virtues of Faith, Hope and Charity, stencilled on china in every Victorian cottage. Not to be despised – belief, hope, charity and justice, providence, improved quality, more capacity, more choice, more competition, and an evolving system (which meets the calls of the future which are still to be articulated by those who come after us).

This stresses again what Hayek says about learning to choose, and its practice. And which Mill stressed – notably, that private charity, or philanthropy, has particular value because it is more discriminating and flexible than the State, and because it constitutes a moral and a social discipline for those who make these contributions willingly and out of conscience and concern. As Mill said in *On Liberty*, 'It is the privilege and proper condition of a human being, arrived at the maturity of his faculties, to use and interpret experience in his own way ... The human faculties of perception, judgement, discrimination, feeling and even moral preference are exercised only in making a choice. He who does everything because it is the custom, makes no choice. He gains no practice either in discerning or desiring what is best ... He who chooses his plan for himself employs all his faculties.'[6] Of course, as WL Burn comments: 'The free choice carried with it the liability to choose wrongly, but that was not merely part of the price but part of the value. A man could not learn discrimination except by past failures to exercise it.'[7]

If reform is to be real, it needs democratic consent and ownership among professionals too. There has to be a genuine debate. And with some wit and vigour, in vibrant, honourable, elegantly clear language. We should seek to conduct this discussion in public rather than in the high but private cadences of the Palace of Westminster, the high tables of Oxford and Cambridge, the Inns of Court, or editorial lunches. In this conversation, too, we need the language of the workplace and the market – the language of normal daily life.

We want to achieve several things at once. Better healthcare for all, in a political system which protects politics itself. In an economy which can pay for care. In a culture which values the individual, dynamism and surprise. One which respects that naivety which encourages outsiders to address problems with creative confidence, abandoning preconceptions and asking 'why not?' Which combines inspiration and logic. Which shares a theory of existence in which the unthinkable – the good and the bad – is possible and which requires individual alertness and self-responsibility to ensure the best.

There is no still water in healthcare reform. New ideas appear constantly. We should not underestimate the fact that despite the recent changes in the cultural context of politicians, real change in healthcare will require immense political and intellectual force. This is the key role of direct incentives. In politics, too, fear can be as powerful a driving force as hope. As we confront many new proposals, we need to keep reminding ourselves by asking 'Is this really what we want to do? Will this really achieve the society we want and the care we admire?'

We should consider that the apparently impossible is possible. And we have to find ways of making the possible practical. There are a cluster of interrelated cultural and political issues. None of these raise trivial tasks. Nor are they merely technical questions. They ask us to consider how human beings, how healthcare systems and indeed how political systems operate at the most fundamental levels.

Cultural and political projects fall into two categories, like all works of art. They fall into those that deepen one's view of life, and those which simplify it; those that depict the world as more complicated and interesting than previously thought, and those that depict it as less complicated, and less intriguing. Perhaps less reassuring, more troubling, but more challenging. Here, thinking about the NHS – about the patients as well as about the diseases they have – and alternative structures, I am reminded of what Niels Bohr, one of the fathers of quantum mechanics, said: 'Anyone who can contemplate quantum mechanics without getting dizzy hasn't understood it.' Godel demonstrated that there are a few mathematical questions which are beyond the reach of logical proof – so-called undecidable questions. But not so in healthcare. In quantum mechanics scientists hope to construct a computer which can enter two different but parallel universes and answer each question (and even more than one version of a question) in a different universe. However, we have to make choices in *one* universe, without what quantum mechanics call 'Twilight Zone technology'.

We should remember what John Gardner said of universities. It is equally true of the first principles of healthcare reform, of the mosaic we seek, of what UK healthcare is capable of becoming, and of how society and care can change together.

Gardner said that the university stands for:

1 the things that are forgotten in the heat of battle
2 the values that get pushed aside in the rough and tumble of everyday life
3 the goals that we ought to be thinking about and never do
4 the facts that we do not like to face
5 the questions that we lack the courage to ask.[8]

Some final thoughts. One of the management gurus once said 'If you really want to find out how a system works, try changing it'. Much is only revealed in the process of reform. And, as Scruton has said, 'it is only at the end of things that we begin to understand them'.[9]

Is it an impossibility to move away from the elusive tussle with reform on present lines, and to set in place different approaches? I suggest that the arguments and the evidence we have seen indeed indicate that initiatives (like direct cash payment and the revolution in the optics market) demonstrate that we shall see huge change during the next decade. But to continuing sceptics, consider Karl Liebknecht's appraisal of the 'art of the possible':

> *The extreme limit of the possible can only be attained by grasping for the impossible. The realised possible is the resultant of the impossibilities which have been striven for. Willing what is objectively impossible does not, therefore, signify senseless fantasy-spinning and self-delusion, but practical politics in the deepest sense. To demonstrate the impossibility of realising a political goal is not to show its senselessness. All it shows, at most, is the critic's lack of insight into society's laws of motion, particularly the laws that govern the formation of the social will. What is the true and the strongest policy? It is the art of the impossible.*[10]

We are, above all else, considering the scarcest thing in the world – the days of our lives. Our stepping-stones are chance and choice. It is an adventure, and a traveller's tale, amidst our mortality. Oakeshott tells us that:

> *The pursuit of perfection as the crow flies is an activity both impious and unavoidable in human life. It involves the penalties of impiety (and anger of the gods and social isolation), and its reward is not that of achievement but that of having made the attempt. It is an activity therefore suitable for individuals, not for societies. For an individual who is impelled to engage in it, the reward may exceed both the penalty and the inevitable defeat. The penitent may hope, or even expect, to fall back a wounded hero, into the arms of an understanding and forgiving society. And even the impenitent can be reconciled with himself in the powerful necessity of his impulse, though, like Prometheus, he must suffer for it. For a society, on the other hand, the penalty is a chaos of conflicting ideals, the disruption of a common life, and the reward is the renown which attaches to a monumental folly.*[11]

And the lessons here chime with 'being English', with the *esprit de la nation*. Or, as the character Frank Gibbons, in Noel Coward's *This Happy Breed*, put it:

> *'the people themselves, the ordinary people like you and me, know something better than all the fussy old politicians put together – we know what we belong to, where we come from, and where we're going. We may not know it with our brains, but we know it with our roots'.*[12]

Professor W Macneile Dixon said that:

> *just as none of us can live any life save his own, none of us can wholly transfer his burdens to another's shoulders. We must in some measure in these days think for ourselves, as we must breathe for ourselves, and walk for ourselves. Happier, it may be, are those who can with serenity leave this troublesome business of thinking to others.*[13]

And so we should properly ask whether Utopia – in Nozicks' phrase – is 'where our grandchildren are to live', or whether we can radically improve health services more quickly than that.[14] And if so, how? I have sought to make the dynamist case, and to be specific about an approach which includes practical steps. There are good examples to follow, notably in the UK in eye care.

Of course, as Oakeshott warned us, we often exchange one puzzle for another. And W Macneile Dixon spoke of:

> *this play of arguments and counter arguments [which] stand behind the great unknowables, time, space, substance, change, causation, smiling ironically down upon the to-and-fro excursions of our troubled minds.... [And] With a great show of wisdom we are telling ourselves little, with profound exploring fathomless depths, where all soundings fail.... Not at one stride,* non uno itinere, *as we fondly fancy, shall we reach the truth.*[15]

Michael Oakeshott would have smiled at these words. He, like Macneile Dixon, tells us that life can only be understood by living. And as Professor Kenneth Minogue has said, Oakeshott hoped that we might take off from present experience and rise to what he called 'a conditional platform of understanding'.[16] It remains for the individual, as ever, to confront, to embrace and to relish the threefold challenge that this represents. A reviewer of one of Paul Theroux's travel books once spoke of 'Mr Theroux's journey round himself'. This is the course of all our lives. For the responsibility of each of us is – as the Renaissance emblem-book writers prompted – '*Aspice* (Look!), *Vide* (See!) and, ultimately, *Elige* (Choose!)'.[17]

Notes

1   Massingham HJ (1940) *Chiltern Country.* BT Batsford, London, pp.94–6.
2   Compare this idea with the King's Fund's notion of a static and protected 'local health economy'. The King's Fund approach is described in King's Fund (2002) *The Future of the NHS. A framework for debate. Discussion paper.* King's Fund, London.
3   Shake-speare W (1623) *Plays.* W Jaggard, London. Spinoza B de (1846) *Tractatus Theologico-Politicus* (edited by CH Bruder, Leipzig), III, p.83, quoted by Manning J (2002) *The Emblem.* Reaktion Books, London, p.153. Dower J, President of the Ramblers' Association, quoted by Matless D (1998) *Landscape and Englishness.* Reaktion Books, London, p.252.
4   Jones S (1999) *Almost Like a Whale. The origin of species updated.* Doubleday, London, p.xxvi.
5   See, as a sampler, Mander J and Goldsmith E (eds) (1996) *The Case Against the Global Economy. And for a turn toward the local.* Sierra Club, San Francisco, CA.
6   Mill JS (1859) *On Liberty* (2e). W Parker & Son, London, p.109.
7   Burn WL (1964) *The Age of Equipoise.* G Allen & Unwin, London, pp.115–7.
8   Gardner J (1968) *No Easy Victories.* Harper & Row, New York, p.90. I owe this reference to Professor Russ Vince.
9   Scruton R (2000) *England, An Elegy.* Chatto & Windus, London, p.vii.

10 Quoted by Yeo S in P Corrigan (ed.). *Capitalism, State Formation and Marxist Theory. Historical investigations.* Quartet Books, London, from Bahro R (1977) The alternative in Eastern Europe. *New Left Review.* **106**: 31.

11 Coward N (1934–62) *This Happy Breed.* W Heinemann, London, 6 vols, iv, pp.553–4.

12 Oakeshott M (1962) *Rationalism in Politics: and other essays.* Methuen, London; Barnes and Noble, New York, 1962; new expanded edition, T Fuller (ed.), Liberty Press, Indianapolis, 1991, p.59.

13 Macneile Dixon W (1938) *The Human Situation.* Longmans Green, New York, p.12.

14 Nozick R (1974) *Anarchy, State and Utopia.* Basil Blackwell, Oxford.

15 Macneile Dixon W, ibid., p.125.

16 Minogue K, The history of political thought seminar. In: Norman (ed.), op. cit., p.91.

17 Manning, op. cit., p.36.

Postscript

This book was completed in the autumn of 2002, with some additions during the editing period in January 2003. It is as up-to-date as I could make it, but, of course, there is healthcare news every day. The test of the value of this book will be whether the first principles and understandings set out help the reader to assess these new developments. And whether the analysis stands up to the challenge of the March of Events. As the proofs are returned to the publisher, I note that recent important events have included several to which I believe my analyses prove helpful and appropriate. These events include the following.

1 In February 2003 *The Times* reported that Alan Milburn (Secretary of State for Health) was considering raising extra funds for the NHS by US-style bonds. 'You cannot have a real shift in power from the centre to the local if you do not have a recognition that money is power.'[1] This chimes exactly with my proposals concerning patient fundholding, which will return tax-based funds to the individual, to spend via a mutual Patient Guaranteed Care Association.

2 Dr Liam Fox (Shadow Secretary of State for Health) told the Conservative Party's spring conference on 16 March 2003 that his party would introduce a Patient's Passport 'which will enable patients to move around a number of providers, NHS, not-for-profit, voluntary or independent.' For 'This freedom is essential if we are to see greater plurality and diversity in both the funding and provision of healthcare that we seek … Our Patient's Passport would enable patients to move around the NHS and take the standard tariff funding with them. This would set them free from dependence on block contracts agreed between PCTs and agreed providers.' This sounds like patient fundholding. We await the details.[2]

3 Mr Milburn made an important speech on choice to NHS Chief Executives on 11 February 2003. He said, '… by linking the choices patients make to the resources hospitals receive … we can provide real incentives to address under-performance in local NHS services.'[3]

Mr Milburn re-emphasised patient choice as the driving force of change, whilst at the same time reporting significant advances in capacity. He announced large extensions of the choice scheme, based on the successful London pilot scheme. And, as the expert commentator Stephen Pollard pointed out to a Reform conference in April 2003, this is effectively the voucher.[4] Certainly, it can evolve to become patient fundholding across the spectrum. But this will require individuals to be given the opportunity to take a tax-based fund to a co-operative purchasing organisation.

Next year some 100 000 extra patients will be able to choose the hospital where they are treated. Choice in maternity care is to be extended, and there will be changes, too, in GP registration, enabling people to register with a practice close to their workplace if they wish. The choice scheme is to be extended as follows. First, from summer 2003 to London patients waiting more than 6 months for any form of elective surgery. Second, from July 2003, to West Yorkshire patients awaiting eye operations and to Manchester patients awaiting ortho- paedic, ENT and general surgery. Third, from July to those awaiting cataract operations in the south of England. Fourth, as Mr Blair announced recently, from summer 2004 to all patients waiting more than 6 months for any form of elective surgery. Fifth, from December 2005, with expected extra capacity, to all patients waiting longest for hospital treatment. Capacity will limit choices in some cases – perhaps to one other hospital – but the principle is admitted.

Mr Milburn said that over 1700 of 3800 patients offered choice of early heart treatment at an alternative hospital (having waited more than 6 months for surgery) had taken up the option since July 2002. Over two-thirds of patients who had waited similarly for cataract operations in London had also done so. This is a payments-by-results system in outline. It is a further increment towards patient fundholding.

In addition, Mr Milburn promised a new concordat to extend the relationship between the NHS and the private sector, suggesting that PCTs may be en- couraged to extend purchasing from the voluntary sector. This will extend choice further, accessing greater capacity. The next step should be to enable *all* patients irrespective of health status to take their tax-based fund to a preferred purchaser. And to enable co-operative purchasers to benefit from the new free- doms to seek services from any legally registered provider.

4 The Government published the Health and Social Care (Community Health and Standards) Bill on 13 March 2003. NHS Trusts seeking to become Foun- dation Hospitals will now be called 'public benefit corporations'. The first wave will come from the 32 three-star Trusts that have already put forward prelim- inary applications.[5] The successful applicants will be controlled by a new inde- pendent regulator within five years.

However, this proposal still offers no individual empowerment. The individual consumer of services will have no control through the cumulative and co- operative power of a mutual purchasing organisation such as my proposed Patient Guaranteed Care Associations. Mr Milburn told the House of Commons Health Committee on 5 March 2003 that he had set a target date of 2008 for all NHS hospitals to get Foundation status. And the same policy could be applied to PCTs. However, on present policies, these, too, will remain beyond the reach of incentives driven by the patient fundholder who would be enabled to take their tax-fund to an alternative purchaser and thus to an alternative provider.[6]

5 Gordon Brown, Chancellor of The Exchequer, re-affirmed in a speech to the Social Market Foundation 'that markets are a means of advancing the public interest'.[7] Yet he continues to exclude healthcare, and instead still seeks to spend his way to security. He re-iterated this approach in his budget statement to the House of Commons on 9 April 2003. Yet this approach offers no means for the

individual to command a specific service when they want it, and funding by itself, I suggest, will not achieve the necessary cultural changes.

6 Reform, the campaign for new directions for public policy, published on 7 April 2003 a radical new agenda, *A Better Way*, by Sir Steve Robson, the former Second Permanent Secretary at HM Treasury, and two former Finance Ministers of New Zealand, Sir Roger Douglas and The Hon Ruth Richardson who formed the Commission on the Reform of Public Services.

This challenging report offers similar arguments to my own. It urges giving patients real choice by moving to health insurance. And it firmly contradicts the validity of Mr Brown's approach.[8]

7 The Department of Health's own NHS Modernisation Board, in its second annual report, focused on waiting lists, and Ministers continue to suggest that the test of their health policies will be waiting times. This is an insufficient and even an inappropriate test, although it may be the one most commonly applied. And, in practical terms, potential patients require up-to-date public information about results of the kind that would be insisted upon by a Patient Guaranteed Care Association acting on behalf of its voluntary membership.[9]

8 On 6 April 2003, *The Sunday Times* published a 96-page *Good Hospital Guide*, profiling the main NHS and private hospitals in England, Wales, Scotland and Northern Ireland and 29 of the leading hospitals in the Republic of Ireland, based on data compiled by the independent Dr Foster organisation. In its commentary the first leader said: 'Our *Good Hospital Guide* shows alarming variability in performance among hospitals on mortality rates, waiting times and best practice. True, there have been some improvements, but not enough to justify the avalanche of cash pouring into the NHS. In some areas standards are deteriorating despite the extra billions.' This underlines the query that without incentives and demand-side reform the services cannot be improved sufficiently, despite huge additional investment.[10]

When we consider these reports, we might keep in mind the words of the former Prime Minister, Lord Rosebery, who spoke of 'the character breathing through the sentences.'[11]

JS
14 April 2003

Notes

1 Charter D (2003) Milburn looks at US-style bonds to fund hospitals. *The Times.* **6 February**.
2 Fox L (2003) *The Patient's Passport*, speech to Conservative Party spring conference 16 March 2003. *See* www.conservatives.com.

3 Milburn A (2003) *Choice for all*, speech to NHS Chief Executives, 11 February 2003. *See* www.doh.gov.uk/speeches.

4 Pollard S (2003) *Politics can change*, speech to Reform conference *A Better Way*, London, 7 April 2003.

5 Wright O (2003) Milburn to give up control of hospital coffers. *The Times*. **14 March**.

6 Sparrow A (2003) Defiant Milburn wants all hospitals to be self-governing by 2008. *Daily Telegraph*. **5 March**. *See also* Brown G, Budget statement, *Hansard*, House of Commons, cols 272–289, 9 April 2003.

7 Charter D (2003) Brown vows to reform public services. *The Times*. **3 February**.

8 Robson S, Douglas R and Richardson R (2003) *A Better Way*. Commission on The Reform of Public Services. Reform, London. *See* www.reformbritain.com.

9 NHS Modernisation Board (2003) *The NHS Plan – A progress report. The NHS Modernisation Board's Annual Report, 2003*. Department of Health, London; Wright C (2003) NHS improving but still far from cured, says report. *The Times*. **11 March**; Hawkes N (2003) Extra NHS funds getting through to patients, says Milburn. *The Times*. **2 April**.

10 *Sunday Times, Good Hospital Guide*; first leader, A debtor's budget, *Sunday Times*; McCall A (2003) Death rate is double in worst hospitals. *Sunday Times*, all 6 April 2003.

11 Quoted, Rhodes James R (1970) *Churchill, A Study in Failure 1900–1939*. World Publishing Company, New York, p.34.

Index